STRIKING BACK!

THE TRIGEMINAL NEURALGIA
AND FACE PAIN
HANDBOOK

George Weigel
and
Kenneth F. Casey, M.D.

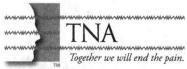

TNA
Together we will end the pain.
TM
TRIGEMINAL NEURALGIA ASSOCIATION
Gainesville, Florida

To those who have persevered and overcome this excruciating condition…
and to the many family members, friends, medical professionals
and caring souls who helped them get their lives back.

DISCLAIMER

The information in this book is intended to help readers better understand trigeminal neuralgia and related face pains and to help those with face pain make an informed decision about their health. It is offered with the understanding that neither the authors nor the publisher are engaged in rendering medical or professional advice. This book is NOT intended as specific medical advice and is NOT intended to substitute for the qualified advice of medical practitioners. If you have trigeminal neuralgia or similar facial pain, we highly recommend that you see a trusted medical professional.

Cover graphic by Kristy Higby, Mercersburg, Pennsylvania
Printed by Whitehall Printing Company, Naples, Florida
Edited by Jane Boles, Gainesville, Florida

Published by

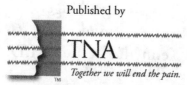

Together we will end the pain.

TRIGEMINAL NEURALGIA ASSOCIATION
925 Northwest 56th Terrace, Suite C, Gainesville, FL 32605

ISBN: 978-0-9672393-2-3

CONTENTS

5: THE DENTAL CONNECTION   63

6: OTHER FACE PAINS: NOT TN, NOT DENTAL, BUT IT STILL HURTS   79

7: MEDICATIONS FOR FACE PAIN   107

14: IT STILL HURTS... NOW WHAT? 259

15: NOT SURGERY, NOT PILLS: THERAPIES BEYOND MAINSTREAM MEDICINE 281

16: ACUPUNCTURE FOR FACE PAIN 319

17: CHIROPRACTIC FOR FACE PAIN 329

18: NUTRITION THERAPY 345

23: HELPFUL LISTS, QUESTIONNAIRES AND OTHER AIDS   445

FOREWORD

A book has many functions. People read for pleasure, because they have to, to learn independently, to prepare for a situation, to ready themselves for a decision. Valid information matters. Information without hyperbole, without bias, is very hard to obtain in our present society. A book has many attributes. It can be well organized, well focused, well written, scholarly and thoroughly researched, pertinent, honest and thorough. Non-fiction must fulfill these criteria. A valid self-help volume must fulfill these criteria from all perspectives.

Such is the case with Striking Back! The Trigeminal Neuralgia and Face Pain Handbook. This alone is a tribute to Mr. George Weigel and Dr. Kenneth Casey for utilizing their superb talents. They have carefully researched the newest information. They have done this with little or no bias. I caution the reader to read this work carefully as some of the areas that the authors discuss in a lucid and careful way will be easily considered un-scientific and wasteful of the time and money to the patient seeking help. Some of the material included will appear inflammatory to many treating physicians because the perspectives and reports, usually not well documented in a serious way, would be discredited by a competent medical observer. Despite this, the authors have, I think rightfully, chosen to include material on such areas as diet and vitamin therapy, magnetotherapy, acupuncture and chiropractic efforts.

Striking Back replaces all previous books without sacrifice of the historical perspectives. There is great attention to important detail. You will read chapters discussing new areas of interest (vide supra!). The book meets the criteria for a useful, well organized and well written compendium of contemporary knowledge about trigeminal neuralgia. It is not only a utilitarian read but an enjoyable discourse on the subject. The section on atypical (type 2) trigeminal neuralgia is especially helpful to sufferers of face pain who have not met prior criteria for operative intervention but who may now be helped. Physicians and dentists, the medical practitioners who see patients so frequently in emergency rooms, physician extenders and nurse practitioners will benefit greatly from this book.

Striking Back is a boon to those who suffer from face pain and those who care for them. The authors, who have worked so hard and so well on this volume, should receive a great "thank you" from all of us.

Peter J. Jannetta, MD

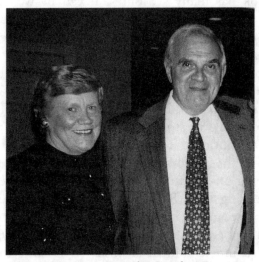

Claire W. Patterson, Founder, President Emeritus, and Director of Institutional Relations and Research, Trigeminal Neuralgia Association (TNA) and Peter J. Jannetta, MD, Vice Chairman, Department of Neurosurgery, Allegheny General Hospital.

PREFACE

George Weigel

Like most people, I had never heard of trigeminal neuralgia until the endodontist mentioned those strange words at the end of a futile second set of root-canal treatments.

"Is it serious?" "Is it fatal?" "What do you do about it?" "What even IS it?" Those were the questions that raced through my mind, sitting there alone in the dentist's chair.

I soon found out that this disorder of the face's main sensory nerve isn't fatal – that is, if you don't count the people who tragically lost hope and killed themselves to escape the terrible agony of it. But one thing that kept jumping out at me as I researched the medical journals was how often doctors referred to trigeminal neuralgia, or "tic douloureux," as "the most excruciating pain known to man."

Great.

I also found out after even more research that there are lots of options for treating TN, and even more importantly, that almost all trigeminal "neuralgians" ultimately find a way out of their pain.

Like many cases of TN, mine sneaked up on me. A few weeks after having a filling replaced on a molar, I started getting a faint, vague pain in that area. It wasn't constant, and for weeks it amounted to no more than a mild bother.

Then the bother slid into hurting, enough so that I was convinced something was wrong. So I did the logical thing. I went back to the dentist.

An exam didn't turn up anything obviously wrong, but my dentist said it was a pretty good bet that the nerve in the tooth was dead or dying from the filling replacement and that a root canal was in order.

Three endodontist visits and $450 later, the pain was worse instead of better. Antibiotics and even some stiff pain-relievers were not helping at all.

By this time, the pain had a strange electric-like quality to it. It would be bad for awhile, then go away. And it didn't hurt just at the tooth. It seemed to hurt underneath the tooth and along the whole right lower jaw up to my lower right "eye" tooth.

The dentists speculated that maybe it was actually the next tooth forward that was the real culprit. So they suggested a second root canal on that tooth. Eager to try anything at that point to get out of the pain, I agreed. Three more visits and another $450 later, it hurt worse than ever.

It was at this point that the endodontist asked a key question. "Can you make the pain happen by touching somewhere on your face?" he asked.

"Yeah, I replied. "As a matter of fact, sometimes when I touch my lip, it sets off pain in my jaw."

Bingo. That classic "trigger" characteristic was what finally convinced the endodontist to conclude: "You know, I think you might have trigeminal neuralgia."

The ordeal of unnecessary root canals is not that uncommon. Since TN is not nearly as common as such other pains as toothaches and temporomandibular joint disorders (TMD or TMJ), people often go through long periods of misdiagnosis or mysterious and frustrating "undiagnosis" until the real problem is unearthed.

My case was particularly tricky because I was only 36 years old when I came down with TN. It usually strikes those age 50 and up. "You're too young to have this," one doctor told me.

For two-and-a-half years I put up with increasingly painful cycles of lightning-like stabs to my right lower jaw. I would tell people it felt as if a dentist had drilled the tops off of my teeth and was shooting jolts of electricity directly onto the raw nerves.

It was hard for people to understand. After all, I looked just fine. No wounds, no swelling, no deformities. Even all the tests came back normal. So how could someone who looked so healthy hurt so badly?

By this time, I was convinced the neurology journals were right. If there were any pains any worse than this one, I surely didn't want to meet them first-hand.

I was used to getting hit with 90-mph baseballs in 30-degree weather as a former catcher in college, but compared to the pain of TN, that pain was nothing.

TN pain hurt so badly that one day I found myself curled up in bed, alternating between tears of agony and holding my breath while waiting for the worst spikes to subside.

Toward the end, I was having more than 100 attacks a day. Most of them lasted 20 seconds to two minutes each. Sometimes a dull ache followed the spikes for 20 minutes or so. Other times the pain would disappear just as suddenly as it came on.

Touching my lip was no longer the only trigger for the pain. A light wind would do it. So would saying, "Hello," when answering the phone. Brushing my teeth was guaranteed agony every morning and every evening. After awhile, the pain didn't even need to be triggered. It would just come on by itself as if it had a mind of its own.

None of the anticonvulsant medications doctors prescribed helped much at all. All they did was make me groggy and forgetful.

Seeing me enduring this kind of pain was hard on my wife and kids. My wife was so understanding yet so frustrated at being unable to do anything to stop the attacks. The final straw was when the TN got to the point where I couldn't even read my kids a bedtime story without having to stop several times in the middle for 30- to 60-second pain breaks.

Finally, my wife told me what I already figured was the inevitable. I needed surgery.

The procedure that seemed like the best bet to me at my age was something called a "microvascular decompression," a brain surgery that's aimed at moving a blood vessel off the trigeminal nerve near where it connects to the brain stem.

I wasn't sure a vessel compressing the nerve was my problem – even an MRI exam couldn't pick that up – but that's the leading theory behind most cases of TN. Through contacts at the Trigeminal Neuralgia Association, I found out about an excellent neurosurgeon at Johns Hopkins Hospital in nearby Baltimore, Md. (Dr. Benjamin S. Carson Sr.) and underwent a nearly 5-hour surgery that stopped the pain in its tracks.

Dr. Carson said he found an unusually large artery that had wrapped itself around my trigeminal nerve and had even attached itself onto it. He separated the two and placed a sliver of neck muscle and Gelfoam between the nerve and artery to keep them apart.

I haven't had any of those lightning attacks since.

One thing that became apparent during my ordeal was the lack of good comprehensive, plain-English information about this wretched condition. Almost all of the precious few materials I was able to find were written by doctors for doctors – most of it filled with big medical words.

Soon after my operation, I resolved to start a support group in my hometown area of Harrisburg, Pa., and then to put together the kind of book that I went looking for, but couldn't find, when I first came down with TN. I started the support group in 1994. You're holding Part II of my resolution.

It's been gratifying to hear from people all over the world who have been helped by my first book. Armed with the information and ideas, thousands of people have found a route to pain relief. No longer do we need to suffer in silence or ignorance.

If you're reading this book because you've got TN, my advice is to learn all you can about it, keep in mind that there's no one treatment that's best for everyone, and hang in there because practically all "neuralgians" find relief one way or another.

May this book be the ray of hope and guidance you need to find that relief.

PREFACE

Dr. Kenneth Casey

In part, this book reports the success of the Trigeminal Neuralgia Association. Its members have shown many how to find, interpret and use medical information for the good of self and society.

I have spoken often, and believe, that this group can be the prototype for the next revolution in medicine – the age when the patient and doctor talk and decide together what is the best course of action. TNA can help lead other support groups toward a unified, informed patient lobby in the coming fight for good outcomes.

This book represents the result of continued attention to face pain, in all its forms. The final answers are not contained in these pages, but the appropriate questions to prompt that work are here.

We hope you all find something that gives you a sense of peace, because you are the reason for trying to find the best way to care.

Fouche is quoted as saying, "It was worse than a crime, it was a blunder."

All of us, when we are entrusted with the care of our own health, seek to find out the most pertinent and most up-to-date information. We seek information from our physicians, we seek information from family members, and we seek information from self-help books, magazine articles and all manner of other current publications.

A problem with a good deal of information that we gather is that we are unable to put it into perspective for a specific problem and unable to prioritize it as to its relevance to our day-to-day living. We can often be accused of having the necessary information and simply not acting on it.

For those individuals who bravely suffer with face pain, knowledge is a tool. In that sense, this book is a tool aimed at helping face pain sufferers find a way to "fix" their problem.

My co-author, George Weigel, and I have seen trigeminal neuralgia and other face pains from two different perspectives.

George had trigeminal neuralgia himself and for years has helped face pain sufferers understand and cope with the pain as a support-group leader.

As a neurosurgeon with a special interest in face pain, I have seen and treated hundreds of trigeminal neuralgians and face pain sufferers as patients.

By combining these perspectives, we attempted in this volume to explore the facts and theories about causes and treatments but also to address the human side of what it's like to cope with some of the worst pain known to mankind.

In several chapters, a good deal of effort is spent explaining – in clear, certain terms – what might be the origin of face pain and how that origin or cause might apply to those who pick up this book. In addition, effort is spent on explaining why conflicting theories of face pain may have some common thread in the realm of treatment.

You'll find information on both traditional and non-traditional approaches to the management of face pain as well as tips from other patients.

From a medical perspective, this book serves a valuable purpose in bringing together a variety of different disciplines on the subject of face pain. Individuals from the field of dentistry, neurology, neurosurgery and general medical care are among those who contributed.

At the same time, the most important points of view come from those patients who have experienced face pain and who have sought to establish an uneasy relationship with that face pain through a variety of different means. Any and all of these means should be available to those who suffer from face pain and to the families who suffer with them. This book serves as a way to draw that knowledge together.

Another important section deals with support groups. It is through the nature of these groups that individuals can gather information quickly, disseminate that information among themselves and, perhaps more importantly than anything else for those of us as medical professionals, to test the veracity of the information gathered in the real work place of face pain care.

All too frequently, as medical professionals, we will devise a treatment which, on paper, appears to be quite safe and useful but which, unfortunately, in use turns out to be impractical for day-to-day living.

Through the Trigeminal Neuralgia Association and the individual efforts of the patients in this book, we have a compendium of facts that have been tried and proven in the battle against face pain.

I think the mistake, then, is to ignore the information we have on face pain and that the blunder is to allow others to dictate to someone in face pain a course of action that may not be appropriate for that individual.

ACKNOWLEDGMENTS

The names you'll find mentioned throughout these pages only begin to cite the many people who had a hand in making this book possible.

First and foremost is Claire Patterson, the phenomenal woman who has devoted her life to spreading the word about trigeminal neuralgia treatments and in the process founded the Trigeminal Neuralgia Association. Without her and TNA, there would be no network of TN support groups, no push for more and better research, and certainly no book like the one you're now holding.

Also critical to the effort has been Dr. Peter J. Jannetta, the Pittsburgh neurosurgeon who developed and popularized the microvascular decompression surgery that has helped end the pain of so many "neuralgians." Perhaps just as importantly, Dr. Jannetta is the one who "challenged" Claire to go do something about that great void of information on TN.

Numerous other outstanding doctors contributed key information to the book as well as devoting careers to helping fight TN. Tops on that list are current and past members of TNA's Medical Advisory Board: Dr. John Alksne, Dr. Ronald Apfelbaum, Dr. Nicholas Barbaro, Dr. Ronald Brisman, Dr. Jeffrey Brown, Dr. Kim Burchiel, Dr. Jeffrey Cohen, Dr. Steven Graff-Radford, Dr. Henry Gremillion, Dr. Stephen Haines, Dr. Mark Linskey, Dr. James Nelson, Dr. Bruce Pollock, Dr. Albert Rhoton, Dr. David Sirois, Dr. John Tew, Dr. Ronald Young, Dr. Joanna Zakrzewska, and Dr. Richard Zimmerman. These are some of the world's top TN clinicians, and they all added their years of wisdom to these pages.

Special thanks also go out to others who provided important details in particular specialties: Dr. Roger Hinson and Dr. Erin Elster on chiropractic; Dr. Chun-In Jerry Lin on acupuncture; Dr. Allen Neims on complementary and alternative medicine therapies; Emily Jane and Dr. Gerald Lemole on nutrition; Dr. Jerry Bouquot on NICO, and Dr. Toby Newton-John and Sherri Connell on coping with pain.

Literally dozens of other doctors, researchers and practitioners provided additional help. You'll see their names as you read through the chapters. We should all be grateful for their advice and findings.

One other doctor needs to be singled out for a special thank you, because without him, one of the authors (G.W.) would have been in too much pain or too drugged to write a coherent sentence. Thanks, Dr. Ben Carson of Johns Hopkins Hospital in Baltimore, Md., for giving back a life.

Medical professionals weren't the only ones who added valuable insights and important information. TNA Chairman Roger Levy added TNA's perspective on a variety of issues, and TNA President Michael Pasternak offered numerous excellent contacts and research suggestions. The rest of TNA's Board of Directors has not only been highly supportive of this book but also very proactive in a host of other TN educational pushes. Cheers to Brian Cronin, Ken White, Gwen Asplundh, Cindy Ezell, Mike Hirsch and Ev Pinneo.

Then there were the other absolutely crucial contributors – those who know TN and face pain first-hand. These are the people who motivate the doctors to find a better way, who help others understand what pain can do to a life and who so often show how strong and brave ordinary people can be when they're backed against the wall.

Many of these face pain sufferers have gone on to become TN support group leaders around the country and world. Their experiences and those of their group members were largely responsible for the entire Chapter 19, "Tips from the Veterans." If one of those tips helps you, thank those who have "been there, done that" and who made the effort to share what they learned.

The real experiences of the many real people quoted in this book put a human face on "Striking Back" and made it more than a narrative of symptoms and treatments. Their stories show what it's like dealing with this demon, from singer Norma Zimmer's compelling description of her TN pain to Sue Remmey's uplifting experience with prayer to Lynn Mason's moving account of learning that her young daughter had TN.

All of this great input would have benefited no one without making it into book form. Mike Hirsch at Whitehall Printing Company in Naples, Fla., was the "angel" who made that happen when he heard about the printing dilemma at a TNA conference in Orlando. He volunteered his company to get the job done. Mike's son, Jeff, and the Whitehall crew expertly produced what became the world's first patient-oriented book on TN and related face pain.

New York editor Rodman P. Neumann volunteered to handle the rather daunting job of laying out the first book. The TNA staff took care of the huge task of tracking down and updating the numerous resources listed in Chapter 24.

Thanks also go to Pennsylvania artist Kristy Higby, who did the striking cover art, and to Florida artists David Peace and Margaret Barry, who provided a variety of medical illustrations that helped make complex neurological concepts easier to understand.

On a personal note, extra-special thanks are due the authors' families for sacrificing time so this book could see the light of day. Now we can help with the dishes again!

Finally, thanks to the families and loved ones of neuralgians for their understanding and patience. It's not easy having this pain, but it's also not easy seeing a loved one hurt so much and being so powerless to do anything about it. Your encouragement often helps more than any pill (although effective pills are nice, too).

If you're still in pain, hang in there. You'll find an answer. If you're still working on it, may God bless your days and guide your way to a speedy answer.

CHAPTER 1

LIKE A LIGHTNING BOLT

"This is the kind of pain you wouldn't even wish on your worst enemy."
—Claire Patterson, TRIGEMINAL NEURALGIA ASSOCIATION founder

The pain hits suddenly, like a jolt of lightning to the face. Again and again the pain stabs, sometimes for a few seconds, sometimes for a few minutes, and then it's gone, just as abruptly as it came.

Jabbing. Shock-like. Searing. Spearing. Shooting. These are words people use to describe a painful condition known as "trigeminal neuralgia" or "tic douloureux." It's sometimes described as the most excruciating pain known to man – and few people who have experienced it would disagree.

"Women who have gone through childbirth without anesthesia will tell you that trigeminal neuralgia is much worse," says San Diego neurologist Dr. James Nelson.

Despite the striking potency of this pain, trigeminal neuralgia (TN as we'll call it) isn't particularly well known. Most people have never heard of it – until they or a relative come down with it. But actually this disorder of the face's main sensory nerve isn't as rare as it might seem.

Studies estimate there are somewhere between 15,000 and 50,000 new cases each year in the United States. At that rate, assuming an average 8-year bout with TN, that means somewhere between 120,000 and 400,000 Americans are coping with TN at any given time.

In 1990, researchers at the Mayo Clinic in Rochester, Minn., looked at 40 years' worth of medical records in that city and found that TN affected about one in every 25,000 of its citizens, mostly those age 50 and up.

Many doctors believe the rate is much higher than that, based on the number of patients they see and the fact that TN is often misdiagnosed – a problem we'll discuss in greater detail in Chapter 2.

When other similar or related face pains are considered, the numbers balloon even further. An estimated 1.7 million Americans are believed to suffer from some sort of face pain, with 50,000 to 60,000 new cases per year.

It's difficult to get an accurate handle on exactly how widespread the problem is because patients may be seeing so many different types of practitioners for treatment of TN and other face pain, including family doctors, dentists, oral surgeons, neurologists, neurosurgeons and chiropractors.

TN also happens to be a disorder that's not required to be reported to government agencies, so there's no national data base kept by agencies that track specific health problems.

One thing *is* more certain. Because TN is primarily a disorder that affects older Americans, it's likely to become more common as our life spans increase.

Not just an aging disorder

TN isn't something that strikes only those age 50 and up, though. Nearly one in 10 cases occur in people under age 40. The earliest documented case involved a 13-month-old, raising the specter that in rare cases, people are born with this pain.

WHEN TN FIRST APPEARS	
Age at onset	Percent
0-10	rare
11-20	0.5%
20s	3%
30s	6%
40s	18%
50s	29%
60s	28%
70s	12%
80s	2%

— Source: "Pain and the Neurosurgeon: A 40-Year Experience" by Drs. J.C. White and William H. Sweet (1969)

TN is a pain that has no boundaries. It's an equal-opportunity problem that has affected people from all walks of life for centuries. Jefferson Davis, the Confederacy's only president, had it. So did Russian composer Sergei Rachmaninov, who ached for 20 years before getting relief from a French dentist and hypnotist in 1930. Author Gloria Steinem also has been treated for TN pain, the late actor Norman Fell ("Three's Company") had surgery to get rid of his TN, and Lawrence Welk's "Champagne lady," Norma Zimmer, has battled the pain with a variety of therapies since 1981.

The reported incidence of TN is nearly equal among men and women, although a few studies have tilted slightly toward more women – even when the figures are corrected for women's greater numbers in the overall population. However, many more women than men undergo surgery for TN – in some practices by a ratio of three women to every man.

How the pain behaves

TN pain is usually triggered by a light touch to the face – things like scratching the nose, shaving, putting on makeup, eating, brushing teeth, even a light breeze. The attacks typically run in cycles with pain-free periods or "remissions" of weeks, months or even years between the cycles. Over time, the pain-free periods tend to become shorter and fewer.

Sometimes the pain comes out of nowhere with no trigger at all. While a classic attack is sudden and sharp and then gone altogether, sometimes a low-grade ache or burning pain will persist in its wake for an hour, maybe more.

Gwen Asplundh of Pennsylvania gives a good description of what her pain used to be like: "Sharp, excruciating pain in my left upper and lower jaws would come for a few minutes or longer, off and on, and then fade with a strange burning sensation on my tongue on that side. Chewing food was out of the question. Communicating was accomplished with written notes since speaking was too painful. And brushing

---

TN SNAPSHOT

• Americans with TN:	40,000-50,000
• New cases per year in U.S.:	15,000-50,000
• Odds of getting TN:	1 in 25,000
• Average age of onset:	55
• Average age patient seeks surgical intervention:	63
• Side of face involved:	61 percent right side 36 percent left side 3 percent both sides
• Gender breakdown:	Slightly more females than males
• Average number of trigger points:	1.4
• Most common area of trigger points:	around the nose and lip
• Season when attacks start:	fall, 35 percent winter, 24 percent spring, 24 percent summer, 17 percent
• Family history of TN:	5 percent

— Sources: *Journal of Neurology; Trigeminal Neuralgia Association; University of Cincinnati Medical College; Mayo Clinic, Rochester, Minn.*

my teeth became a thing of the past. I prayed I wouldn't sneeze. The pain lessened when I lay down, but every time I swallowed, it hit again. I can remember trying to take as long as I possibly could between swallows."

Sometimes the sharp attacks occur amid a backdrop of a constant, low-level ache that some doctors refer to as "atypical trigeminal neuralgia."

The emerging belief is that this more constant pain isn't "atypical" at all but rather a variation of classic TN or an additional and harder-to-treat symptom developed by those who have had TN a long time.

A quick TN anatomy lesson

This disorder affects the trigeminal nerve, the largest of the body's 12 sets of cranial nerves. Everyone has two trigeminal nerves, one for each side of the face.

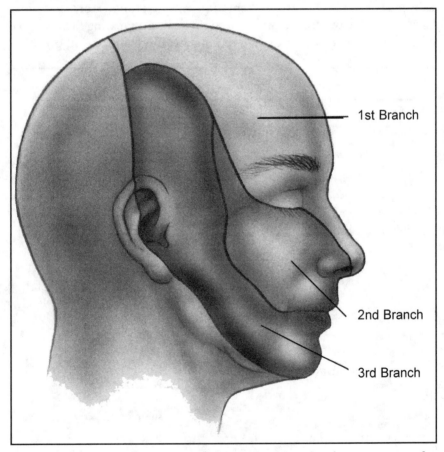

The three branches of the trigeminal nerve each serve a distinct region of the face.   (Sketch by David Peace, University of Florida)

The nerves come out of the base of the brain – a region called the "pons" – and then fan out in three main branches to supply sensation throughout the face.

The name "trigeminal" comes from the Latin word "tres," which means three, and "geminus," which means twin. "Neuralgia" is a Greek word stemming from "neuro" (nerve) and "algia" (pain).

The bottom or "mandibular" branch of the trigeminal nerve serves the lower jaw, including the lower teeth, lower lip, side and front of the tongue, lower gums and part of the ear.

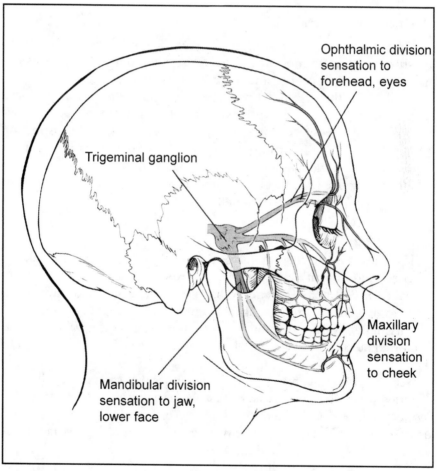

The trigeminal nerve splits at the trigeminal ganglion into three main divisions, which in turn split off into many other smaller branches that supply sensation throughout the face.

(Sketch reprinted with permission of the Mayfield Clinic, University of Cincinnati)

The middle or "maxillary" branch serves the upper jaw, upper teeth and gums, upper lip, cheeks, palate, sinuses, temples and most of the nose.

The upper or "ophthalmic" branch serves the forehead, eyes and bridge of the nose.

Because the trigeminal nerve is the fifth cranial nerve, doctors refer to pain as "V1," "V2" or "V3." The "V" refers to the Roman numeral for five, and the numbers correspond to the branch where the pain is located. "V1" refers to pain in the upper branch, "V2" refers to pain in the middle branch, and "V3" refers to pain in the lower branch.

What trigeminal nerves do

The trigeminal nerves are responsible for the sensations of touch, temperature and pain in most of the face. A separate branch of the trigeminal nerve also controls the muscles used in chewing.

Until 1829, the trigeminal nerve was thought to be part of the facial nerve, another cranial nerve that controls most muscles of the face. We now know the two nerves are separate. That's an important distinction because people often mistakenly think that surgery involving their trigeminal nerve will cause their face to sag or contort.

When the trigeminal nerve malfunctions as it does in TN, it can be extremely painful, though not fatal.

A TN history lesson

TN is not a new affliction. It was described as early as the first century by Greek and Roman physicians, who called it "cephalalgia." The Persians described it 900 years ago and even suggested that it might have something to do with an artery being near a nerve.

Carvings at Wells Cathedral in England dating to the 1200s show the contorted faces of men suffering from agonizing facial pain thought to be TN.

German physician and TN sufferer Johannes Bausch and his colleagues recorded what is believed to be the first Western written description of TN in the 1660s. A decade later, British physician John Locke gave a detailed description of TN when the wife of England's ambassador to France, the Countess of Northumberland, came down with it.

When French surgeon Nicolaus Andre described five cases of it in 1756, he called the disorder "tic douloureux," meaning "painful spasm." TN also picked up the name "Fothergill's disease" in 1773 when English physician John Fothergill described 14 cases to the Medical Society in London.

It's also been called "trifacial neuralgia" and "epileptiform neuralgia." In less medical terms, TN has been called the "suicide disease" as a result of those who killed themselves to escape the pain in the days before good treatments were available. One neurologist puts it, "the king of face pain."

From blood-letting to boiling water

Early treatments included blood-letting and trying to excise demons. Since the 1600s, physicians have used more than 40 different preparations in an effort to stem TN pain.

Among them: arsenic, quinine, bee and cobra venom, various metals, opiate drugs, various purgatives (agents that induce bowel movements), the vitamin thiamine and even hemlock.

Other treatments included applications of tar to the face, steam treatments, searing the surgically exposed nerve with a hot iron, galvanic therapy (steady low-level doses of electric current), and even dipping the hand on the painful side into boiling water.

At the turn of the 20th century, doctors tried radiation and X-ray therapy. When that didn't work very well, they had patients inhale trichlorethylene, a short-lasting anesthetic that also has some pain-relieving properties. It was widely used for TN between 1918 and 1942. We know that chemical better today as the toxic pollutant TCE.

Meanwhile, surgeons tried injecting boiling water, alcohol, wax, osmic acid, chloroform and other chemicals into the face. When all else failed, they cut the nerve to disconnect the pain – first the nerve's branches in the face and by the early 1900s, near the nerve's main connection to the brain.

Before early surgeons figured out that the facial nerve and the trigeminal nerve were two different nerves, they sometimes cut the wrong branches. That meant their patients ended up having paralyzed faces instead of pain-free ones.

TN IN A CLASSIC...

"Didn't that Dough-Boy, the steward, tell me that of a morning he always finds the old man's hammock clothes all rumpled and tumbled, and the sheets down at the foot, and the coverlid almost tied into knots, and the pillow a sort of frightful hot, as though a baked brick had been on it? A hot old man! I guess he's got what some folks ashore call a conscience; it's a kind of Tic-Dolly-row they say — worse nor a toothache. Well, well; I don't know what it is, but the Lord keep me from catching it."

From Herman Melville's 1851 classic book "Moby Dick"

Surgical break-throughs

Early open-skull operations completely disconnected the trigeminal nerve. That not only caused complete numbness but also chewing difficulties. Surgeons soon discovered they could relieve pain without causing chewing problems by sparing the nerve fibers that controlled the jaw muscles.

Then in the late 1920s, neurosurgeon Dr. Walter Dandy of Baltimore's Johns Hopkins Hospital noticed during these open-skull surgeries that blood vessels often seemed to be touching TN patients' trigeminal nerves. In a series of 215 patients, he found about half had offending vessels.

Those observations led him to advance the theory that TN might be caused by a blood vessel causing damage to the trigeminal nerve. For many years, it was thought that the carotid artery – the main artery of the neck – was the most likely culprit.

However, Dr. Dandy did not go the next step and attempt to move offending vessels off the nerve. He continued with the tried-and-true method of cutting the nerve.

Dr. Dandy did refine the technique by proving that patients could get pretty good pain relief without a lot of numbness if only some of the sensory nerve fibers were cut. He claimed that was possible because the nerve fibers responsible for pain and those responsible for touch separated close to the brainstem. Up until then, surgeons assumed that "good numbness" was needed to get "good relief."

It wasn't until the 1950s that Cleveland neurosurgeon Dr. William J. Gardner confirmed Dr. Dandy's findings and eventually performed the first surgery to move an offending vessel off of the nerve.

Dr. Dandy, Dr. Gardner and others in that time period were working with a major handicap, however. Their observations of the spaghetti-sized nerve were with the naked eye. In a 1962 report on his first 18 surgical patients, for example, Gardner was at a loss to explain why six of those patients had TN but no apparent nerve-compressing blood vessels.

A significant break-through came in 1966. Using a new operating microscope that greatly magnified and illuminated vessels and nerves, Dr. Peter J. Jannetta – then a resident at UCLA – noticed that vessels not only were contacting the nerve but seemed to be compressing the cranial nerves of people suffering from TN and facial spasms.

He proclaimed these compressions to be the cause of TN. The trick, he said, was finding them.

Instead of the more accepted procedure of cutting or damaging the nerve to relieve pain, Dr. Jannetta proposed moving the offending vessel off of the nerve and inserting a soft material to separate the two. Today, Dr. Jannetta's "microvascular decompression" technique is one of the leading surgical treatments for TN. The surgery is sometimes called the "Jannetta procedure."

Neurosurgeons today also treat TN with less invasive procedures, such as injecting glycerol, selectively damaging the nerve with a heated electrode and short-circuiting the pain with a tiny balloon that's temporarily inflated against the nerve. All are done by use of a needle inserted through the cheek.

The newest surgery uses beams of cobalt 60 radiation to selectively damage the nerve. Known as "radiosurgery," it involves no cutting or needles at all. Chapters 9 through 13 discuss each of these surgeries in detail.

Treating it with medicines

While surgeons were zeroing in on ways to stop the pain without disconnecting the trigeminal nerve, pharmaceutical science was turning up new medications to control the pain without surgery.

In 1942, the first reports appeared showing that doctors were having success in using the epilepsy drug phenytoin (Dilantin) to control TN pain. It was the first drug that effectively helped TN sufferers without major drawbacks.

An even more effective drug – carbamazepine (Tegretol) – was introduced in 1962. Also mainly an epilepsy drug, carbamazepine was found to give good relief to 70 to 80 percent of TN patients. It is still used today by many doctors as their top choice in TN medicine.

Another drug – baclofen (Lioresal) – joined the arsenal in the early 1980s, nearly a decade after its introduction as a muscle-relaxant. Baclofen usually isn't as effective as carbamazepine, but it has fewer side effects and is often helpful as an "add-on drug" when carbamazepine alone is not doing the job.

The late 1990s and early 2000s brought a wave of new medicines – mostly introduced as anticonvulsants – that swelled the list of possible TN helpers to 18.

Oxcarbazepine (Trileptal) and gabapentin (Neurontin) are the most used of the newcomers. Oxcarbazepine is very similar in makeup to carbamazepine and regarded as being potentially as effective but with fewer likely side effects. Gabapentin has been effective both as an add-on medication as well as a possible solution for those with more constant or burning pain.

Lamotrigine (Lamictal), topiramate (Topamax) and levetiracetam (Keppra) are other recently introduced anticonvulsant drugs that have been used with some success for TN and related face pains. Medications are discussed in detail in Chapter 7.

Research also is under way looking into other classes of drugs that might help face pain, including so-called "channel-blocker" medicines and drugs that target the pain-reading parts of the brain.

Besides these leading medical and surgical treatments, many other treatments sometime give relief to some people, at least temporarily. These include acupuncture, chiropractic, self-hypnosis, hot-pepper cream and various herbal and nutritional regimens, to name a few. We'll discuss these so-called "complementary and alternative medicine" treatments in Chapters 15-18.

The bottom line is that there are many ways today to attack TN. If one treatment fails, there's always something else to try. And there's also the hope that research under way today will uncover new and better treatments tomorrow. There's no reason anymore for TN to be called the "suicide disease."

CHAPTER 2

JUST WHAT IS TN ANYWAY?

"There is no other way to describe it except that somebody has driven a knife in your face, and it's connected to an electrical outlet."
—Diane Pendleton, a TN "veteran" from Pennsylvania

One of the most frustrating aspects of trigeminal neuralgia – for both the patient and doctor – is the difficulty of diagnosing it in the first place. Unlike many afflictions, there is no blood test, X-ray or other test that tells you that what you've got is TN.

This is a condition that's diagnosed almost exclusively by the patient's description of the symptoms. And those symptoms are very striking and distinct – at least in classic cases of TN.

There are five key hallmarks of TN, although not everyone always has all five. They are:

1.) *Sharp pain attacks* that come and go abruptly rather than being a constant ache.
2.) *Pain is confined* to the area served by one or more branches of the trigeminal nerve, namely the lower jaw, the upper jaw/cheek area and the eye/forehead area.
3.) *Pain is almost always limited to one side* of the face (95 to 98 percent of the time), and the pain does not cross over the midpoint of the face. (Pain from the right trigeminal nerve is confined to the right side of the face, and pain from the left nerve is confined to the left side.)
4.) *The pain is usually provoked* by a light touch of the face or a breeze, especially around the eye, nose and/or lips, or a movement of the face, such as talking, eating or yawning. In other words, the pain is typically "triggered."
5.) *The pain seems to run in cycles* and may even disappear for weeks, months or years before returning.

Where and how TN strikes

Although TN almost always occurs on only one side the face, it may affect more than one branch of that side's trigeminal nerve. In fact, the most common case is one in which the patient suffers pain in both the cheek and lower jaw – the lower two branches of the three-pronged nerve.

Second most common are cases in which the patient has pain in either the cheek or the jaw alone.

About 15 percent of patients have pain in both the cheek and eye/forehead region, and about 13 percent of patients report pain in all three branches.

Often, the pain starts in a single branch but progresses to other branches as time goes on.

The same is often true with the trigger zones that set off pain attacks. Patients may not notice any trigger zones early on, but eventually they may find that touching the tip of their nose or upper lip almost always sets off a pain episode. These one or two zones may expand into third or fourth trigger zones over time.

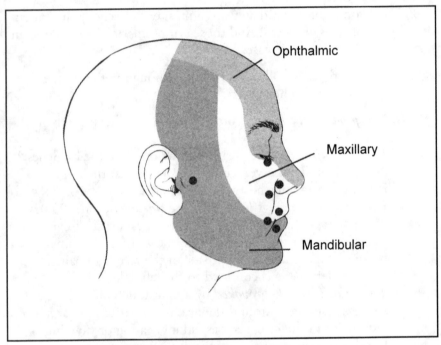

The dots show the location of common "trigger points" for TN pain.
(Sketch reprinted with permission of the Mayfield Clinic, University of Cincinnati)

The trigger zones are most often in the same branch of the nerve as the pain. But about 10 percent of the time, triggers in one branch set off pain in another branch. In up to 20 percent of the cases, there are no triggers at all.

Many patients find that the trigger zones don't always stay the same. They may "move around." One time the lip or nose may be the main trigger, but another day it seems to be a spot on the cheek.

Many patients also report having their worst episodes during stressful periods in their life. What's uncertain is whether stress actually triggers TN episodes or just makes the pain *feel* worse.

There's no doubt, though, that there is a strong connection between mental and physical health. This connection is discussed in detail in Chapter 20.

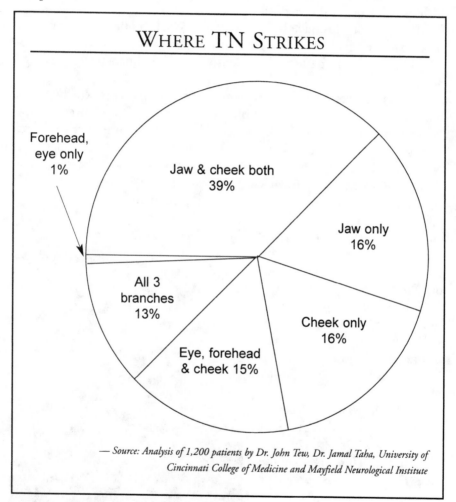

WHERE TN STRIKES

Forehead, eye only 1%

Jaw & cheek both 39%

Jaw only 16%

All 3 branches 13%

Cheek only 16%

Eye, forehead & cheek 15%

— *Source: Analysis of 1,200 patients by Dr. John Tew, Dr. Jamal Taha, University of Cincinnati College of Medicine and Mayfield Neurological Institute*

How people react to TN pain

To avoid triggering attacks, many people stop using cosmetics, stop shaving and avoid washing their face or taking showers. Some stop talking. Some miss work. Some don't go anywhere or do anything for fear of triggering an attack.

Some avoid the dentist like the plague. Some cover their head and face to guard against breezes. If the pain is bad enough, some even stop eating or drinking. Thus secondary threats to TN are problems such as tooth decay, dehydration and weight loss.

"Really any change in input into the trigeminal system can trigger an attack," says Dr. John Alksne, chief of neurosurgery at the University of California's San Diego Medical Center.

Many neuralgians have been impaired enough by the severe pain that they have even had to quit working.

With TN, when patients are asked where they hurt, they unfailingly *point* to the spot.

"In almost every other facial pain syndrome, patients will be found massaging the painful area or rubbing it or applying heat or cold," says neurologist Dr. Donald J. Dalessio of the Scripps Clinic and Research Foundation in La Jolla, Calif. "But in trigeminal neuralgia, exactly the opposite occurs. The patient goes to great lengths to avoid any stimulation of the face or mouth whatsoever."

"I can recognize immediately when a TN patient walks in my door," says Dr. Joanna Zakrzewska, an oral-medicine specialist at England's Barts and the London Queen Mary's School of Medicine and Dentistry. "You can tell by their expression, by how they move."

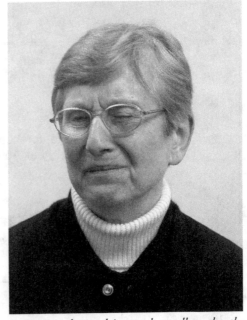

If that doesn't give away the diagnosis, witnessing an attack in progress makes it painfully obvious.

"At the beginning of a severe attack of pain, the patient freezes," says Dr. Zakrzewska. "Often the hand rises to the face but rarely is the face touched. The face contorts— hence the term 'tic'—and some patients cry out in pain. Anyone witnessing such a severe attack is also very upset."

A trigeminal neuralgia attack usually makes the person wince on the painful side. Sharp, sudden attacks may even result in a jerk of the head, as if the person has been stabbed by an invisible knife.

(*Photo by George Weigel*)

"Sometimes the pain would be so excruciating that I would just be brought to tears," said Diane Pendleton, a neuralgian from Pennsylvania in a local newspaper account of her TN pain. "There's nothing you can do but hold on. Sometimes the pain would just take off on its own when I was doing nothing to provoke it. All of a sudden I would have these sharp pains that felt more and more like knife stab wounds."

Pendleton says she even tried slapping herself to try and "stun" the pain away. "It got to the point where the pain of slapping myself was nothing compared to what I was trying to get rid of," she says.

"'It feels like a hot poker sticking in my face.' That's probably the most common description I hear," says Dr. Benjamin S. Carson Sr., a neurosurgeon at Johns Hopkins Hospital in Baltimore. "Or, 'It feels like an electrical wire being rammed into my face.'"

Dr. Carson also is struck by the emotional impact the disorder has on patients. "The unpredictable and random nature of the shocks is completely unnerving to the victim and frequently will break down their resistance," he says.

HOW A TN PATIENT APPEARS TO OTHERS

- Suddenly makes distorted facial expressions.

- Suddenly jerks or turns head in pain.

- Posture is guarded to protect one side of face or a cloth is used to shield face from wind outside.

- Is reluctant to touch face or let others touch face.

- Tends to be very still, withdrawn and quiet during painful cycles.

- Is reluctant to sit in air-conditioned rooms or to go outside, especially on breezy days.

- Is reluctant to go to social events, especially those involving talking and eating.

- Is reluctant to brush teeth, wash face, shave or use cosmetics.

- Seems to have a reduced appetite or even skips meals.

- Constantly feels worn out.

That unforgettable first attack

Very often the TN patient vividly recalls that first attack and everything surrounding it.

When you ask them, "When did it start?" the patient will say, "It was June 15, 1996, it was 8 o'clock in the morning, and the sun was out." The whole scene is fixed in their minds.

That's the way it happened with singer Norma Zimmer, who has appeared for many years on the Lawrence Welk Show, Robert Schuller's Hour of Power, The 700 Club with Pat Robertson and at Billy Graham Crusades.

"It was during a singing engagement for Dr. James Kennedy in Grand Rapids, Mich., on Oct. 13, 1981, that I first experienced the horrible lightning-like shocks to my face," Zimmer recalls. "I was just concluding the beautiful song, 'How Great Thou Art,' when the hideous pain struck.

"It hit me three times, nearly knocking me off my feet. I immediately broke out in a cold sweat. I staggered off the stage, where I fell into my husband Randy's arms. That was the start. For 10 years, off and on, the excruciating shocks of trigeminal neuralgia continued to plague me."

Zimmer was unable to take carbamazepine (Tegretol, Carbatrol). Dental work, chiropractic therapy and acupuncture didn't help either. She spent years trying to avoid triggering attacks while getting temporary relief from physical therapy.

"For several years I continued to sing," says Zimmer, "but the shocking pain would strike as many as 10 times during the concerts, making it almost impossible to continue. The pain only lasted for a second, so I could manage to go on. But the stress of wondering when it might hit was terrible."

Zimmer eventually turned to surgery.

"I will never forget when it began," another neuralgian wrote anonymously in an Internet account of her TN. "Mine began the 24th of May, 1992. My sons were in school, and I was busy around the house, when out of the blue this incredible pain went shooting across my face. It seemed to go from my ear right to my back upper teeth. I *had* to sit down. It was gone in seconds, but it came again, and again. I was terrified, scared to move, scared to even breathe. I didn't want to do anything that could make it happen more often than it already was."

The writer soon learned this mysterious pain was TN, and true to form, it came and went in cycles until surgery ended the ordeal.

A warm-up for the real thing

Other times, TN starts out vaguely before eventually growing into the "real thing." In up to 18 percent of TN cases, the earliest signs are dull, general aches that may persist for weeks or months and come on without being triggered.

Eventually the dull ache turns into the sharp, fleeting attacks that are more common to TN. But until then, the pain is diagnosed as some other problem or treated as a mystery.

Sir Charles Symonds first noticed this progression in the late 1940s. In 1980, Dr. R.G. Mitchell coined the term "pretrigeminal neuralgia" to describe this "warm-up" pain.

Normally the same medications used to treat full-blown TN are effective in controlling the pain of pretrigeminal neuralgia – if a doctor or dentist is able to figure out that's what's going on.

Once you've got the "real thing," though, the severity and frequency of the attacks tend to increase over time. In the early stages, remissions may occur for weeks or months at a time. But then the pain almost always comes back – often more ferocious then before.

Over time, the breaks between these up-and-down cycles tend to get shorter, and the attacks tend to happen more often. Some patients ultimately find themselves having dozens of attacks per day with few or no remissions.

Diagnosis difficulties

Given the striking symptoms of classic TN, you'd think this would be an easy condition to diagnose even without some sort of test to nail it down. That's not the case.

Diagnosis of TN can be difficult for a variety of reasons. The quandary of "pretrigeminal neuralgia" is just one of them.

For starters, TN is not all that common, so some doctors and dentists may be only vaguely familiar with it. Some may have no first-hand experience with it at all. Their only exposure may have been a brief mention in medical or dental training years ago.

"One of the biggest problems is that as doctors we only see what we know," says Dr. Henry A. Gremillion, director of the Parker E. Mahan Facial Pain Center at the University of Florida College of Dentistry. "And we only treat what we see."

Second, common medical practice is to zero in on the most likely problems first and then move on to less likely problems after the likely ones have been ruled out. And there are dozens of disorders besides TN that involve orofacial pain, ranging from simple tooth problems to jaw-joint pain to sinus infections.

Third, patients sometimes don't always give fully accurate descriptions. Since most people have never even *heard* of TN, they're attempting to describe something for which they have no reference. That's why so many patients go first to their dentist insisting they've got some kind of tooth problem. "Toothache" is something most everyone knows. Or they may go to a doctor and complain about their "sinuses acting up."

Because of the quirky nature of the pain, patients may tell their doctor or dentist that the pain is constant or near constant when they're really having acute attacks separated by brief periods of relief. Or they may describe the pain in vague terms, such as "bad" or "terrible."

Sometimes it's hard for patients to give any description at all because talking triggers the pain. When that happens, doctors and dentists can usually stop the pain long enough for a patient history to be taken by giving a local anesthesia injection or anesthetic eye drops. Or patients resort to writing their answers.

Perhaps trickiest of all is when the patient seems to have a mix of symptoms that doesn't really fit into any one particular diagnosis "box." For instance, a patient may have one-sided, sharp, stabbing pains that come and go but also lower-grade, burning pain all the time – and no apparent trigger points.

Many of these cases – sometimes called "atypical trigeminal neuralgia" or "atypical facial pain" if the symptoms stray far enough from classic TN – are now thought to be variations of or later-stage cases of TN. (More on this in Chapter 4: "TN or Not TN?") Whatever they're called, these kinds of cases are even more difficult for front-line medical professionals to decipher.

Further complicating things is how TN's tendency to spontaneously remit gives false feedback.

Example: A dentist suspects that poorly fit dentures are the cause of a patient's jaw pain. So the dentist makes new dentures, and soon after, the pain goes away. Case solved. Or is it? What can happen in TN is that the pain coincidentally goes away around the time of the denture replacement – or the dental work temporarily disrupts a triggering zone. A few weeks later, the TN and its triggers act up again, and the "mystery pain" is back.

Unnecessary treatments

As a result of these diagnosis difficulties, it's not uncommon for patients to bounce around from doctor to doctor having root canals, tooth extractions, sinus surgeries and various other medical and surgical treatments until their TN is ultimately diagnosed. This may go on for years.

A survey of more than 7,600 TN patients by the Gainesville, Fla.-based Trigeminal Neuralgia Association found that more than half of those surveyed were diagnosed initially as having something other than TN. Nearly 90 percent of these people had pain for more than a year before they were accurately diagnosed, and 13 percent said they went 10 years or more before a doctor ultimately nailed down a TN diagnosis.

During this frustrating period, patients often wonder if the pain is "all in their mind" because treatments may not be helping and tests continue to show nothing abnormal. "One doctor *told* me it was all in my head," said Fred Lehman, a former neuralgian from Pennsylvania who ultimately got relief from a microvascular decompression surgery.

Drs. Steven B. Graff-Radford and Robert L. Merrill of Cedars-Sinai Medical Center and UCLA School of Dentistry in Los Angeles found that nearly two-thirds of 61 patients they questioned not only had been wrongly diagnosed initially but also wrongly treated. They turned up numerous misguided treatments, such as pulled teeth, root canals, oral surgery, braces and dental splints. Some patients reported multiple root canals, multiple tooth extractions and even root canals done twice on the same tooth.

In a similar 1988 study, University of Cincinnati neurosurgeons Dr. John Tew and Dr. Harry Van Loveren found that one-third of their 1,100 surveyed TN patients had teeth that were needlessly pulled.

Since secondary branches of the trigeminal nerve supply feeling to the teeth, it's no coincidence that tooth pain is often confused with TN pain. And since tooth- and gum-related problems are far more common causes of face pain than TN, it's a good idea to see a dentist or oral specialist early on to rule out dental causes. These causes are usually readily picked up by exam and X-ray.

"Dental problems can give rise to symptoms similar to trigeminal neuralgia or even play a part in its development," wrote Dr. Zakrzewska in her *"Trigeminal Neuralgia"* medical text (W.B. Saunders Co., 1995). "Patients should, therefore, be encouraged to have a full dental and oral examination." (For more on the dental connection to TN and other face pains, see Chapter 5.)

Education and awareness

On the bright side, misdiagnosis and misguided treatments are becoming less common every year. Unnecessary tooth-pullings and root canals are down markedly in the last 10 years, and patients are getting effective medications much earlier instead of wading through an average of seven to 10 medicines before ending up with one that helps.

Much of the progress stems from recent improved awareness of TN by the front-line practitioners – dentists and family doctors. Since 1990, a key part of the Trigeminal Neuralgia Association's mission has been to go to physician and dental conferences to raise awareness and provide educational materials to practicing professionals. TNA also has been offering its own biennial educational conferences since 1996, including training sessions for medical professionals.

Another aid is a recent change in U.S. public health policy that focuses greater attention on pain in general. New national rules took effect in 2002 requiring all health-care facilities under the aegis of the U.S. Joint Commission of Healthcare Organizations to make pain assessment a priority.

What that means is that most hospitals, health-care networks, long-term-care facilities and the like now must ask patients about their pain, record it and aggressively treat it. The change essentially makes pain assessment a fifth "vital sign" along with temperature, pulse, blood pressure and respiration.

The rules also recognize patients' rights to have their pain properly addressed, require periodic pain reassessments and require facilities to educate patients and their families about pain-relief measures.

At the same time, patients themselves are becoming better informed. Two factors are likely behind that – the rise of the Internet age with its volumes of information just a keystroke away, and a growing network of TN support groups across the United States, Australia and parts of Europe. That kind of ready information has made it possible for people to hunt down possible explanations for their symptoms on their own.

"In our experience in the last five years, more patients are diagnosing themselves than are being diagnosed by their doctors," says Dr. Peter Jannetta, the neurosurgeon who developed the microvascular decompression surgery in the 1960s and who still specializes in TN treatment at Allegheny General Hospital in Pittsburgh.

Diagnosing by description

So what are the keys to zeroing in an accurate diagnosis of TN? The main way is still the old-fashioned patient interview.

That old medical-school axiom, "Listen and the patient will tell you the diagnosis," really applies here. A careful interview should turn up lots of clues to differentiate TN from other conditions, such as:

• *The nature of the pain.* TN pain is sharp, stabbing, jolting and often has an "electrical" quality to it. Tooth pains, facial-muscle pain and sinus problems are more aching and constant, while migraines and cluster headaches are more throbbing or pulsating.

• *How the pain comes on.* TN pain is typically triggered by a light touch to the face and then disappears between attacks.

On the other hand, chewing is a common aggravating factor of temporomandibular joint disorders (TMD or TMJ). Tapping on a particular tooth will usually elicit pain in a dental problem. And a jaw muscle that hurts when it's rubbed may indicate myofascial pain, a jaw-muscle problem.

• *Times the pain occurs.* Some pains, such as hypertension headaches and sinus infections, tend to be worse in the morning. Other pains, such as toothaches and cluster headaches, often are worse at night.

---

10 TIPS ON GETTING A SPEEDY, ACCURATE FACE-PAIN DIAGNOSIS

1. Check with the family. Have any relatives ever had similar symptoms? What was their diagnosis? Their treatment?

2. Try to assess, as best you can, where the pain originates. Does it feel like a toothache? Or does it feel more like a muscle pain or a nerve pain? Is it coming from one particular tooth or more than one – and maybe even the nose or cheek? This can determine whether to first call a doctor, dentist or some other specialty.

3. Ask around to get names of highly regarded doctors and dentists, if you don't already have one. As in any field, some are better than others. Ask friends, family, neighbors, co-workers, other medical professionals and professional organizations such as local dental associations and medical societies for recommendations. Ask especially for experts in face pain.

4. Write down your pain experience so far. When did it start? Were there any precipitating or connected factors, such as a fall or trauma? Has the pain changed at all since you first got it?

5. Be ready to describe the location of the pain. Exactly where does it hurt? Is it always in the same spot? More than one spot? Does it move around? Is it worse in some spots than others?

6. Be ready to describe the nature of the pain as precisely as possible. Have several words ready that best describes it. Is it sharp? Stabbing? Burning? Achy? Electrical? Hot? The more descriptive you can be, the more it will help the doctor.

Continued on next page...

...Continued from previous page

7. Be ready to describe how the pain acts. Is it steady or does it come and go? When do you get it? How often do you get it? How long does it last? Does anything set it off? What makes it better? Worse? Does your body position make any difference?

8. Do some research. Check the Internet, the library or bookstores. Mention your symptoms to friends. Something you run across may strike a very familiar chord and at least raise a diagnosis worth considering. If nothing else, you'll begin to get familiar with the terms and possibilities.

9. Take the person closest to you along to the appointment. That person may have noticed something or be able to provide a clue that may help the practitioner. It's also a second set of ears to ensure you understood everything that was discussed (particularly helpful if you're on medication for the pain).

10. Don't hesitate to see another practitioner if the first one doesn't have a good answer or if the initial therapy isn't working. Doctors and dentists tend to look first for what they know best. If you've unwittingly picked the wrong type of practitioner for your condition, you may end up with an ineffective treatment – or worse. Particularly avoid destructive procedures such as root canals or tooth extractions unless there's good evidence to support it.

Sources: American Pain Society and Dr. Joanna Zakrzewska, Department of Oral Medicine, Barts and the London, Queen Mary's School of Medicine and Dentistry, England

Although TN attacks can happen any time, they're less common once you're asleep for the night. The exception is that some people (up to 40 percent) say they sometimes awaken in pain when they turn on the painful side of their face.

• **Things that aggravate or ease attacks.** Daily doings can sometimes be linked to pain and provide a clue diagnosis.

Drinking alcohol, for example, can bring on a round of cluster headaches. People suffering from migraines usually are sensitive to light and loud noises.

Light breezes that blow across the face or vibrations strong enough to be picked up by the teeth are two factors that TN patients often mention as attack-provokers. And some notice that their TN attacks come on when the air pressure changes, such as before a storm, when flying in an airplane or when visiting an area with a significantly different altitude.

Ruling out other problems

A careful medical history and examination should help sort out the TN and TN-related cases from altogether different disorders. Classic TN cases should be fairly easy to diagnose in experienced hands, but the murkier cases may involve seeing several types of medical specialists to either rule in or rule out the possibilities.

Dr. Parker E. Mahan, a dental professor emeritus at the University of Florida, says the starting point is figuring out whether the pain is originating in the trigeminal nerve or is merely being transmitted *through* the nerve from some other part of the body.

"All other tissue – bone, teeth, muscles, skin, glands – send signals through the nerves," he says. "So it's important to ask, 'From whence does the pain come?'"

A problem in any of those tissues could be causing face pain that mimics TN to some degree. These can include dental problems, jaw-joint problems, arthritis, blood-vessel disorders, facial tumors, sinus infections and even Lyme disease, a tick-transmitted infection that can lead to nerve damage.

Kate Borland of Virginia, for example, saw numerous doctors before one did a sinus CT scan that picked up some congenital problems in her sinus cavity. "I had multiple extra air sacs inside my sinuses, both sides of my nose and all across my forehead," she says. "They were trapping air, and any change in barometric pressure sent me into orbit. Most people have impaired nasal breathing. I had pain."

Sinus surgery cleared out these air sacs and finally ended the deep boring pain… "the one where I wanted to reach into my head and rip out the nerve," as Borland puts it. However, she still has a different type of constant face pain that she believes is related to a badly misaligned upper vertebrae. "My own conclusion is to keep an open mind and remember that the cranial nerves can be irritated for a variety of reasons, just like any other nerves in the body," she says. (Chapters 4, 5 and 6 will go into more detail on other face-pain disorders.)

When tests and exams aren't available to zero in on suspected problems, sometimes the only way to rule out something is by trying the therapy that's usually effective for that problem.

If it works, you're in luck. If not, you've at least ruled out one of the possibilities and can move on to the next possibility. This type of "trial-and-error" can be frustrating for both the patient and doctor (not to mention expensive), but sometimes it's the only way to get to the root of the problem – particularly in the non-classic cases.

Tests that doctors often do

When TN is suspected, most patients are referred to a neurologist, a specialist who's been trained in the medical treatment of nerve-related disorders. In addition to taking a detailed patient history, neurologists also normally will conduct a neurological exam.

This exam includes pin-pricks to test for numbness; coordination tests of the hands, fingers, arms and legs; checks to be sure the patient's gait is steady, and simple strength tests to determine if hand and leg muscles are working properly.

The point of this exam is to rule out – or discover – the involvement of other disease, particularly multiple sclerosis. In a small percentage of cases, TN pain is a result of MS plaques occurring on the trigeminal nerve. Normally, patients know they have MS before they develop face pain, but occasionally face pain *is* the first symptom.

Another test usually done is a magnetic resonance imaging (MRI) scan. An MRI unit is a painless test that uses powerful magnets and computerized images to produce a "photograph" of the body's interior structures. Unlike X-rays, it does not use radiation.

MRI pictures are clear enough to get a good look at tumors and abnormal blood vessels – two other problems that can cause face pain – as well as plaques on the nerve caused by MS. These pictures also normally show the trigeminal nerve itself. And researchers are close to perfecting enhanced MRI pictures that are good enough to see blood vessels that may be compressing the trigeminal nerve – the presumed cause of most TN pain. (See Chapter 8 for more on the MRI's use in helping to make a decision about surgery.)

If an MRI is not possible or available, the next best test is a computed tomography (CT) scan. This imaging system can pick up larger tumors and some blood-vessel problems, but it's not sensitive enough to reliably detect small tumors, multiple sclerosis lesions or blood vessels compressing the nerve.

Some doctors say carbamazepine (Tegretol, Carbatrol) is so effective and specific to TN pain that it can be a diagnostic aid itself. In other words, if that medicine helps, you've probably got TN or a variation of it. If not, it might be time to go back to the drawing board. However, others caution that up to a third of patients who really do have TN may not respond at all to carbamazepine. They say that while carbamazepine's effectiveness might be helpful as a clue, a TN diagnosis shouldn't automatically go out the window just because it *doesn't* work.

Changes in sensation?

Usually there is no *major* loss of facial sensation with TN. If there is, that may be a sign of a tumor, aneurysm (bulging, weak area of a blood vessel) or other abnormal growth in the head or face.

Dr. Dalessio says it's not unusual, however, for TN patients to mention a slight "numbness or deadness of the face or a feeling that part of the face has been anesthetized by Novocaine. Pain may or may not be associated with these sensations, which may come and go, last for a day or two or more, or sometimes become permanent."

Finnish neurologist Dr. Turo J. Nurmikko suggests TN patients may not be imagining this slight loss of feeling. Using sophisticated measuring devices, he did in-depth testing on 26 TN patients for temperature sensation, fine touch and pin-prick sensation. The results showed that 15 of the 26 patients had at least one abnormal measure.

Dr. Nurmikko concluded that small-scale changes often do occur that aren't as apparent under routine testing as they are when detailed measurements are used.

A family connection?

One other point worth exploring is family history. There is some evidence that TN may run in families.

Dr. Jannetta estimates that 5 percent or more of TN sufferers have a family history of the condition.

"I presume this occurs because we inherit our parents' blood vessels as well as other physical characteristics," he says. "Familial trigeminal neuralgia is commonly on the same side and generally starts at a younger age in succeeding generations."

Dr. Jannetta and others also have reported that bilateral TN – the rare occasion of having TN on both sides of the face – seems to be more common in patients who have a family history of TN.

"Although there's some heredity at work, it's not great enough odds for an offspring to worry about," adds Dr. Albert Rhoton, a neurosurgeon and TN specialist at the University of Florida College of Medicine.

Kids with TN

Diagnosing TN can be tricky enough when dealing with older adults. When it strikes young children, it's so unusual that doctors may not even think to consider it.

That's what happened when Suzanne Mason of Michigan began displaying the classic symptoms of trigeminal neuralgia.

Piercing attacks would hit her with a suddenness that would make her head jerk, then just as suddenly disappear. The pain always was on the same side of the face – in her case, the left, never the right.

For awhile, she'd seem to get better, only to have a new wave of attacks return, sometimes 60 of them a day. Everything pointed to a textbook case of TN, except for one thing. Suzanne was only 13 months old when the attacks started.

The medical literature says TN is primarily an older person's condition, something you get in your 50s, 60s or 70s – maybe in your 40s. But toddlers or young children? No way. It just isn't supposed to happen.

TN in young people is very rare, but it can and does happen. In the few cases in which surgeons have operated, they've found the same problem that's usually found to cause TN in adults – a blood vessel compressing the trigeminal nerve.

Cases of TN in young children were recorded in the United States as early as 1921 when one surgeon reported severing the trigeminal nerve of a 10-year-old boy to stop his pain.

In 1982, Cleveland neurosurgeon Dr. Robert F. Spetzler reported performing what is thought to be the first microvascular decompression on a child. The surgery relieved a 10-year-old boy of his TN pain.

Luann Carpino of Arizona – whose son, Nick, began having TN attacks at age 3 – thinks there may be more kids with TN than is realized. "I know they're out there," she says. "But I think a lot of them are still being misdiagnosed."

In her son's case, TN wasn't diagnosed until Nick was videotaped having an attack at age 7.

"We showed the tape to the neurologist and he said, 'That looks like tic (douloureux), but it can't be,'" recalls Carpino. "The doctors were really hesitant to diagnose TN because of Nick's age."

The Masons also went through numerous specialists over three years before Suzanne happened to have a major attack in front of two neurologists at the University of Michigan.

"All of a sudden she grabbed her face and started screaming and got real red and hot," says Lynn Mason. "That convinced them, but no one believed it."

Not only is diagnosing TN in kids tricky because it's so unusual, but kids often aren't able to verbalize the problem as well as adults.

"Nick was always pulling at his face when he was a baby," Carpino says. "He would often hold himself rigid and do off-the-wall things like rock himself back and forth. We thought he was just colicky.

"Finally, when he was about 3 and old enough to talk, he told us his face hurt and that it was 'hot' and 'tingly.' We realize now that the rocking probably was a distraction technique when he was having an episode."

Now 18, Nick has been managing his pain with gabapentin (Neurontin).

"One of the areas that I, as a parent, was not prepared for was the onset of puberty and how this impacted TN – both physically and emotionally," says Carpino. "Nick dealt with a lot of depression and grief. We had no idea this would happen. Also, the pain episodes changed in frequency due to puberty."

Lynn Mason remembers that Suzanne also pulled on her face a lot as a baby and "cried all the time. When they're young, they have no way of letting you know what's wrong."

When Suzanne was finally diagnosed with TN at age 5, she had a microvascular decompression surgery done by Dr. Jannetta in Pittsburgh. It was only partially successful.

After three more years of good periods and bad periods, the pain really flared, and Suzanne went back to Pittsburgh for a second microvascular decompression at age 8. That limited her pain to just an occasional twinge.

A junior in college as of this printing, Suzanne still gets daily "tingling" sensations but no pain, and she takes a low dose of oxcarbazepine (Trileptal) to prevent any break-throughs.

"Having this disorder is bad enough for an adult," says TNA founder Claire Patterson. "It's hard to imagine how a child could cope with it."

CHAPTER 3

WHAT'S CAUSING THIS TERRIBLE PAIN?

"Pressure on the nerve leaves a short-circuiting effect."
—San Diego neurologist Dr. James Nelson

Up until the 1980s, most papers and textbooks listed the cause of TN as unknown or unclear. A few still do. That's because not everybody agrees on exactly what's causing the pain. Not everyone even agrees what TN *is* and what might really be something else with similar symptoms.

Many of the particulars about TN have been mired in controversy over the years. Among the questions that have perplexed researchers and TN sufferers alike:

- Why is the pain so severe?
- Why does it come and go so suddenly?
- Why does light touch trigger it?
- Why are the trigger zones often not in the same area that hurts?
- What makes the pain go away on its own for weeks or months or even years at a time?
- Why don't the usual pain-killing drugs work?
- Why does it tend to affect older people?

There's even disagreement when it comes to deciding exactly what kind of problem TN is. Is it a disease? A disorder? An injury? A set of symptoms with several different causes? Or maybe a condition medicine just hasn't yet fully figured out?

To begin to understand what's going on inside when TN strikes, it helps to know a little about how the trigeminal nerve works when it's healthy and functioning normally.

How nerves work

The job of nerves in general is to report contact with the world around us. They're the body's messengers that make it possible for the different parts of the body to work together as one coordinated unit. Nerves make sure the heart beats as needed, they signal your legs to move faster when you're about to miss the bus, and they let you know when there's something crawling around on the back of your hand.

Nerves do all of this by way of billions of minuscule nerve endings or "receptors" that are stationed throughout the body. These receptors constantly monitor the environment in, on and around the body for changes. They then report this contact with the world back to the brain.

Each receptor has a very specific job. Some report only when there's heat, some report on cold, some report only light touch, some monitor for pin pricks, some monitor for pressure and so on. A receptor whose sole purpose in life is to monitor heat in the left little finger, for example, only springs into action when there's a significant enough change in heat in the left little finger to alert the body.

Each of these receptors is connected to a nerve fiber – a tiny strand of tissue whose job is to carry signals from the receptor. When enough of a change in the environment occurs that a receptor activates, a chemical change occurs in the cells of the nerve fiber connected to it. This sets off a chain reaction called a "nerve impulse" that's somewhat akin to an electric current.

Instead of electricity, nerve fibers use body chemicals (sodium, potassium and chloride) to move nerve impulses. As these biochemicals move through microscopic channels across nerve-cell membranes, the impulse is handed from cell to cell down the length of the nerve fiber.

The road to the brain

A nerve fiber isn't one long, continuous strand that goes the whole way to the brain, however. Fibers are a lot like highways that sometimes come to an intersection. To continue down the right road, impulses have to jump from one fiber to another across microscopic gaps called "synapses." At each synapse, the body has a chance to modify the receptors' messages. That can mean reducing a message's pending impact on our consciousness or increasing our awareness of it.

This is actually a very clever gatekeeper system to filter out changes that aren't worth alerting the brain. The nervous system sets certain thresholds of change that need to occur in order to continue to send the impulse. If the threshold isn't met, the signal ends, and the brain isn't "bothered" by every little change. This is why you may not experience pain from a tiny scratch or feel a speck of dust that lands on your head.

Without this sort of filtering system, the brain would be overwhelmed by all of the minor sensations bombarding our bodies every second.

The last stop is the brain itself, and it, too, has a built-in system of "checks and balances" that grades the nerve signals and decides which are "normal" and which need some sort of response by the body.

This grading system is what allows us to decide, for example, whether that hot tub of water is just perfect, hot enough that we need to wriggle our feet around a little first, or so hot that we'd better get our foot back out right away.

Up to a point, we can also decide to "overrule" a sensation. That's why we can tolerate heat from a heating pad. It's hot, but we're aware that it's intentional and that it's not immediately threatening. And so we put up with it and even adjust to the initially uncomfortable feeling. Introduce that same degree of heat from a sudden, unexpected source, on the other hand, and we might jump back with pain.

We're even able to temporarily snuff out quite intense pain signals for an overriding good or protective reason. For example, a person who twists an ankle and falls in the middle of a road may be able to hobble out of harm's way while suppressing the pain signals the ankle is sending out. When the emergency's over, the pain then comes through loudly and clearly.

The thresholds and grades that determine how we'll react also are able to adapt to changes in our body and the environment around us. For example, a warm shower normally feels good, but use the same temperature of water on newly sun-burned skin and suddenly you feel burning pain. Or use that heating pad on your back for *too* long and the sensation goes from comforting warmth to unbearable heat.

A sample impulse

Here's the way it's all supposed to work. Let's say the receptors in your finger tips have picked up a sudden change in heat. An impulse is sent along the nerve fibers in that region, the "gatekeeper" cells are convinced it's definitely significant, and now the thalamus (the "central switching station" of the brain) gets the impulse.

This is where you first perceive or "feel" something hot. The thalamus then alerts the cerebral cortex, another part of the brain whose job it is to locate the source of the problem, assess any damage going on and fire off new impulses that tell your hand and arm muscles to get your fingers off of the hot stove.

The cerebral cortex also will dispatch white blood cells to fight potential infection, activate nutrient reserves that are needed to start the healing process and send out "stop-pain" signals once the threat is under control.

Incredibly, all of this internal communication takes place in milliseconds.

One other thing the thalamus does is alert the limbic center of the brain, which determines your emotional response to sensations such as the hot-stove incident.

Depending on factors such as your mood, past pain experience and social setting, your reaction and even perception of the pain could vary greatly. At home by yourself, you may jump up and down after touching the hot stove and yell a few choice words at the profuse pain. Around dinner guests, you might say "ouch" and calmly go for some ice cubes. Around a date you're trying to impress, you might just grin and bear it.

The limbic system also creates a memory of this episode and etches a link in our mind between hot stoves and pain so we learn not to touch one again.

This kind of elaborate pain-sensing system is quite different from other mammals, which respond to all painful stimuli with pre-conditioned responses. It's also an important piece in explaining the TN puzzle and a possible avenue for getting pain relief, as we'll talk about in Chapter 20, "Coping With Face Pain."

Like a phone cable

People typically envision a nerve as a spaghetti-like strand of tissue that branches out into a few smaller tentacles. Actually, a nerve is more like a phone cable that's really a bundle made up of many smaller individual phone lines, or in this case, nerve fibers.

Each of the thousands of fibers in a typical nerve has its own specific purpose since each is attached to one of those narrowly focused receptors.

This is what allows the same nerve to tell the difference between a feather tickling our cheek and a pin pricking it. Each trigeminal nerve, for example, has an estimated 125,000 individual fibers – some that signal heat, some that signal pain, some that signal light touch and even some that control the jaw muscles we use when chewing.

Nerves come in different sizes depending on the number and types of fibers they contain. The more complex the nerve's duty, the more fibers it has and the bigger it is. Since the trigeminal nerve performs such a complex duty and has so many fibers, it's the biggest nerve in our head.

The fibers themselves also differ in size and number, depending on the types of message they carry and how fast those messages need to travel. Fibers that sense pain, for example, are larger than those that sense light touch. There are even different types of pain fibers – some that spring into action quickly (i.e. the so-called "A fibers" that give the brain sharp, immediate feedback when you hit your thumb with a hammer) and some that kick in for the longer term (the "C fibers" that carry that aching, throbbing pain that may last minutes or hours after you whacked your thumb).

The body strategically assigns more fibers to parts of the body where close monitoring is most important. Thus your face has a lot of receptors; your back has relatively few. Skin generally has more receptors and nerve fibers than muscle, which has a layer of skin protecting it. And organs have even fewer receptors and fibers because they are protected by skin, muscle and bones. This strategic placement of receptors explains why a pin prick in the face hurts worse than one in the derriere.

Many of the nerve fibers and the nerve itself are sheathed by a fatty, protective substance called "myelin." This is an especially important characteristic of nerves when it comes to TN and related face pain, as you'll see shortly. But first, a closer look at exactly what the trigeminal nerve does.

The trigeminal nerve's duty

The trigeminal nerve is one of the body's 12 sets of cranial nerves. Cranial nerves are those that exit directly from the brain stem and, with one exception, serve only the head and neck region. Thirty-one other sets of spinal nerves arise from the spinal cord and supply movement and sensation to the rest of the body.

Some nerves are for sensing only, some are for moving body parts only, but most are mixed nerves that do a bit of both. That's the case with the trigeminal nerve. It not only picks up all sorts of sensations throughout the face but also controls movement in most of the muscles used in chewing. That motor function explains why chewing is often a trigger for TN pain – it's all under the trigeminal domain.

Our two trigeminal nerves are important because they are responsible for almost all sensations in the face from the forehead to the lower jaw, including heat, cold, pressure, touch and, of course, pain. The right trigeminal nerve serves the entire right side of the face, and the left one serves the left side.

All of the trigeminal nerve fibers and branches come together at a "bulge" in the nerve called the trigeminal or "Gasserian" ganglion. This is where the nerve enters the skull. The nerve then travels inside the skull and connects to a part of the brain called the "pons."

When the nerves are working properly, their pain function is absolutely essential because that's what alerts us to any problems that might pose a threat to the face, whether it's a simple toothache, a festering infection or a life-threatening tumor.

THE 12 PAIRS OF CRANIAL NERVES

1.) Olfactory (smell)

2.) Optic (vision)

3.) Oculomotor (movement of eyes and focusing)

4.) Trochlear (movement of eyes)

5.) Trigeminal (sensation in face, jaw muscles used in chewing)

6.) Abducens (movement of eyes)

7.) Facial (facial muscles, scalp, taste)

8.) Acoustic (or vestibulocochlear) (hearing, balance)

9.) Glossopharyngeal (taste, muscles used in swallowing, sensation in pharynx and middle ear)

10.) Vagal (movement and sensation in pharynx and larynx; sensation in abdominal organs; monitors heart rate, blood pressure and digestion)

11.) Accessory (muscles in pharynx, larynx, upper neck and upper throat)

12.) Hypoglossal (movement of tongue)

"Pain is much like a fire alarm system in your house," says Emily Jane Lemole, a Pennsylvania health counselor. "It tells you something is wrong in the body."

When the pain-signaling system itself malfunctions, however, a person may experience pain even though the threat has passed or even though there was no real threat in the first place.

Pain can even be purely psychological – no physical cause but still no less real to the person feeling it.

What's going wrong

Everyone agrees, at least, that in TN, the trigeminal nerve is "misfiring" – sending pain signals when it shouldn't.

Most also agree that loss of or damage to the nerve's protective coating – the myelin – is related to the problem. The disagreement starts when it comes to explaining why the myelin is abnormal and what's causing the nerve to misfire.

The most widely accepted view is that myelin damage results from a chronic irritation of the nerve – usually a blood vessel compressing it in the first 4 millimeters of the trigeminal nerve as it connects to the pons (the "root" of the nerve, in other words).

Blood constantly pulsating through the vessel causes the vessel to beat on the myelin, the explanation goes, eventually wearing down the myelin to the point where the nerve begins to malfunction.

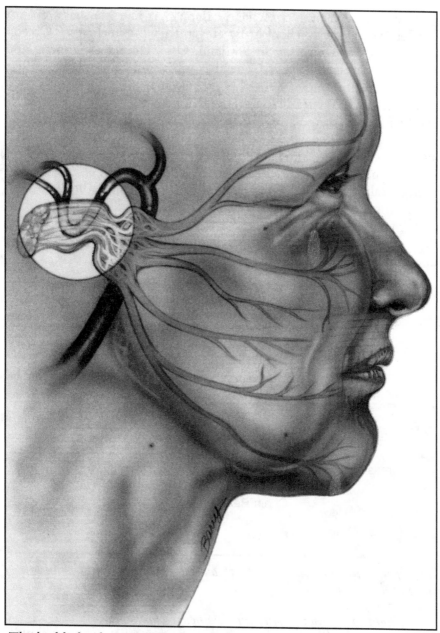

The highlighted area inside the circle shows where inside the head a blood vessel is often found to be compressing the root of the trigeminal nerve. (Sketch by Margaret Barry, University of Florida)

Recent research by Drs. Z. Harry Rappaport and Marshal Devor at the Tel Aviv Medical School in Israel, Dr. Kim Burchiel at the Oregon Health Sciences University in Portland, Ore., Drs. Peter Jannetta and Kenneth Casey at Allegheny General Hospital in Pittsburgh and others sheds new light on exactly how TN pain occurs.

This research equates TN with what happens when a plugged-in electrical wire loses its insulation. When the bare strands touch, they spark, short-circuit, and the wire stops working like it should. In TN, the damaged nerve fibers are like bare wires, and light touch is like the kick of the cord that sets off sparking and short-circuiting.

In a healthy nerve, a gentle touch of the lip or a slight breeze on the cheek would create an impulse that's sent to the brain by nerve fibers that sense light touch. But in a nerve with damaged myelin, impulses are thought to "jump" or "leak" from light-touch fibers to pain-signaling fibers, thereby sending an altered signal to the brain.

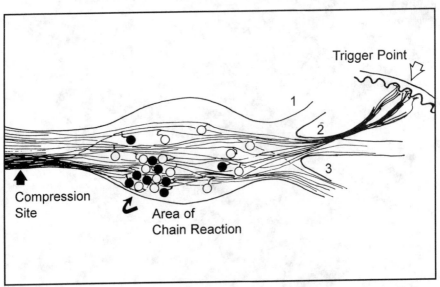

This sketch illustrates the theory of how a light touch from the middle or second division of the trigeminal nerve can set off a misguided chain reaction of pain.

The light touch should only activate neurons that respond to light touch (represented by the open circles). But when neighboring neurons that respond to pain (represented by the filled circles) are hypersensitve due to nearby compression damage from a blood vessel, they also may activate.

(Sketch reprinted with permission of Dr. Z. Harry Rappaport, Tel Aviv University Medical School)

Much of this fiber-jumping is thought to occur either at the Gasserian ganglion, the point on the trigeminal nerve where the three main branches and all of their respective fibers come together, or at the point of vessel compression near the nerve root, where the pain and light-touch fibers are closest to one another.

In other words, a sensation that starts out as an innocuous impulse on a light-touch nerve fiber crosses over into a neighboring pain fiber, turning that impulse into a pain signal instead. The brain then misreads the gentle touch of the lip or slight breeze on the cheek as pain. "It's like tuning your radio to one station and getting another," says Dr. David Sirois, chairman of the New York University College of Dentistry's Department of Oral Medicine.

This creates major havoc in the nervous system and brain. Suddenly, all sorts of intense, conflicting signals are coming in from the face. The entire nerve pathway seems to be reacting to what started out as a very minor and very focused signal. Instead of a limited and proper reaction to a minor stimulus, many wrongly recruited nerve fibers are firing off by themselves.

The pain-processing parts of the brain don't know what to make of this. The logical brain responses don't work because the incoming signals aren't accurately reporting what's taking place. Confused, the brain calls other parts of its pain-response arsenal into action.

It's much like what happens if you leave an inflated blood-pressure cuff on the arm for too long. At first, you might experience a bit of discomfort in the lower arm. After awhile, the upper arm begins to ache a bit. Finally, you might even begin to get a bit queasy. The pit of your stomach feels a bit hollow. Then the shoulder, chest and whole arm hurt. The brain has regionalized the signal and "called out the reserves."

"Irritable" nerves

When a nerve is injured – from whatever cause – it often becomes overly sensitive or "hyperexcited." Recent research suggests that happens, at least in part, because the body tries to compensate for the injury by creating new channels for biochemicals to carry signals through the nerve. (Impulses travel when sodium, potassium and chloride move through these channels from one nerve cell's membrane to another.) It's as if the body builds several new "highways" to carry traffic that no longer can travel over the damaged original highway.

The result is that nerve fibers tend to "overreport" or fire off signals at the slightest provocation. That creates a situation in which things that didn't upset the nerve now do.

Nerve injuries also may interfere with the brain's ability to send "stop-pain" signals, hindering a switch-off of the pain once an attack such as TN starts.

Nerve monitoring in animal studies has confirmed that background nerve activity goes up when myelin is injured. That means it might not take much of a stimulation to trigger a TN pain attack – sometimes even a stimulation that's not noticed at all.

Once an attack is triggered, it may not stop until the nerve has completely worn itself out and is physically incapable of firing anymore.

Drs. Rappaport and Devor believe what finally stops attacks is that the nerve discharges all of its potassium, sodium and calcium – the elements the body uses to create nerve impulses in the first place. Until the supplies of those body chemicals replenish themselves, the nerve is incapable of firing again.

Both the rate at which these chemicals replenish and the levels needed to cause the nerve cells to ignite in the first place (those threshold levels that we talked about earlier) vary from person to person and time to time. Drs. Rappaport and Devor say that may explain why one person with a compressing blood vessel ends up with terrible TN pain while another person with a similar compression might not.

This might also explain why some patients are able to "overload" their pain. Some patients say they endure one big attack when they start to eat and then get a pain-free window of 10 or 15 minutes to finish the meal before another attack occurs. It's not unusual for neuralgians to go hours between attacks.

According to Drs. Rappaport and Devor, the massive attacks of TN deplete the nerve of nerve-firing chemicals, and there isn't enough left to ignite a new chain reaction – until later.

The only mystery here is why a person can still feel a light touch right after a pain blowout but that light touch no longer triggers pain. If the chemicals are depleted, in other words, how can the nerve fibers send any signals?

Another possible explanation is that the gatekeeper system in the nerve cells and brain – after being overwhelmed initially by the wave of pain signals – resets the threshold levels to quell the errant, overly sensitive nerve firings. Eventually, the thresholds return to normal levels, setting the stage for a possible new attack.

This scenario is much like putting out a fire. A fire flares and burns out of control until the fire company has time to respond and put it out. But if the cause of the original fire isn't eliminated, the blaze will rekindle after the firefighters are back at the station.

The remission cycles

Not only do TN attacks hit for a few seconds to a minute or so and then go away for hours at a time, most neuralgians experience much longer periods where they have no attacks at all. Sometimes people go months or even years between "cycles" of TN attacks.

The leading explanation here is that the nerve has temporarily healed itself by generating new myelin. Nerves are capable of repairing themselves, but the repair rate can vary over different times and can vary from person to person. Thus one possible reason why some people are more prone to TN attacks than others is that they don't repair myelin as quickly.

When myelin repair falls behind, a full-blown TN cycle may occur. When repairs "catch up," a pain-free interval may result. And when partial repairs are made, the theory goes, that's when a person may experience a "rumbling" type of pain.

The suspected role of aging

The whole theory of a blood vessel compressing and injuring the trigeminal nerve may answer why TN seems to strike primarily those in their 50s and up. Vessels often harden and elongate with age, and our brains even "sag" (like other parts of the body), thereby causing a vessel/nerve contact where there was none before.

"My experiences and those of my colleagues have clearly shown that vascular compression of the trigeminal nerve is present in virtually all patients with TN," says Dr. Jannetta, who was one of the earliest proponents of the vessel theory. "The one major exception is in patients with multiple sclerosis."

In those cases, MS itself causes the body to attack and destroy myelin. When myelin destruction occurs at the root of the trigeminal nerve – the same location where vessel compressions are usually found – people get the same kind of pain. (More on MS-related face pain in Chapter 4.)

Some people also are just more prone to trigeminal nerve injury because of the makeup of their blood vessels. That's apparent just by looking at the back of people's hands. Notice how some people have unusually large, protruding and "wiggly" vessels while others have barely visible vessels? Odds are the first group also has similar kinds of blood vessels throughout the body, including inside the head. All it takes is for one tortuous vessel to be in the wrong place – namely up against one of the trigeminal nerves – for agonizing pain to result.

Dr. Jannetta says the characteristic of our blood vessels is something we often inherit, which is a likely reason for TN's slight propensity to run in families. And in rare cases, as we discussed at the end of Chapter 2, some children are born with blood vessels compressing their trigeminal nerves.

Compressions of all kinds

In cases not involving MS, Dr. Jannetta says the cause of TN is an artery or vein – sometimes more than one – squeezing the nerve. He says he has found vessels large and small growing onto the nerve, hiding behind the nerve and even wrapping themselves around the nerve like miniature snakes.

Sometimes vessels can be completely embedded within the trigeminal nerve fibers, "gouging the dickens out of the nerve," as Dr. Jannetta puts it.

Sometimes several vessels combine to squeeze the nerve in a "vessel sandwich."

Just where and how these vessels compress the nerve determine the nature and severity of a person's pain. Dr. Jannetta, who has treated

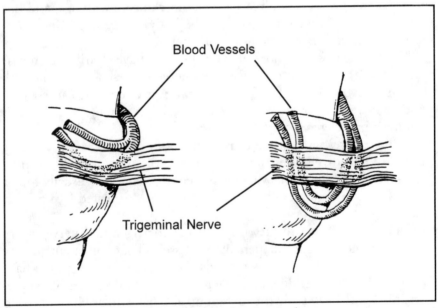

Examples of how blood vessels can compress the trigeminal nerve.
(Sketch by Ron Filer, used with permission of University of Pittsburgh)

thousands of face-pain patients over nearly 40 years, says he can usually predict where he's going to find an offending blood vessel during surgery just by his patients' description of the location and nature of their pain. He's even developed a series of training sketches for surgeons that show various types of compressions surgeons are likely to encounter.

After seeing what happens to people when their trigeminal nerve is compressed, Dr. Jannetta began to explore what happens when other cranial nerves are compressed. He found a variety of links to other problems, ranging from high blood pressure to sleep apnea to diabetes.

"When nerves are compressed, they're injured, and you get a caricature of what the nerve does normally," Dr. Jannetta explains.

In the case of the pain-sensing trigeminal nerve, the "caricature" is extreme agony. In the case of the acoustic nerve that's responsible for hearing, the caricature is ringing in the ears. In the case of the facial nerve, it's one-sided facial spasms. (See the accompanying chart for other suspected compression-related conditions.)

"Compressions can cause a compendium of problems," says Dr. Jannetta.

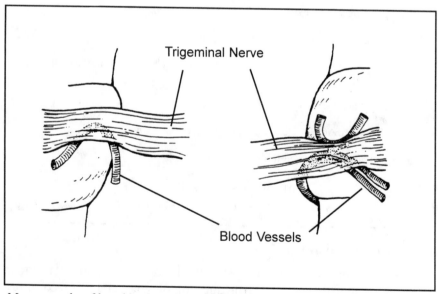

More examples of how blood vessels can compress the trigeminal nerve.
(Sketch by Ron Filer, used with permission of University of Pittsburgh)

PROBLEMS WITH OTHER COMPRESSED NERVES

When the trigeminal nerve is compressed by a blood vessel, severe pain can result. But what happens when other cranial nerves or parts of the brain are compressed? Below are conditions that may result when the following nerves are compressed:

Olfactory nerve:	loss of smell
Optic nerve:	blind spots
Oculomoter nerve:	quivering or paralysis of eye muscles or drooping of eyes
Trochlear nerve:	quivering or paralysis of eye muscles
Trigeminal nerve:	face pain, cluster headaches or spasms of jaw muscles (if motor fibers are affected)
Abducens nerve:	quivering or paralysis of eye muscles
Facial nerve:	spasms or paralysis of face muscles
Acoustic nerve:	ringing in ears, dizziness, balance problems, hearing loss
Glossopharyngeal nerve:	throat pain or difficulty swallowing
Vagal nerve:	difficulty swallowing
Accessory nerve:	torticollis(uncontrolled neck contractions that turn the head)
Hypoglossal nerve:	difficulty moving tongue
Nervus intermedius:	cluster headaches, deep ear pain
Left medulla:	high blood pressure
Right medulla:	type II diabetes, high cholesterol

— *Source: Drs. Peter Jannetta and Kenneth Casey, Allegheny General Hospital, Pittsburgh*

Is it always a compression?

One of the nagging issues that still divides doctors – particularly neurologists vs. neurosurgeons – is the question of whether a vessel compression is *the* one and only cause of TN.

After all, most neurosurgeons who perform microvascular decompression (MVD) surgeries have gone inside people's skulls looking for an offending vessel to move out of harm's way, only to find none. The medical journals have reported anywhere from 1 percent to 16 percent of surgeons' MVD procedures turn up no evidence of a compression. (The 1 percent to 3 percent range is the recent norm.)

Doubters also point to cases in which surgically corrected compressions didn't relieve people's pain, and they mention cadaver studies in which some deceased people were found to have vessels against their trigeminal nerves, yet never complained of pain.

Doctors in this camp argue that an open-skull procedure is needlessly risky for a condition that's not fatal and also treatable by other less risky operations and treatments.

Dr. Jannetta says when MVDs fail right off the bat, it's because the surgeon missed a compression spot or failed to adequately insulate the vessel from the nerve.

Surgeons sometimes don't find vessels, he says, because they may not be looking in all the right places. In other words, they might simply miss seeing a very small offending vessel in an unlikely or hard-to-examine area. He says that as a surgeon's skill and experience with MVDs rises, the number of "nothing-found" cases drops.

Another occasional finding is that the nerve itself is scarred or not getting adequate blood. Those problems can interfere with the trigeminal nerve's function and produce the same kind of symptoms that a compressing blood vessel can.

As for the cases in which people have had vessels on their trigeminal nerves but no pain, Dr. Jannetta says it takes more than mere contact to cause TN trouble. It takes an actual compression, he says.

London neurosurgeons Dr. Peter J. Hamlyn and Dr. Thomas T. King sought to settle this debate in 1992 by comparing the vessel situation of TN patients to that of an equal number of people who had recently died.

Drs. Hamlyn and King studied 41 TN patients who underwent MVD surgery. They also examined the trigeminal nerves of 41 people who had died within 17 hours previously and who did not have TN. The deceased subjects were matched for age and sex with the TN patients, and they underwent the exact same operation as the living TN patients. Resin was pumped into the deceased subjects' vessels to simulate a living condition.

The results: Of the 41 living TN patients, vessel contact of the nerve was found in 37 cases at operation. In all but one of the 37, the nerve appeared distorted, and a groove was noticed in the nerve when the vessel was lifted off it. In other words, the vessel appeared to be compressing the nerve, not just contacting it.

Neurosurgeons also say they often find a grayish discoloration of the nerve at the point of compression, suggesting damage to the nerve's myelin sheath.

In the cadavers, only four of 41 had a vessel contacting the nerve. "No cases of compression were found," Drs. Hamlyn and King reported. "Vessels similar to those found in the (TN) cases were absent, and no grooves or distortions were seen."

Their conclusion: "Even simple contact occurs only occasionally in the normal individual... It appears that grooving of the nerve is specific to trigeminal neuralgia."

Tumors and cysts

Tumors and cysts also can be a cause of TN. In a 14-year Mayo Clinic study, about 10 percent of the nearly 3,000 TN patients treated there were found to have brain tumors. Most other studies have reported much lower rates, down around 2 to 4 percent.

The most common type of tumor found in the Mayo Clinic study was a meningioma, a tumor of the brain's membrane lining. Neuromas, tumors of nerves, also can cause TN.

Tumors and cysts can cause TN pain either by compressing the trigeminal nerve directly or by pushing blood vessels against the trigeminal nerve. That may happen, for example, when an acoustic neuroma occurs on the acoustic (hearing) nerve that's near the trigeminal nerve. As that tumor grows, it takes up more space in the brain and may push a nearby blood vessel onto the neighboring trigeminal nerve.

Fortunately, most masses can be readily detected by CT or MRI scans and readily addressed by surgery, radiation, chemotherapy or some combination of the three.

The "AAA" of anatomy problems

Three other anatomical problems that can lead to TN are aneurysms, arteriovenous malformations and arachnoid tissue.

Aneurysms are weak areas of blood vessels that allow the vessel to bulge and possibly rupture. If this bulging allows pulsating blood to injure the myelin of the trigeminal nerve, it can cause the same problems as a "normal" blood vessel that's worked its way up against the trigeminal nerve.

This problem is often difficult to detect, but when aneurysms are found, they can be stabilized with surgical clips.

Arteriovenous malformations, or "AVMs," are abnormal blood vessels that grow randomly. Sometimes they grow up against the trigeminal nerve and cause compression injury to the nerve's myelin sheath. AVMs are prone to sudden rupturing, and they can be fatal when that happens. Fortunately, AVMs are usually detectable by imaging, and they can be surgically removed or destroyed by radiation.

In even more rare instances, a scarred or abnormally thickened arachnoid layer of the brain can cause a compression injury to the trigeminal nerve. Surgery to remove the scarring or thickened tissue can solve this source of pain.

Some other things that could be causing TN

If it's not villainous vessels, MS lesions *or* abnormal growths at the root of the pain, what else could it be?

Some have suggested that one other possibility may be a degenerative process that comes with aging of the nerve. Others have suggested that unknown toxins might be behind at least some cases.

Brain injuries can also cause pain that acts like TN. If the thalamus is injured, for example, it can give people a false sensation of pain even when there is no reason for it in the area that seems to hurt. No matter where pain originates, it's always perceived in the brain. So if the pain-processing parts of the brain are injured by trauma or stroke, they can malfunction and create a host of problems.

Some researchers previously speculated that a persistent viral infection of the trigeminal (Gasserian) ganglion could be a possible cause. However, recent research has found no evidence to back up that possibility.

There have even been a few reported cases of TN appearing as a rare side effect of an overdose of the heart drug digoxin.

Also, disabling conditions such as stroke can actually cause the nerve to die at certain points, creating a facial pain similar to TN called "trigeminal neuropathy." (More on this type of pain in Chapter 4.)

Practitioners of complementary and alternative medicine have their own theories as well.

For example, chiropractors attribute at least some cases of face pain to misaligned vertebrae putting damaging pressure on the spinal root of the trigeminal nerve. They say the answer to that is realigning the upper cervical spine. (More on this in Chapter 17.)

Acupuncturists believe the cause is an imbalance in the body's natural flow of energy. They seek to correct the pain by inserting needles at various points of the body in an attempt to rebalance that energy flow. (More on this in Chapter 16.)

A few in the field of oral surgery believe that jaw-bone infections following root-canal and other oral surgery can sometimes injure trigeminal nerve branches and cause severe TN-like face pain. They say the answer is cleaning out "bony cavities" in the jaw and treating with antibiotics. (More on this in Chapter 5.)

And some doctors and nutritionists have proposed that lack of Vitamin B-12 and possibly other nutritional defects prevent the body from building the myelin needed to head off TN pain. They say that Vitamin B-12 shots or megadoses – plus other nutritional changes – may stop pain without surgery or medicine. (More on this in Chapter 18.)

CHAPTER 4

TN OR NOT TN?
VARIATIONS ON THE THEME

"Words matter, because what you describe will make a difference in treatment"
—Dr. Kim Burchiel, chief of neurosurgery,
Oregon Health Sciences University

People in pain don't always care much what label their pain is given. They know they hurt, and their main goal is just to get rid of the pain. And fast.

But it's critical to nail down an accurate diagnosis – to put a person's pain in the "right box" – because similar symptoms may have different causes that therefore call for different treatments. Barking up the wrong tree not only leads to ineffective treatments but may even make the pain worse.

As we discussed earlier, diagnosing a case of classic trigeminal neuralgia *should* be easy, but in real life, it doesn't always turn out that way. The going gets even tougher when symptoms don't fit into that neat, little, five-point TN diagnosis box mentioned at the beginning of Chapter 2.

What happens when someone says they have those sharp, stabbing, electric attacks but also a constant burning, throbbing, aching pain?

What if they don't have *any* sharp stabs – just a constant ache?

What if there's numbness along with the pain?

What if there are no pain triggers?

What if the pain started out acting like classic TN but is now changing into something different… a more burning, constant pain?

What if the pain creeps outside the trigeminal nerve's territory, maybe into the back of the head, the neck or the shoulder?

What do you tell someone like Carol Preston of Texas, who describes her pain this way: "It's like having a cattleprod put directly into your ears, and then when that does not get stopped, it moves all over your face – one prod of electrical shot after another, never knowing when or where it will attack, in sleep or awake, with no warning." She's also had slurred speech, dizziness and hypersensitivity to noise.

What do you call these cases?

Are they all TN? A blend of TN and one or more other conditions? Or something else altogether?

It must be "atypical?"

Perplexed by these mixed-symptom cases, doctors began referring to them as "atypical trigeminal neuralgia." That term dates back to 1927 when that definition was given to pains similar to TN that didn't quite match the definition of classic TN.

"Atypical" cases are marked by pain that's described more as "aching," "burning" and "throbbing" as opposed to "sharp," "stabbing" or "electric-like." Many times, people have both – a constant or near-constant aching pain with fleeting stabs superimposed over them.

So-called atypical TN seems to affect women far more often than men. People often have no memorable first attack as is usually the case with the sharp and sudden onset of classic TN. "Atypical" pain also may or may not have trigger zones that set it off, it's more likely to affect both sides of the face than classic TN, and slight numbness or other sensory loss often accompanies it.

If these symptoms stray far enough from TN – especially when the pain goes beyond the areas served by the trigeminal nerve – the diagnosis may change to the even murkier tag of "atypical face pain."

While these names attempt to distinguish one type of pain from another, they do little to define the problem or the underlying causes. They say more about what the pains are *not* than what they *are*.

Another shortcoming is that these names don't define the boundaries among the three conditions. For instance, when someone has both sharp, stabbing pains and constant, aching pain, at what point do we call it "atypical TN" instead of classic TN? And at what point does a case of "atypical TN" become "atypical face pain?"

The definitions matter because the effectiveness of treatments vary depending on the nature of people's pains. Anticonvulsant medications, for instance, usually work best against sharp, stabbing pains while antidepressants and anti-inflammatory medicines tend to be more effective against burning, aching, constant pain.

Sorting out the "atypicals"

The most effective way to sort out these variations is by the patient's description of them.

In medicine, doctors most of the time are able to figure out a diagnosis just on the patient's history and descriptions alone. Physical exams and tests are done most of the time to confirm the suspicions.

In the case of TN and related face pain, the first big hurdle is to separate the nerve-related cases from everything else. Our faces can hurt for lots of reasons, ranging from tooth problems to sore jaw joints to inflamed sinuses to blood-vessel-related problems such as migraines. Tests such as dental exams, X-rays and MRIs are helpful at confirming most of the conditions outside the realm of TN and nerve pain.

Once the nerves are implicated (usually by a combination of the patient's descriptions and ruling out other possibilities), the aim is to figure out which nerve is the problem, exactly where on the nerve the problem is occurring and what's behind it.

That can get tricky because the face's nervous system is so interconnected and complex. Remember, 12 different sets of nerves are all performing different duties throughout the head. Sometimes two or three different nerves branch out into one body part, each responsible for its own function.

For example, the middle branch of the trigeminal nerve serves part of the ear canal and the lining of the inner ear, but it doesn't go deep into the ear. The glossopharyngeal nerve picks up where the trigeminal nerve leaves off in the rest of the ear canal and eardrum. Still other parts of the ear are served by the *nervus intermedius,* a branch of the geniculate nerve.

So when a person says his or her ear hurts, any of these nerves could be involved. The more precisely a person can locate and describe the pain, the better the chance of zeroing in on the right problem at the right place. These clues can be subtle but important.

A variation on the TN theme?

Doctors and face-pain researchers are especially interested in the exact nature and location of nerve problems for another reason. They believe this may explain the cause of many of these so-called "atypical" cases.

You'll recall that the leading explanation for classic TN is a blood vessel compressing the trigeminal nerve near where it connects to the pons (brainstem). It's now widely accepted that that kind of injury in that spot produces sharp, stabbing attacks in the face.

But what happens if a blood vessel compresses the nerve farther out from the root? What happens when different parts of the nerve are compressed by different blood vessels, in differing angles, under differing pressures or for differing lengths of time? Or what happens when the nerve is injured in other ways, such as by a viral infection or trauma?

The emerging opinion – at least among neurosurgeons – is that you get a whole spectrum or continuum of pains. One type of nerve injury may cause mostly sharp pain in the lower jaw, another type may cause mostly burning pain in the cheek. Two different compressions at two different spots might explain mixed symptoms.

Dr. Peter Jannetta, the Pittsburgh neurosurgeon, calls these "variations on the theme" of classic TN. In other words, the underlying problem is the same; it's the differences in how and where the nerve is injured that accounts for the pain variations, he believes.

Dr. Jannetta says that when he operates on people with so-called "atypical" pain, he almost always finds blood vessels compressing the trigeminal nerve – just as in those with classic TN symptoms.

In one new study on this question, Dr. Anthony M. Kaufman at the University of Manitoba in Winnipeg, Canada, compared the surgical results of 156 consecutive people who had microvascular decompression operations. One-hundred-twenty-nine of these people had classic TN, and the remaining 27 had so-called "atypical TN."

Kaufman and his colleagues discovered blood vessels compressing the trigeminal nerve root in every case in both groups. The only difference was the classic TN patients had slightly better results. Eighty-two percent of the classic TN patients reported complete pain relief or at least 75 percent relief, while only 74 percent of the "atypicals" had that level of relief.

Kaufman's conclusion: both TN and "atypical TN" are forms of the same problem, namely a blood vessel compressing the trigeminal nerve root.

What's injured… and for how long?

Dr. Kim Burchiel, chief of neurosurgery at Oregon Health Sciences University in Portland, also believes so-called "atypical" cases are really variations on the TN theme.

He suggests that the type of face pain a person feels is related to the type of nerve fibers that are injured. When small "fast-pain" fibers are injured (the ones that spring into action immediately when the bee stings your face), the resulting pain is sharp, stabbing and electrical, as in classic TN. But when slower fibers that carry heat and delayed-reaction pains are injured (the ones that cause a throbbing ache for hours after the bee did his damage), the pain is more of an aching, burning pain more akin to "atypical" TN.

Dr. Burchiel also believes that a more constant, burning face pain occurs when the motor branch of the trigeminal nerve is compressed by a blood vessel. That's the section of the nerve that regulates chewing. And he's found that veins are more frequently the compressing vessels in his "atypical" TN cases than arteries.

How long *any* vessel is allowed to compress the nerve might be the most significant concern. Blood vessels that beat on nerves year after year may cause a chronic injury that not only changes the nature of a person's pain but also makes it harder to treat.

"My own belief is that the nerve is becoming more damaged over time," says Burchiel. "It's my impression that TN is a progressive disorder. It may start out with textbook symptoms, and medicines may help. But over time, it becomes less and less textbook and become less and less responsive to medication."

One of the most common changes TN patients describe is that sharp, stabbing pains tend to pick up an underlying and more constant burning pain that lingers after a lightning attack. Over time, that kind of aching, lingering pain can actually become the predominant type of pain.

Dr. Jannetta often sees other changes in long-time neuralgians. "In time, patients with TN pain will get more frequent pain that will tend to last longer and in some cases will begin to awaken them from sleep," he says.

Attacks that once happened three or four times a day start happening 10 or 12 times a day – or more. Pain that used to rate an 8 on the 1-10 scale at the neurologist's office becomes a 10 – or a 20. Higher and higher doses of medicine may be needed to stop pain from breaking through. And those pain-free remission periods start shrinking, or disappear. That kind of progression doesn't always happen, but it's certainly not unusual.

Neurosurgeons say that if a damaging compression takes place long enough, the nerve may be injured beyond repair. Nerve fibers may even begin to scar together. That, they say, may explain why surgery success rates aren't as good for so-called "atypical" cases and for those who have waited more than seven years to have surgery to move a blood vessel off of their trigeminal nerve. (Details on that surgery – microvascular decompression – are discussed in Chapter 13).

Dr. John Alksne, chief of neurological surgery at the University of California in San Diego, equates this with other, more familiar chronic injuries.

"If you have a rock in your shoe for 15 minutes," he says, "you take it out and you're great. If you have a rock in your shoe and you go on a 20-mile hike, you're going to have a sore on your foot that's going to take some time to heal. If you have a rock in your shoe for 10 years, that sore may never heal."

If this thinking is correct, it raises new implications about whether – or when – it makes sense to consider surgery. We'll discuss that "nerve-wracking" issue in Chapter 8.

When do variations become something else?

Not everyone is convinced that all of these "atypical" cases are really different versions of TN.

Many neurologists, in particular, are skeptical about lumping too broad a set of symptoms under one supposed name or cause. Most neurologists can tick off examples of patients they've treated who have undergone ineffective surgeries – or worse yet, ones that made the pain worse or harder to control.

Dr. J. Keith Campbell, professor emeritus of neurology at the Mayo Medical School in Minnesota, says so-called "atypical" cases are not nearly as well understood or managed as classic TN cases – either by medications or surgery. He believes that the more the symptoms stray from classic attacks into the murkier constant pain, the less likely it is the person is suffering from TN.

When the pain is constant without any sharp spikes or triggers, it's time to consider a different diagnosis, Dr. Campbell says. "I don't think these are a subdivision of TN at all," he says. "I think these are a separate problem altogether."

Some of these possibilities are discussed in Chapter 6, "Other Face Pains: Not TN, Not Dental, But It Still Hurts."

Another possible explanation is that "atypical" cases may sometimes involve nerve injuries other than a compressing blood vessel, such as by the bacterium that causes Lyme disease, the viruses that cause shingles and AIDS, head trauma and complications from surgeries that attempted to stop face pain.

Although these account for a very small percentage of total face-pain cases, they might well explain the majority of ones that affect the trigeminal nerve but don't fit into what we call trigeminal neuralgia.

Changing the names

Some doctors and researchers believe it's best to scrap the old "atypical TN" and "atypical face pain" names altogether and rethink the entire way we classify TN and related face pains.

Dr. Burchiel is one who believes "atypical" is not only a murky, catch-all term, it can be somewhat "pejorative." "It's like saying, 'What's wrong with you? Why can't you have something that's more typical?'"

He also argues that these kinds of pains really *are* fairly typical – we just didn't have a better name for a problem we couldn't explain.

"I refuse to make a diagnosis of 'atypical,'" says Dr. Steven B. Graff-Radford, a face-pain expert at Cedars-Sinai Medical Center in Los

Angeles. "I'd rather say, 'I have no idea. Will you go see someone else? I'll give you a list of other people who might be able to help you.'"

Worst of all, if most or even some of these so-called "atypical TN" cases really are compression-related variations of classic TN, they may be more treatable surgically than earlier thought.

By not linking them to TN, "there is a danger that patients with otherwise treatable facial pain will be discarded on the heap of the 'atypical,'" Dr. Burchiel says.

Dr. Burchiel has proposed a new classification system that divides all trigeminal nerve-related face pains into one of seven different disorders.

He's also devised an 18-question survey that matches the patient to the disorder. Those questions can be found in Chapter 23.

Following are the seven types of face pains that Dr. Burchiel proposes:

Trigeminal neuralgia, type 1 (TN-1). This is pain in areas served by the trigeminal nerve that comes on spontaneously and is more than 50 percent sharp, stabbing, come-and-go attacks.

Trigeminal neuralgia, type 2 (TN-2). This also is pain in areas served by the trigeminal nerve that comes on spontaneously, but more than 50 percent of it is a constant pain as opposed to sharp and fleeting.

Trigeminal neuropathic pain. This is pain that originates in the trigeminal nerve due to unintentional injury, such as trauma.

Trigeminal deafferentation pain. This is pain that occurs when parts of the nerve are injured to the point where they're completely disabled, such as complications from surgeries done to selectively injure the trigeminal nerve in an attempt to treat TN pain, i.e. glycerol injections, radiofrequency lesioning, balloon compressions, neurectomies and the like.

Post-herpetic neuralgia. This is face pain that follows an attack of shingles (herpes zoster).

Symptomatic trigeminal neuralgia. This is pain that's secondary to another condition, primarily multiple sclerosis and tumors.

Atypical facial pain. This is face pain that has no known physical cause and is thought to be psychogenic – generated by the brain itself.

Let's take a closer look at each:

TN-1 and TN-2

TN-1 is essentially what has been called classic TN, only it expands the definition to include an underlying burning component. As long as the predominant type of pain is that sharp, stabbing, come-and-go type, it's TN-1.

People in this class are most likely to have a blood vessel compressing their nerve at its root, and they're most likely to respond to antinconvulsants such as carbamazepine (Tegretol, Carbatrol) and oxcarbazepine (Trileptal). They're also presumed to have a compression in its earliest (and perhaps most "fixable") stage – or at least at a stage where chronic injury hasn't yet taken its toll.

TN-2 covers most cases of what have been called "atypical TN." This would include:

- People who used to have primarily sharp, stabbing, fleeting pain but who now have more constant, burning, aching pain.
- People who always have had more aching, burning, constant pain than sharp stabs.
- People who have *no* sharp stabs and no pain triggers, so long as the burning, aching pain is confined to areas served by the trigeminal nerve.

TN-2 cases are presumed to be caused by a compression, except that the compressions are occurring to the nerve's motor branch, are affecting more heat- and delayed-pain-carrying nerve fibers than "fast" pain fibers, or have simply created long-term, chronic injury anywhere along the nerve's course.

TN-2, the theory goes, is many times a later version of TN-1.

If that's correct, TN-2 cases also should be treatable by microvascular decompression surgery – if the compressing blood vessels are moved off of the nerve before scarring or other unfixable long-term damage has occurred.

TN-2 pain also may respond well to carbamazepine (Tegretol, Carbatrol) and oxcarbazepine (Trileptal) – at least the sharp, stabbing components of the pain. The anticonvulsant gabapentin (Neurontin) sometimes helps both sharp and burning pain, and serotonin-blocking antidepressants such as amitriptyline (Elavil), imipramine (Norfranil, Tofranil) and nortriptyline (Pamelor) often help the more constant, burning pain component.

Steroids, other anti-inflammatory medications, local anesthetics and many of the non-surgical, non-medication therapies discussed in Chapters 14-18 also may help. Example: Carol Preston, the Texan with the mixed symptoms, got help by a combination of narcotics and craniosacral therapy.

Trigeminal neuropathic pain

By definition, a "neuropathic" pain is pain resulting from a damaged nerve. Under Dr. Burchiel's proposal, trigeminal neuropathic pain would be pain in the trigeminal nerve and its branches caused by *unintentional* injury.

This would include such injuries as facial trauma in a car crash or other accident; nerve injury from a difficult tooth extraction, root canal or other dental procedure; complications from a sinus surgery or other ear, nose or throat operation, and side effects of stroke or diabetes.

Since the nerve itself is injured, it doesn't even take a stimulus to cause pain. The nerve itself reports pain messages to the brain – usually on a constant basis. This type of pain is usually described as "dull," "burning" or "boring," although people often also have occasional sharp and fleeting pains that are triggered.

These sharper attacks are usually set off by the slightest, lightest touch – a result of the nerve being super-sensitive from the injury. The difference between these triggers and those in TN, though, is that the trigger is in the same spot where it hurts. In TN, the trigger zones are usually different from where it hurts... for instance, a light breeze on the cheek may set off a lightning-like attack in the lower jaw.

There's usually a sensory disturbance that goes along with neuropathic pain. It may be numbness or it may be a tingling or "pins and needles" feeling. The nerve is still working, but in an errant way. And the brain is attempting to understand, cope with and adjust to these errant signals.

Like other parts of the body, nerves don't always heal "back to normal" either. They may resprout a tangle of poorly developed nerve endings called "neuromas" at an injury site. Neuromas don't function properly and usually send errant messages to the brain.

Sometimes neuropathic pains or "neuropathies" heal themselves in time, but other times they are permanent.

Dr. Burchiel says it's important to separate these cases out from TN-1 and TN-2 because they are not caused by compressing blood vessels. Therefore, microvascular compression surgery is unlikely to help, and the selectively destructive procedures such as glycerol injections, radiofrequency lesioning and balloon compression may even make the pain worse.

Neuropathic pain seems to strike women far more often than men – or at least women report it more often. Dr. Graff-Radford says research indicates that the female hormone estrogen seems to play a role in this type of pain. He says animal studies suggest that increased estrogen causes an increased reaction to nerve injury, including increased sensitivity to touch and greater pain. Since women have higher estrogen levels than men, that may explain why women are more prone to neuropathic pain.

We'll discuss some of the options of treating this and the following other variations of TN in the next three chapters. Some of the so-called "complementary and alternative medicine" (CAM) therapies discussed in chapters 15-18 also may help.

Trigeminal deafferentation pain

This also is a pain stemming from an injury to the nerve, only in this case sections of the nerve are disabled or no longer working at all.

This category would consist mainly of people who are left with various pains and/or numbness that follow surgical procedures that attempted to solve a nerve problem. This includes:

- Neurectomies, procedures that remove nerves.
- Injections, including alcohol or glycerol delivered to the Gasserian ganglion.
- Rhizotomies, procedures that use heat, extreme cold, electricity or similar measures to selectively injure a nerve.
- Mechanical injury, such as how surgeons temporarily inflate a tiny balloon to squeeze the trigeminal nerve against the skullbone.
- Radiosurgery, procedures that use radiation to injure nerves.

These procedures are discussed in more detail in Chapters 9-14. But the point here is that some injuries and procedures that seek to help trigeminal pain can create their own kind of pains and abnormal sensations as a consequence.

As we'll discuss later, the idea of these surgeries is to stop people's pain with little or no troubling after-effects. But when it doesn't work out that way, one of two problems can result. One is that the original pain is gone, but now the person has a new and sometimes painful condition to address. The second is that this new abnormality exists in addition to the original pain, which either wasn't helped or came back after temporary relief.

Dr. Burchiel says it's imporant to break out this type of pain because it's different in quality than the original TN pain, it's a different degree of nerve injury and it may require different treatments.

Deafferentation pain is generally continuous and has an aching, burning quality – usually with numbness, tingling and/or hypersensitivity in the affected area. Some people describe it as a "burning numbness."

Symptoms may even go beyond the trigeminal system. This is because the brain can't respond as it wants because of the "disconnected circuits" and starts trying to find other ways to cope with this irregular situation. As a result, it may start activating other systems, much like the blood-pressure cuff that we mentioned in Chapter 3 can lead to arm pain, shoulder pain, chest pain and even queasiness if left on too tightly for too long. It's kind of the brain's way of "calling out the reserves" when the usual, more focused way of dealing with problems isn't working.

As with neuropathic pain, undergoing additional surgeries on the nerve is usually not going to help and may even make things worse. Deafferentation pain may, however, respond to some of the same medications and therapies used to treat neuropathic pain.

Deafferentation pains may get better with time, but like neuropathic pain, they also may become permanent.

One of the most troubling examples of this type of face pain is a condition called "anesthesia dolorosa." This is a seemingly impossible combination of both dense numbness and severe pain in the same area following an injury to that area.

Two explanations are behind it. One is that the injury destroyed the nerve fibers responsible for carrying touch signals while letting the nerve fibers that carry pain signals intact. The other is that even though the injury has numbed or disconnected the nerve, the brain is still "reading" signals from memory. In other words, in the absence of new signals from the nerve, the brain is processing signals it has been trained to remember. That's the same phenomenon behind "phantom-limb pain" – that feeling of arm or leg pain that people get even after they've lost that arm or leg. Anesthesia dolorosa might be thought of as "phantom face pain." We'll discuss treating this in more detail in Chapter 14.

Post-herpetic neuralgia

Sometimes face pain can occur as an after-effect of a condition known as "shingles."

Shingles is an infection of the herpes zoster virus that causes a painful, blistering rash that can last two to five weeks. This is the same virus that causes chicken pox.

After chicken pox heals, the virus resides harmlessly and quietly on sensory nerves for decades. Then suddenly, it can come alive again as shingles.

"Everyone who gets shingles has been exposed to chicken pox," says San Diego neurologist Dr. James Nelson. "The virus gets you when you're a child... Sixty years later, it may decide to come out."

Shingles outbreaks are more common as our immune systems become less effective with age. That's why shingles tends to happen almost exclusively to those over the age of 50. It also may affect others whose immune systems have been suppressed, such as through illness, cancer chemotherapy or some other stress. Outbreaks also sometimes follow TN surgeries.

Once triggered into action, the virus travels from the nerve cells to the skin, where it shows up as an annoying and usually painful rash. The small, crusting blisters of this rash most often occur in a band around the ribs or chest, but the rash also may show up on the neck, face, arms, legs or inside the mouth.

Dr. Nelson says pain in the affected area is often the first sign and may be the *only* sign for the first four to seven days before the rash shows up. In those first days, shingles may be mistaken for other problems – back pain, kidney infection, heart problem and the like.

The rash itself usually heals within a month, and that's the end of it for four out of every five people. However, in as many as one in five of the outbreaks, the virus causes enough scarring damage to the nerve that pain can result for months or even years. This pain is called "post-herpetic neuralgia."

In the face, the herpes zoster can affect any of the nerves. When it affects the glossopharyngeal nerve, throat pain can result. When it affects the acoustic nerve, hearing problems can result. When it affects the facial nerve, a drooping or paralyzed face may result. When it affects the trigeminal nerve, face pain results. The most common region that face pain strikes is the eye and forehead – the region served by the upper branch of the trigeminal nerve.

The odds of getting post-herpetic neuralgia rise with age. One study found that about half of those who got shingles over the age of 60 ended up with post-herpetic neuralgia and that nearly three-quarters of those over the age of 70 got it.

Post-herpetic pain tends to be more constant than classic TN. People describe it in different ways. Some say it's sharp and jabbing, at least some of the time. Some describe it more as a "burning" pain. And others say it's "deep and aching" or "dull and boring."

Along with the pain there is often skin sensitivity and sometimes an itching or numb feeling.

Dr. Nelson says there is some evidence to suggest that post-herpetic neuralgia can be limited if anti-viral medicines are given very early in the outbreak. The challenge there is getting a quick diagnosis, which as we mentioned above, is often hindered by the lack of the telltale rash until several days into the outbreak.

The good news is that more than half of the time, this type of face pain goes away on its own. It may be a matter of months for some people, but others may have it for years before it finally resolves. In up to 40 percent of the cases, though, post-herpetic neuralgia does not go away and requires ongoing pain treatment.

It's rare for shingles to occur more than once. Once you get it and get over it, you're not likely to get it again.

Symptomatic trigeminal neuralgia

This is a category of TN pain that's secondary to another condition, primarily multiple sclerosis and brain tumors.

MS is a condition that's also thought to be viral in origin. In this case, the virus attacks and scars the myelin sheath (the protective coating) around nerve fibers within the brain and/or spinal cord. When these areas of damage or "lesions" occur along the root of the trigeminal nerve, patients get pain that's very similar to that caused by compressing blood vessels. For people who come down with TN in their 20s, 30s and early 40s, MS is a condition that should be considered.

Neurosurgeon Dr. Ronald Brisman of Columbia Presbyterian Medical Center in New York reports that nearly 5 percent of TN cases are related to MS.

TN isn't a particularly common problem for those with MS, though. Dr. Brisman says that only about 2 percent of all MS patients also have TN.

Usually, an attack of TN is not a person's first indication that they have MS. By the time an MS sufferer gets TN attacks, he or she normally already has been diagnosed with MS and is having movement difficulties, weakness or numbness of arms or legs, dizziness, unsteadiness, double vision or other MS symptoms. Doctors estimate that TN pain is the first symptom of MS in only 5 to 8 percent of the cases.

A magnetic resonance imaging (MRI) test usually is able to pinpoint if MS is behind a person's face pain.

Those with MS are three times more likely to have pain on both sides of their face than TN patients without MS. As many as three in 10 MS/TN patients have both-sided pain, Dr. Brisman reports. Overall, only 2 to 5 percent of all TN cases are "bilateral," or occurring on both sides of the face.

When bilateral TN occurs – whether from MS or other causes – the attacks act independently of one another. Most patients report that the pain is more severe on one side than the other. In bilateral cases, the second side typically begins hurting from five to nine years after beginning on the first side.

Dr. Brisman finds that MS patients are more likely than non-MS patients to have dull, burning and constant pain rather than just the sudden stabs of classic TN. And these patients are more likely to develop TN earlier in life than TN patients in general.

If medications don't help, glycerol injections and balloon compression surgeries work most of the time. Radiosurgery and radiofrequency lesioning also are options.

In about 2 to 4 percent of TN cases, tumors can cause face pain. These growths can either shove blood vessels against the trigeminal nerve or put pressure directly on the nerve themselves.

The most common TN-related tumors are meningiomas (tumors of the brain's membrane lining), acoustic neuromas (tumors of the nearby auditory nerve) and sinus tumors. These cases are usually solved by attacking the tumors – either removing them surgically or shrinking them with radiosurgery.

Once the tumors are gone, the pain usually resolves. In some cases, blood vessels still must be surgically moved away from the nerve after the tumor has been removed or irradiated.

In rare cases, TN pain can occur when an abnormal, extraneous blood vessel called an "arteriovenous malformation" (AVM) compresses the trigeminal nerve.

AVMs can be clipped out of the way, surgically removed or obliterated by radiosurgery. Again, once the AVM is addressed, this symptomatic TN pain goes away.

In even rarer cases, face pain can occur as a result of a mixed connective tissue disorder that's affecting the trigeminal nerve.

The three specific disorders that sometimes cause symptomatic TN are: lupus (an inflammatory disorder that can affect a variety of body tissues); Sjogren's syndrome (most often a disorder of the body's moisture-producing glands), and scleroderma (a hardening of tissue caused by an overproduction of collagen).

These conditions are usually treated by steroids and/or medications that suppress the body's immune system. Face pain that stems from them can be treated with anticonvulsants such as gabapentin (Neurontin), carbamazepine (Tegretol, Carbatrol) and oxcarbazepine (Trileptal) or with tricyclic antidepressants.

More details on connective tissue disorders are in Chapter 6.

Atypical facial pain

This last of Dr. Burchiel's proposed seven types of face pain is this one, which he defines as one that has no known physical cause and is apparently psychosomatic or psychogenic in nature.

This doesn't mean the pain is "not real." It's *very* real to the person experiencing it. The difference is that this pain has its origin in the brain itself, in areas we refer to as the "psyche." That involves a different part of the brain's circuitry, particularly the anterior cingulate cortex and part of the thalamus.

"This category is perhaps the most difficult for patients with facial pain, and some clinicians, to accept," says Dr. Burchiel. "However, to not acknowledge that some patients do suffer from predominantly psychogenic pain flies in the face of clinical experience. An unwillingness to recognize these patients also does them a great disservice, since the lack of appropriate referral for psychological support and counseling prolongs their suffering, and referral for inappropriate invasive procedures can make them worse."

Dr. Burchiel says what he would call "atypical facial pain" really *is* very atypical and unusual. He says he's only had one person with this type of pain.

He adds that it's important to make this type of diagnosis only after thorough psychological testing.

The patient history is the main clue that psychological testing might be worth pursuing, Dr. Burchiel says. He says this type of pain may have some of the same characteristics as TN-1 or TN-2, but patients may also complain about the pain moving around, occurring on both sides of the face, spreading outside the region served by the trigeminal nerve and maybe even affecting other body regions altogether.

This type of pain affects women more often than men and also often coexists with depression, fibromyalgia and/or chronic fatigue syndrome.

CHAPTER 5

THE DENTAL CONNECTION

*"In trigeminal neuralgia, the site of the pain does not
coincide with the source of the pain."*
—Dr. David Sirois, New York University College of Dentistry

It's not unusual for people to report that their TN pain seemed to start around the time they had dental treatment. There's good reason for the assumption – the nerves supplying our teeth are the same as those that transmit TN pain. The same nerve that's telling our brain there's piercing, electrical pain in the face is also the one that alerts us to a toothache.

That doesn't mean that dental treatment *causes* TN.

For one thing, hundreds of thousands of people have dental work every day, and only a minuscule few ever end up with TN. So at the very least, it would seem that dental disease or treatment isn't a common link.

When lingering pain *does* follow root canal or other dental treatment, it can be one of a variety of disorders – but not trigeminal neuralgia, says Dr. David Sirois, chairman of the Department of Oral Medicine at New York University's College of Dentistry.

"I firmly and adamantly do not believe dental procedures cause classic TN," Dr. Sirois says. "That's not to say people don't have post-procedure (treatment) pain. But that's a different kind of (neuropathic) experience."

His point is that it's important not to mislabel dental conditions as TN because both the cause and treatment approach for TN is fundamentally and dramatically different from dental-related pains, such as pulpitis (an infection in a tooth's pulp), periodontal pain (inflamed or abscessed gums) or "dry socket" (a local infection that may follow a tooth extraction).

Dental pain due to dental disease is usually fixable. Even damage to a nerve during a dental procedure usually heals in time. But all of the dental treatment in the world won't help a bit if the pain really *is* TN being caused by an offending blood vessel compressing the trigeminal nerve. Root canals won't stop it, mouth appliances won't stop it, and removing teeth won't stop it. Just ask TN patients who have had whole rows of teeth removed to no avail.

On the other hand, dental disease as a cause of face pain should not be overlooked. No one wants to take hefty doses of anticonvulsant medications or undergo nerve surgery if they really do have a dental problem.

We'll look at a few dental-related chronic pains later in this chapter, but first, let's look at how to separate out the cases that really are tooth problems.

How tooth pain factors in

When it comes to things that make faces hurt, tooth pain is far and away the most common. When someone develops an acute pain in the face, 95 percent of the time it's tooth- or gum-related, such as tooth decay or inflammation, says Dr. Bradley Eli, director of the San Diego Headache and Facial Pain Center.

Tooth problems are usually straightforward conditions to diagnose, he says. X-rays and dental exams are very effective at picking up causes such as broken teeth, dental caries ("cavities") and gum disease. The exception is very slight tooth cracks that sometimes are hard to detect yet still significant enough to cause pain.

"The problem that comes up is when there is no abnormality," says Dr. Sirois. "That's when the dentist may proceed to do treatment you don't need. And that can make things worse."

A survey of 12,000 face-pain sufferers by the Florida-based Trigeminal Neuralgia Association found that 55 percent of people ultimately diagnosed with TN (or a variant of it) had earlier had some sort of unsuccessful dental procedure in a failed attempt to relieve pain.

Dentists say that patients often are in such pain that the patient insists on having a root canal or practically begs to have a tooth pulled. (A root canal is a procedure in which a dentist drills a hole in a tooth and removes the inflamed nerve from the inside of the tooth. The nerve chamber is then sealed with a rubber substance. This is done primarily to stop pain caused by tooth pulp tissue that has become infected and inflamed.)

Complicating the problem is that not all cases of TN are "full blown" right from the beginning. Some people start out with milder or non-triggered pain or with a combination of sharp and burning pain – neither of which sounds off an obvious TN alarm. Those who start out with so-called "pre-TN" instead of a sharp, immediate onset are particularly hard to diagnose early on and are more likely to undergo failed dental treatment.

Also confusing in TN is that although the *source* of the pain is most likely the trigeminal nerve root inside the head, the *site* where it seems to hurt is the structures supplied by the trigeminal nerve: the jaw, cheek, forehead or even the teeth themselves. It's no wonder, then, that both patients and front-line practitioners assume something must be wrong with the jaw, cheek or forehead and go looking to "fix" something there.

"Most people aren't even aware of TN," says Dr. Henry Gremillion, director of the University of Florida's Parker Mahan Facial Pain Center. "And so when they drink a cold iced tea or bite down on something hard and get a sharp, lancinating pain, they think something's wrong with their tooth."

Flushing out tooth problems

"A typical scenario is that a patient goes to the dentist complaining of a tooth or jaw pain," says Dr. Steven Graff-Radford, a face-pain specialist at Cedars-Sinai Medical Center and UCLA School of Dentistry in Los Angeles.

"As time progresses, it becomes trigeminal neuralgia," Dr. Graff-Radford says. "Unfortunately, dentists don't know this will progress, yet they have the patient knocking on their door every day asking, 'What are you going to do about this ache?' And the dentist doesn't see anything wrong with the tooth, so in desperation he does a root-canal treatment."

"While that action is understandable, it's a big mistake," says Dr. Graff-Radford.

He maintains that dentists should never do any irreversible treatments unless a definite dental cause can be pinned down by exam or X-ray. Otherwise, he says, dentists should manage the pain with medications or with temporary nerve blocks until the true cause of the pain is found.

"If you had a pain in the toe," says Dr. Graff-Radford, "the doctor wouldn't pull the nerve out. Never. Not in a million years. But as dentists, we do this all the time."

Dr. Sirois says one good clue to help separate the tooth pains from the TNs is the quality and behavior of the pain. Nerve pains such as TN typically have a sharp, electrical, brief quality to them. These pains usually come on suddenly and then go away. Inflammatory tooth pains, on the other hand, are typically more dull, boring, aching and deep and are reliably provoked by touching or tapping the tooth.

The type of medicines that help also can provide a clue. Pains related to inflammation usually respond to anti-inflammatory medicines or painkillers – often even over-the-counter medications such as ibuprofen and naproxen. TN is almost never helped by those types of medicines.

The bottom line in these kinds of cases is that dental work really didn't cause TN to occur. A case of TN already was brewing, and that – not actual tooth pain – is what sent the person to the dentist in the first place. Unfortunately, it was treated as something else.

The "straw that broke the camel's back"

A second scenario is that dental work is the aggravating factor that finally sets off a case of TN in the works. The premise here is that the trigeminal nerve and its myelin sheath already have been damaged, but not yet to the point where pain attacks have begun.

As the damage builds, the nerve fibers become more prone to firing off at the wrong time, more prone to sending those misguided pain signals to the brain, more prone to losing their ability to shut off signals. They become more sensitive or "hyper-excited," as Cincinnati neurosurgeon Dr. John Tew puts it.

In other words, the stage has been set. Sooner or later, that first burst of pain is going to lash out. For many people, it's something simple, such as brushing their teeth, putting on their makeup or taking a bite of a sandwich that sets off their first attack.

For some, though, the triggering or precipitating event is a visit to the dentist. It doesn't have to be major work either, says Dr. Gremillion. In its injured, super-sensitive state, the trigeminal nerve might go haywire at the slightest "insult."

Dr. Gremillion says that the local anesthetics that dentists use to numb an area before fixing a cavity can even act as a trigger. He says these are mild "neurotoxins" – agents that irritate nerves. Most of the short-acting anesthetics also contain epinephrine, he adds. Epinephrine is a vessel-constricting chemical that's used to prolong the numbing effect, but it also can trigger nerve pain.

"You can even traumatize the nerve with the needle itself," Dr. Gremillion says.

If the needle and anesthetics don't set off the pain, the high-speed vibrations from a dental drill provide way more sensory input than any bite of sandwich. Even some of the acids used in restorative and teeth-whitening work can be enough to irritate a sensitive nerve ending.

It's easy to see why dental work would get the blame when TN attacks start in the dental chair or soon afterward. But most likely what happened was the work didn't cause the pain, it was merely the proverbial "straw that broke the camel's back."

New pain but not TN

The third scenario is the real pain really did result from dental work, but it isn't trigeminal neuralgia. It's one of the conditions that Oregon neurosurgeon Dr. Kim Burchiel, in the previous chapter, proposes calling "trigeminal neuropathic pain."

Any time a dentist drills into a tooth, there is potential for direct physical injury to the nerve endings as well as a possibility of introducing bacteria that can lead to an infected, inflamed nerve. These types of problems are uncommon, and even when they occur, they usually heal or can be treated.

Occasionally, though, injured nerve endings can sprout a tangle of new, poorly developed nerve fibers called "neuromas." It's somewhat similar to how trees send out a web of weak, young branches above where a big branch has been lopped off. Neuromas don't function like normal fibers, and they can send all sorts of chronic, errant messages to the brain, ranging from "crawling, tingling" feelings to pain signals of injuries that don't exist. Neuromas are usually treated with medications since additional surgery might worsen the problem.

When bacteria infect a nerve and cause a painful inflammation, it's called "neuritis." People sometimes confuse this pain with TN because it can be intense and stabbing at times. However, the quality tends to be more of a burning pain, and it's also generally constant and throbbing as opposed to come-and-go like true TN. Neuritis may respond to anti-inflammatory and antibiotic medication.

These problems don't mean that a dental procedure was performed inappropriately. Sometimes the nervous system just doesn't heal properly, even following a seemingly minor insult. Unfortunately, there is no way to tell ahead of time which individuals or procedures pose an increased risk of persistent neuropathic pain.

Dental pain and TN

A fourth scenario is the most perplexing of all. It's entirely possible for a person to have both a brewing case of TN *and* a dental problem at the same time. That can really confuse the situation when a dentist is sure he or she fixed an obvious problem, yet an abnormal pain continues – or gets worse.

The solution to that is to "peel away" at the problem by addressing definite problems with specific treatments first and then seeing what problems are left. It may take a visit to more than one type of specialist to nail down a diagnosis of co-existing conditions. Fortunately, this is a rare situation but one that shouldn't be discounted.

Dental problems to consider

There are at least six dental or oral pains that sometimes mimic TN and other face pains. These should be considered and ruled out before moving onto other possibilities.

1.) *Hypersensitive tooth.* As we age, our gums often recede, exposing the root surface of teeth. The root lacks the protective enamel covering, and the exposed surface can be much more sensitive to touch and temperature changes.

When we eat or drink something hot or cold or touch a sensitive area with a toothpick, that may set off a sharp pain that feels like a nerve-related pain.

It is a nerve pain. But it's not TN. It's called a "hypersensitive tooth" or "dentin hypersensitivity." The key difference between this and TN is that this pain hurts right where it was triggered.

Contributing factors are hard tooth-brushing, eating a lot of acidy foods and grinding teeth. Fluoridated toothpastes and mouthwashes may help, and so might using toothpaste made especially for sensitive teeth. In some cases, a dentist may apply a dental adhesive to cover the exposed dentin.

2.) Severe, deep pulpitis. When dental decay advances far enough, the bacterial infection can infect and inflame the pulp tissue of the tooth. If untreated, the pulp begins to die. This condition, known as "pulpitis," isn't always painful, but when it is, it can hurt severely.

Pulpitis pain tends to come on suddenly and then throb for anywhere from minutes to hours. Sometimes the person isn't even exactly sure of the pain's origin because the throbbing aches may radiate out into the cheek, ear and even temple. Lying down often makes it worse.

Because this pain may come and go in waves, it may be confused with TN. It's almost always easily discovered on a dental exam, though. One tap in the right place, and it's acutely apparent where the pain is coming from. The response to tooth stimulation and an X-ray can be used to detect the decay and inflammation. When irreversible, the condition is generally treated by either root canal or by removing the tooth.

3.) Cracked tooth. Hairline cracks can occur in teeth from biting into a hard object or from some sort of trauma to the mouth. They're not always easy to detect, and the pain often isn't localized. Vertical cracks (by far the most common type) aren't very easy to fix either.

Cracks can make teeth sensitive, cause pain and allow infections to get into the pulp. Dentists may detect cracks by using magnification during an exam and also by using dye. (The dye seeps into cracks.)

Adhesives may protect a cracked tooth and possibly prevent the crack from worsening, but this isn't a good, long-term solution. Sometimes crowns are placed over a cracked tooth to support and protect it, but this doesn't always relieve the pain if an irreversible pulpitis already has occurred. In that case, a root canal or removal of the tooth could be needed.

4.) *Periodontal pain.* When plaque and tartar accumulate, the resulting inflammation can lead to detachment of the gums and bone loss, which in turn leads to the formation of pockets between the gums and tooth. It also can lead to receding gums. While periodontal (gum) disease is usually chronic but not painful, it can become acutely inflamed and painful sometimes.

This pain can be severe and is usually triggered by biting and chewing. The person can usually tell exactly where the pain is coming from, but the pain may radiate out in the jaw. Upon exam, the area is tender to the touch and usually red and inflamed.

Inflamed pockets can be cleansed, irrigated and treated with antibiotics in the early stages. But advanced periodontal disease may not respond to this conservative treatment and may have irreversibly damaged the supporting bone. Sometimes this may even affect the pulp of teeth.

5.) *Vascular orofacial pain.* This is a somewhat newly defined condition and one that's not universally accepted. It's believed to be related to constricted blood vessels supplying the teeth and tissues in the mouth. It's unclear what may be the underlying cause, but the pain comes in episodes and is a throbbing type of pain that can occur anywhere in the mouth.

It most often strikes people in their 40s and 50s and is often accompanied by tearing of the eyes, nasal congestion and sometimes nausea. Over-the-counter pain-killers such as ibuprofen and naproxen usually help, and tricyclic antidepressant medications are usually effective at heading off new episodes.

6.) *Acute alveolar osteitis.* Commonly known as "dry socket," this condition is a local infection in the socket following a tooth removal. This throbbing pain usually begins within two to three days following the extraction.

Irrigating the socket and applying an antiseptic dressing usually solves the problem.

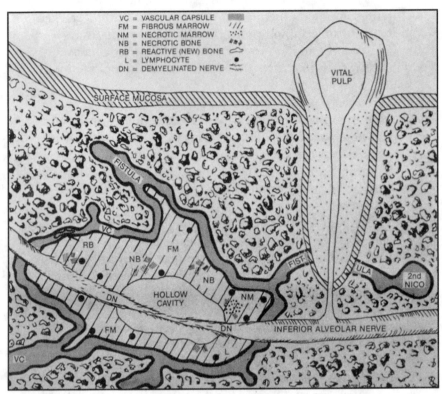

VC = VASCULAR CAPSULE
FM = FIBROUS MARROW
NM = NECROTIC MARROW
NB = NECROTIC BONE
RB = REACTIVE (NEW) BONE
L = LYMPHOCYTE
DN = DEMYELINATED NERVE

This sketch shows how a bony cavity in the jawbone can affect nerve branches.
(Used with permission of Dr. Jerry E. Bouquot,
The Maxillofacial Center, Morgantown, West Virginia)

The "bony-cavity" theory

NICO – an acronym for "neuralgia-inducing cavitational osteonecro-sis" – is a very controversial condition in which pockets of jawbone ostensibly become damaged and die, resulting in damage to the nerve branches that pass through these areas. The bone death or "bony cavi-ties," as they're sometimes called, can occur from loss of blood flow to the jawbone or as the result of a festering, low-grade, non-pus-produc-ing infection of the jawbone.

When nerve damage follows the bone damage, the pain either may be dull and achy – like so-called atypical TN or sharp and stabbing like clas-sic TN.

An estimated 5 to 10 percent of NICO cases are originally misdiag-nosed as TN, say Dr. Jerry E. Bouquot, director of research at The Maxillofacial Center for Diagnostics and Research in Morgantown, W.Va., and Dr. Robert E. McMahon, a clinical investigator for the

Indiana University Medical Center in Indianapolis, Ind.

Another 67 percent of the cases ultimately found to be NICO were originally misdiagnosed as "atypical TN" or "atypical face pain," Drs. Bouquot and McMahon report.

They say NICO often goes overlooked because it's not an easy condition to detect. Dr. Bouquot says bone X-rays need to be viewed in a dark room under magnification, and even then it takes an experienced eye to spot NICO damage. Thin-slice bone scans give a more accurate view, and a new ultrasonic device called a "Cavitat" also may aid in detecting the damage, he adds.

The dental mainstream counters, however, that NICO is "overlooked" because most dentists simply don't subscribe to the entire underlying theory. They say these small bony cavities are common even in people who don't have pain and that there's no evidence to back up claims that these cavities are causing pain.

Dr. John E. Dodes and Dr. Marvin Schissel, in their book *"The Whole Tooth"* (St. Martin's Press, 1997), say oral pathologists have looked at the same tissue blocks that have been diagnosed as NICO and found them to be perfectly normal.

"There is no scientific evidence to support these assertions or the diagnostic and treatment methods based on them," Drs. Dodes and Schissel wrote.

How NICO happens

Oral surgeons have known about bone infections and their role in killing bone tissue since at least the 1850s. Bony cavities can occur for a variety of reasons.

Infection is just one way, such as following tooth abscesses and gum infections, tooth extractions or other oral surgeries. Because bone death and related nerve damage often take time to develop, NICO pain may not show up until years afterward.

Bone also can die when its blood supply is cut off or diminished. That can happen in the case of trauma to the face or in cases of blood-vessel disorders, narrowing of the arteries, frequent use of vessel-constricting medications, viral damage or even alcohol and nicotine abuse.

In other words, you don't have to have a history of a pulled tooth, root canal or oral surgery for NICO to occur. The underlying cause can be more subtle.

"Any process which diminishes blood inflow or outflow from the bone can produce this disease," says Dr. Bouquot. He estimates that NICO occurs in about one out of every 2,200 to 5,000 adults, affecting some 68,000 Americans at any given time.

About three-quarters of NICO sufferers are between the ages of 35 and 64, and about three-quarters of them are women. On average, these people have suffered pain for six years before ultimately being diagnosed with NICO, according to Dr. Bouquot's research.

Bony cavities don't always lead to pain, though, and they can occur in other bones besides the jawbone.

Extreme damage can occur to bone with little or no pain. "In the hip, for example, it is not unusual for a patient's first sign of disease to be the complete collapse of the joint," says Dr. Bouquot.

He suggests that pain is more likely to happen in the jawbone because no other bone in the body has such large sensory nerves.

NICO isn't evident from an inspection of the patient's teeth, jaw or gums. Usually there is no apparent swelling or redness. However, touching or pressing on the affected area usually hurts, especially on the more-sensitive cheek side of the jawbone.

Besides X-rays and bone scans, oral surgeons may use a series of local anesthetic injections to confirm and locate the area of NICO damage.

Since the damage seldom heals itself, the current recommended treatment is to cut into the bone and surgically scrape out the infection and dead tissue – a procedure known as "curettage."

Antibiotic medications also are typically used. And in cases where poor blood flow is suspected as an underlying cause, anticoagulant medications may be used.

At surgery, Dr. Bouquot says it's common to find hollowed-out areas of bone, "spongy" or "chalky" bone, and discolored, frayed and even severed nerve branches in NICO cases.

In two studies of face-pain patients who underwent curettage for suspected NICO problems, two-thirds got at least a 75 percent relief of their pain. Drs. Bouquot and McMahon followed 103 patients for an average of 4.6 years and found that 59 percent had no pain and nearly 14 percent had at least a 75 percent improvement. Most of the rest either were improved somewhat or not at all, but 3 percent of the patients reported worse pain after the procedure.

Dr. Bouquot says about a third of those with NICO get their pain back or end up with new pain in different sites later. Why? Most likely because the underlying causes such as a defective immune system or poor blood flow to the jawbone are still at work.

Dr. Bouquot and others researching NICO say this condition may not be behind a majority of face pains, but they say there's enough of a link that it's an avenue worth checking out.

"We suggest that all facial neuralgia patients be carefully examined for (NICO) with the use of radiographic techniques and anesthetic techniques," Dr. Bouquot recommends.

The other side of NICO

Surgery for NICO and the premise behind it remain highly controversial. Only a minority of dentists accept it.

Dr. Sirois, for example, says there is a big difference between finding small bone cavities and implicating them as a cause of face pain. He says it's a bit like concluding that having a driver's license leads to speeding. While it's necessary to have a license in order to speed, it doesn't *cause* speeding; plus there are lots of people with licenses who do not speed.

"Considerably more work needs to be done to show either a mechanism or causal linkage between bone cavities and pain," Dr. Sirois says.

Dentists also point out that just because pain goes away after a curettage procedure doesn't mean the bone cavity caused the pain. Curettage, by its very nature, "denervates" or desensitizes the trigger zones enough to prevent attacks for awhile. Once the area heals and the nerves are back to full sensitivity, pain usually returns.

Dentists are particularly concerned about patients whose pain is made worse by the procedure. Sometimes the nerves and tissue never completely heal, and the patient can be left with permanent pain.

Says Dr. Sirois: "The benefit-risk needs to be carefully weighed, and better studies need to be done to more accurately understand the mechanism, diagnosis and prognosis of proposed NICO treatment."

Fillings as triggers?

Another controversial link to face pain is silver fillings – the materials dentists use to fix tooth cavities. Mercury and other metal fillings in particular have been fingered as potential oral villains.

A few dentists – concerned that mercury can cause face pain and other health problems – have gone so far as to suggest that people with mercury fillings should have them removed. The prevailing professional standard is that such recommendations are unethical and not indicated since no convincing evidence exists that mercury fillings cause face pain. Replacing the fillings for cosmetic purposes is accepted, but claiming that their removal will cure a disease is considered crossing the line.

Dr. Eli says that even if someone is concerned about mercury exposure, the process of vaporizing the fillings to remove them would expose the patient to more toxic effects than letting them alone.

There have been a few reported cases, however, of metal fillings of different materials reacting to create a mild electric current capable of triggering TN pain. Such "galvanic" electrical currents between differing metals is known to occur, but it's rare.

Dr. William Cheshire at the Mayo Clinic in Jacksonville, Fla., ran into one case of this and reported it in a June 29, 2000, letter to the New England Journal of Medicine. Dr. Cheshire wrote that his 66-year TN patient had a recent root canal that slightly repositioned a tooth with a silver filling closer to a tooth with a gold-alloy crown. When the patient ate tomatoes and other acidic foods, she got a metallic or "battery-like" taste in her mouth and experienced low-grade jolts that were enough to set off excruciating TN attacks.

Dr. Cheshire said this triggering stopped after the patient had the silver filling replaced with non-metallic porcelain. He theorizes that when the two dissimilar metals came into contact with acidic saliva, it created a galvanic cell that produced a localized electrical current.

That also happened to Ivan Guevara of California. He was diagnosed with TN about a year after having a root canal and was on carbamazepine for six months. While searching the Internet for explanations for his pain, he ran across a dental-journal article about oral electricity caused by two differing types of metal fillings.

Guevara found that his root-canal tooth had been filled with amalgam and bolstered by a gold crown. "In March 2003, I had the amalgam replaced with a (non-metal) composite," Guevara said. "The neuralgia disappeared, and I have not taken any medication for nine months."

A 1996 report in the journal General Dentistry described another similar case involving a 35-year-old woman who developed pain after a tooth next to a gold-crowned molar was patched with a silver filling. Her dentist was able to stop the pain by adding a small amount of resin between the two metals.

Keep in mind that this phenomenon is rare and that replacing fillings is expensive. It also can lead to further tooth and nerve damage – possibly without helping pain at all or even making it worse. If a galvanic current is suspected as a cause of face pain, a tooth can be easily and temporarily sealed with a resin solution to test whether "insulating" the tooth helps the pain.

Dental care with TN

Given the agony that can be set off by anything ranging from a dental drill to a toothbrush, it's no wonder so many neuralgians shy away from dental care of any sort.

Big mistake, dentists say. If you stop brushing, stop flossing, stop going to the dentist, that's only going to lead to more and worse tooth problems. And eventually, that will mean more drastic, invasive work like root canals and extractions that simpler steps could have headed off.

If you've got TN, talk to your dentist about ideas he or she may have to help you keep up with home dental care. "Your dentist can show you how to use topical anesthetics," says Dr. Sirois. "There are also a variety of sprays, gels and solutions that can be dispensed."

Some pointers on dental care without triggering pain blowouts:

- *Time that care.* "Attend to your teeth at the time of day when your TN medication is most effective," advises Dr. Gremillion. That may vary from person to person, but most TN medicines reach peak effectiveness about an hour after you take them. Whether it's then or a particular time of day when the pain is usually least, do your brushing and flossing then.
- *Soften the toothbrush.* Sometimes switching to the softest-bristle brush you can find might be enough to make brushing bearable. Some neuralgians also tolerate electric toothbrushes better than manual brushing.
- *Try a gum-numbing cream.* Some people are able to brush their teeth by first wiping their gums with a topical anesthetic such as Anbesol or Orajel. These numb the area for about 10 minutes.
- *Switch to a non-irritating toothpaste.* Some toothpastes are "grittier" than others. Tartar-control toothpastes, for example, are more irritating than others. Try a brand made for sensitive teeth.
- *Brushing alternative.* If toothbrushes of any type are just too painful at any time any way, try ultrasonic or irrigation tooth-cleaning systems that avoid brushes altogether. Or try wiping your teeth clean with a soft cloth.
- *Decay-fighting liquids.* A fluoride tray (a rubber mouthpiece that fits over the teeth to apply fluoride cream) or a high-concentration fluoride toothpaste can help strengthen tooth enamel. Antibacterial/antiplaque mouthwashes such as

Biotene or Peridex also may help cut down on the factors that cause of tooth decay.

- *Substitute saliva.* If you've got a dry mouth (a possible side effect of some TN medications), consider using "substitute salvia" such as Salivart. Saliva is the mouth's natural cleanser. A lack of it can increase tooth decay.
- *Avoid teeth whiteners.* Whether they're applied by a professional or bought over the counter, most of these products contain acids that are corrosive and irritating to the teeth and their nerves.

Going to the dentist

Few things strike more fear into the heart of a typical neuralgian than the thought of going to the dentist. It's not the needles and drills that scare them. It's the fear that something, *anything* – maybe even the little dental pick or the hygienist touching the lip at the "wrong" place – will set off flailing waves of pain. A simple cleaning to a neuralgian often strikes the same terror chords as a root canal to anyone else.

Here's where a patient and understanding dentist can help a lot.

"Look for a dentist who is a team player and who recognizes that you are a key player," says Dr. Gremillion.

"Take it slow," advises Dr. Sirois. "Start on one side and see how it goes. You don't have to get the whole cleaning done at once."

Some other tips for keeping dental work as painless as possible:

- *Go to the dentist when you're not hurting.* Make sure your dentist knows you have TN so he or she will be flexible to schedule your appointments (maybe even on short notice) during periods when your pain goes into remission. This will also help the dental staff to understand in case you have to cancel in case TN pain flares up right before an appointment.
- *Be well medicated.* If you don't have remissions or must have dental work done during an active pain cycle, consult your doctor so you're on an optimal dose of medicine. He/she may want to temporarily boost the dose a few days ahead of time to prevent a pain break-through. Also try to schedule your appointment during the time of day when you're least likely to get pain or when your medication is at peak effectiveness.
- *Topical anesthetics.* Most dental patients need numbing compounds mainly for tooth repairs, crown work, extractions and the like. But for a TN patient, even teeth-cleaning and exams

may bring on pain. Topical sprays or gels can be used to temporarily numb the gums.

- *Touch the sensitive area last.* If there's a trigger zone that usually sets off the pain, ask the dentist or hygienist to examine and clean everything else first.
- *Switch local anesthetics.* If you need treatment, discuss with your dentist the type of anesthetic to be used. Florida dentist Dr. Gerald Cioffi likes to use long-acting Marcaine for his TN patients – even though he keeps the work as quickly as possible – because it can desensitize the trigeminal nerve for up to 10 hours. Dr. Gremillion also recommends Marcaine *without* epinephrine, the agent that constricts vessels but can irritate nerve endings. "You may need to ask in advance because the average dentist doesn't keep this particular drug in stock," he adds.
- *Consider the injection point.* Dentists have some leeway as to exactly where they inject a local anesthetic before dental work. Dr. Gremillion says it may help if the injection is given as far away as possible from known, active TN trigger points.
- *A knockout.* If all else fails and you absolutely need dental work, discuss the possibility of a general anesthetic (either intravenously or by inhaled gas) to put you to sleep while the work is being done.

CHAPTER 6

OTHER FACE PAINS: NOT TN, NOT DENTAL, BUT IT STILL HURTS

"Before we start giving a lot of medicines,
we ought to be sure of the diagnosis."
—Dr. Joanna Zakrzewska, London oral-medicine specialist

A lot of things can go wrong that end up causing pain in the face. Dental problems and trigeminal neuralgia and its variants are just two areas we've already discussed.

Our head performs so many different, important duties that it's loaded with more intricate functioning parts than any other part of the body. We've got tiny bones that allow us to hear, muscles large and small to move our face, ligaments and tendons holding the bones and muscles together, minuscule highways of blood vessels to feed all of this living tissue and, of course, tens of thousands of individual nerve fibers that control the whole shebang.

Injury or disease in any of these components can signal the brain that something is wrong. Clench your jaw enough and the overworked muscle gets sore. Develop an infection in your sinuses and your cheek begins to throb. Drink too much alcohol and you get a piercing headache, maybe even a migraine.

It's the job of the nerves to report these kinds of threats and insults to the brain, which then determines what, if any, corrective or protective action is needed. Often these signals show up as pain. Sometimes the nerves themselves or the region of the brain that deciphers pain signals can malfunction, leading to some of the hardest-to-detect conditions.

At least two dozen known conditions and disorders other than TN and dental problems can cause face pain. Some of them have definite, obvious causes and specific, effective treatments. Others are of murkier origin and are tougher to treat.

In some cases, a diagnosis is easily nailed down by exam or test, ranging from X-rays and CAT scans to blood tests. But in other cases, it's the nature of the pain and the patient's description of it that provides the only way to sort out the conditions. That's not always easy either because some face pains aren't very "localized" – the pain radiates out from the point of injury or disease so that a whole generalized area of the face hurts.

Sometimes it's easier for patients to realize what they have by hearing about a set of symptoms that match theirs (as opposed to blindly describing their symptoms and hoping the right doctor will diagnose the right condition). That may lead to a "diagnosis epiphany" – hearing for the first time about a condition that exactly matches yours.

In the rest of this chapter, we'll take a closer look at some of these other non-TN and non-dental problems that can cause face pain.

Cluster headache

Cluster headaches are sometimes confused with TN because they occur in episodes and cycles. An attack builds in intensity over a 5- to 10-minute period and then hangs on anywhere from 15 minutes to 3 hours before going away. Forty-five minutes is the average.

Attacks may occur several times a day or every few days, then there's a remission. These remissions typically last anywhere from two weeks to a year, but in chronic cases, the breaks are less than two weeks – if at all.

Curiously, attacks also tend to "cluster" around seasonal changes, especially near the longest and shortest days of the year. Many people say this pain wakes them from sleep (unlike in TN), often about an hour and a half after they go to sleep. Lying down during an attack usually makes it worse. And many say they get attacks late almost every evening while relaxing (a trait that's earned this condition the nickname "clockwork headache").

People who get cluster headaches tend to use words like "searing," "boring" and "piercing" to describe this pain. Some say it feels "like a red hot poker stuck in my eye." It's definitely not a dull pain.

Like TN, the pain is almost always confined to one side of the face, although in a few cases the pain has been known to switch sides. Pain most often strikes the eye and temple regions and sometimes radiates out into the forehead, cheek, jaw, teeth and even neck. Red eyes, tearing, sensitivity to light, nasal stuffiness and/or runny nose also usually accompany cluster headaches. Some people's foreheads also perspire, and a few become nauseous during attacks.

Cluster headaches (sometimes called *migrainous neuralgia* or *petrosal neuralgia*) are believed to be caused by the dilation of the arteries inside the skull. Other suspected causes are an inflammation of the blood vessels in the sinuses or an inflammation of the trigeminal or facial nerves.

Attacks are often brought on by alcohol, cigarette and coffee use. There's also a possible link to sleep apnea (periodic stopped breathing during sleep) and prior head injury. Unlike TN, light touch does not set off attacks.

Cluster headaches often run in the family, suggesting a strong genetic link to this problem. Nitroglycerin – sometimes used to treat angina attacks – also can trigger a cluster headache, ostensibly because this medication dilates blood vessels.

This is one face pain that strikes men much more often than women. Studies have suggested that men are anywhere from two to five times more likely than women to suffer from cluster headaches. Men typically start getting these attacks in their teens and 20s, while women tend to get them later in life, often in their 60s.

A variety of medications, sprays and injections are used to prevent and treat cluster headaches.

Injections of sumatriptan (Imitrex) are usually effective in quickly knocking down an attack in progress. Tablets of such medications as sumatriptan, zolmitriptan (Zomig) and verapamil (Calan, Isoptin, Verelan) are used to prevent attacks. Steroids also are sometimes used as a preventative, and a nasal spray of the local anesthetic lidocaine and inhaled pure oxygen are other therapies that sometimes help during attacks. Pain-killers seldom help.

When all else fails, nerve-injuring surgeries such as radiofrequency lesioning and glycerol injections (both discussed here in later chapters) may help. Microvascular decompression of the trigeminal nerve (see Chapter 13) along with cutting a portion of the geniculate nerve also has helped some people.

The good news, though, is that unlike TN, this is a pain that often gets better over time instead of worse. Cluster headache sufferers typically get more and longer remissions as time goes along, and the problem may even go away altogether.

Cluster tic syndrome

Cluster tic syndrome is a name given to the coexistence of two different pains at the same time – namely cluster headaches and trigeminal neuralgia (tic douloureux). Fortunately, it's very rare.

This can be a tricky one to diagnose because it has both the sharp, stabbing, come-and-go pains of TN but also the more searing, boring traits of cluster headache.

Treatment may require a combination of the therapies used to treat stand-alone cases of TN and cluster headache. Anticonvulsant drugs may control the sharp pains, while sumatriptan and/or inhaled lidocaine may control the searing pain.

In the long run, the cluster-headache component may resolve itself, while the TN pain can be addressed by surgery or other methods if the anticonvulsant medications fail. In several patients who underwent surgery for cluster tic syndrome, blood vessels were found to be compressing either the trigeminal nerve or facial nerve, or both.

Migraines and facial migraines

A migraine is a very severe and throbbing headache that can last anywhere from a few hours to three days. These can occur anywhere in the head, but when they occur in the face, they're called *"facial migraines."* These are the ones that are most likely to be confused with TN and related face pains.

Migraine pain results from inflamed blood vessels. The inflammation can be triggered by a variety of stimuli, including caffeine, alcohol, stress, the food additive MSG, changes in body estrogen levels, nitrates, changes in sleep habits and bright fluorescent lights, to name a few.

The pain usually occurs just on one side. In facial migraines, the pain typically affects the nostrils, cheeks, gums and teeth.

In some cases, migraines are preceded by a visual "aura," a distorted, flickering view in the periphery of the field of vision. The pain builds gradually until it can become debilitating. People often become nauseous during attacks and highly sensitive to noise and light.

Migraines often run in families, and women are three times more likely than men to get them. Attacks in women are often connected to menstrual periods.

Recognizing and avoiding known triggers is the first line to combating migraines. A recent Canadian study published in Pain Medicine News (January/February 2003) found that regular exercise also was an effective way to prevent migraines. The study also reported that stress management, a healthy diet, relaxation techniques and massage also helped.

For frequent migraines, prescription medicines such as indomethacin (Indocin), propranolol (Inderal) and methysergide (Sansert) may help prevent them. Injections or nasal sprays of sumatriptan (Imitrex) are often effective in easing attacks in progress. At least four other "triptan" medications also are now available: rizatriptan (Maxalt), naratriptan (Amerge), almotriptan (Axert) and zolmitriptan (Zomig).

The U.S. Food and Drug Administration also recently approved a dental splint that may help prevent migraines in some people.

Trigeminal neuritis

Neuritis is an inflammation of a nerve. As we discussed in Chapter 5, teeth commonly become inflamed after a cavity or crack, and that's the main reason for root canals. But what if an inflammation occurs elsewhere on the trigeminal nerve? When this happens, it's called *"trigeminal neuritis."*

Trigeminal neuritis is often described as dull and burning, sometimes with tingling, numbness and/or hypersensitivity in the affected area. It can occur in any area that the trigeminal nerve serves, and it's almost always a constant pain, not fleeting as in classic TN.

The reason for the inflammation can vary. Causes include an injury to the nerve, a bacterial or viral infection of the nerve or a reaction to a toxin or allergen. The post-herpetic neuralgia discussed in Chapter 4 is one example of this kind of pain (a virus-related cause).

Ramsay Hunt Syndrome is another example of a viral-caused neuritis – in this case affecting the facial nerve instead of the trigeminal nerve. This syndrome involves intense ear pain, a rash and sometimes paralysis of the facial muscles. Ramsay Hunt Syndrome can be treated with antiviral medications, and it usually resolves itself, although permanent hearing loss or permanent facial paralysis happens occasionally.

Face pain that accompanies Lyme disease is an example of a trigeminal neuritis caused by a bacterium (more on that below). Diabetics also are prone to getting various types of neuritis, including trigeminal neuritis.

Trigeminal neuritis is usually treated by anti-inflammatory drugs and other medications or injections that are designed to reduce swelling and inflammation. Antibiotics also may be used when a bacterial cause is suspected.

Lyme disease

This is a bacterial version of neuritis that can cause trigeminal nerve damage and lead to TN or TN-like symptoms. The bacterial infection that causes the damage comes from a tick bite.

Ticks pick up the *"Borrelia burgdoferi"* bacterium (and possibly other pathogens) from the blood of wild animals that carry these bacteria. This infection has been known in Europe since 1883, but the first reported outbreak of it in the United States was near Lyme, Conn., in the late 1970s. That's where the name "Lyme disease" and "Lyme borreliosis" originated.

The Lyme bacterium is a nasty invader that attacks just about every type of cell in the body. Thus it can lead to a whole range of symptoms, including face pain when it attacks the trigeminal nerve.

Specifically, the bacteria can erode the outer protective coating of the trigeminal nerve fibers (the myelin), creating damage that's very similar to that done by a compressing blood vessel. Only in this case, the damage is bacterial instead of mechanical.

The early symptoms of Lyme disease are flu-like – things like a headache, stiff neck, fever, muscle achiness and fatigue. The tell-tale sign, though, is a "bulls-eye" rash around the area of the tick bite.

According to the Lyme Disease Foundation in Hartford, Conn., the bite starts out causing a small reddish bump of about a half-inch in diameter. As a reddish rash expands outward from that in a circular pattern, the center remains more of a normal flesh color. The rash can be as small as a thumb or large enough to cover a person's entire back.

As the infection spreads, symptoms can mushroom in a host of ways, including severe fatigue, swollen glands, sore throat, joint pain and swelling, tingling, numbness, severe headaches and muscle aches, face twitching and difficulty thinking.

Depending on what organs the infection attacks, some even more serious symptoms can result, such as muscle paralysis, vision problems, irregular heart beats, breathing difficulties and liver abnormalities. Because of the wide range of possible symptoms, Lyme disease is often a tough problem to diagnose – especially if the bulls-eye rash isn't apparent.

Further complicating the diagnosis is the fact that there is no definitive lab test to pinpoint it. The best tests are several blood tests that indirectly implicate Lyme disease by measuring the antigens the patient's body is producing to fight off infection. Otherwise, Lyme disease is diagnosed by the patient history and exam.

As with post-herpetic neuralgia, the sooner Lyme disease is caught and treated, the less likely that face pain will be a problem.

The ideal situation is to avoid tick bites in the first place by covering up outside and by thoroughly checking your body and hair once inside. Usually the tick has to latch on and be in place for about a day before the infection is transmitted, according to the Lyme Disease Foundation.

If found on the body, the tick should be removed as soon as possible by pulling it out with a pair of tweezers. Attempting to burn it or otherwise damage it before removing it may cause the tick to inject more of the bacteria into the bite site, says Dr. Joseph J. Burrascano Jr. in his report, *"Managing Lyme Disease: Diagnostic Hints and Treatment Guidelines for Lyme Borreliosis."*

Once the infection occurs, Dr. Burrascano recommends using antibiotics as soon as possible for four to six weeks. The longer the infection has had a chance to spread, the longer the antibiotics need to be administered, he adds. In long-present cases, antibiotics might be needed for four to six months.

Since the bacteria attack so many different types of cells, different types of antibiotics may be needed. Some of the ones most often used are doxycycline (Vibramycin, Monodox, Doryx), amoxicillin, cefuroxime (Ceftin), ceftriaxone (Rocephin), cefotaxime (Claforan), and either azithromycin or clarithromycin with hydroxychloroquine or amantadine.

"All patients respond differently, and therapy must be individualized," says Dr. Burrascano. "Some patients will require ongoing maintenance therapy to remain well."

In addition to the antibiotics, some patients are helped by anti-inflammatory pain-relievers, muscle relaxants and antidepressants.

Dr. Burrascano also suggests multivitamins and B complex vitamins, daily helpings of yogurt and acidophilus preparations, and possibly magnesium supplements in the form of magnesium chloride or magnesium oxide.

Pain and stiffness can be treated with physical therapy, exercise, heat, massage and TENS units. And Dr. Burrascano suggests avoiding alcohol, caffeine, smoking and poor sleep habits.

One study of 120 Lyme patients in New Jersey found that about one in four of these patients developed face pain that mimicked TN. Because face pain can happen so often in Lyme disease, researchers believe at least some cases of TN and so-called atypical TN are misdiagnosed Lyme cases.

When the bacteria is brought under control, the pain symptoms usually subside. However, flare-ups are not uncommon, and new tick bites can produce new infections. Just because you've had Lyme disease once doesn't mean you're immune and can't get it again.

A vaccine to prevent Lyme disease also has been introduced, and more specific and reliable blood tests for diagnosing are being developed.

Glossopharyngeal neuralgia

What happens when a blood vessel compresses the glossopharyngeal nerve instead of the trigeminal nerve? It causes pain in the region this nerve serves – primarily the throat and base of the tongue.

This pain is closely related to TN because it's thought to be the exact same cause, just affecting a different nerve. In addition to a blood vessel compressing the nerve, other causes of nerve injury are tumors, multiple sclerosis and possibly a calcified (hardened) ligament.

Glossopharyngeal neuralgia is a sharp, stabbing, shock-like pain that is usually triggered, just as in TN. Common triggers are swallowing, yawning, light touch, sneezing, cold drinks and acidic food and drinks. Attacks typically last one to two minutes, and then the pain goes away.

"The pain may radiate to the ear as well but should always have a tongue or throat component," says Dr. Ronald Apfelbaum, a neurosurgeon at the University of Utah Medical Center.

Less common than TN, glossopharyngeal neuralgia sometimes occurs along *with* TN – giving patients pain in two different regions served by two different nerves. Also, about 12 percent of people with glossopharyngeal neuralgia have it on both sides of the face – a significantly higher number than TN.

Glossopharyngeal neuralgia tends to affect primarily those over age 50 and strikes women about twice as often as men.

One other related problem that's occasionally found in glossopharyngeal neuralgia patients is an irregular heartbeat. The link isn't totally clear, but a blood vessel compressing the neighboring vagus nerve is one suspected explanation. For that reason, doctors sometimes do an electrocardiogram test to check for related heart disorders.

Local anesthetic sprays to the back of the throat usually stop a glossopharyngeal neuralgia attack in progress, and the same anticonvulsant medicines used to treat TN are usually effective in treating this neuralgia as well.

If that doesn't work, microvascular decompression surgery (see Chapter 13) may help if the underlying cause is a blood vessel compressing the glossopharyngeal nerve. Radiofrequency lesioning, in which the nerve is selectively damaged with a heated electrode, also has been used effectively to disable this pain.

As with cluster headaches, the good news is that this neuralgia is one that sometimes becomes less frequent and painful over time. Sometimes it goes away altogether.

Geniculate neuralgia

When a blood vessel or tumor compresses the facial nerve – another of the 12 cranial nerves – geniculate neuralgia can result.

This pain also is very much like TN, except that it strikes deep in the ear – an area served by a branch of the geniculate nerve known as the *nervus intermedius.*. (Another name for this condition is *"nervus intermedius neuralgia."*)

The pain of geniculate neuralgia is sharp, stabbing and electric-like, just like TN and glossopharyngeal neuralgia. Some people describe it as feeling like they have an ice pick in their ear. The pain comes and goes, but attacks may last for minutes or drag on for hours.

A light touch of the ear is a common pain trigger, and so is chewing, swallowing and talking. Some patients also complain of excess salivation, a bitter taste in their mouth, ringing in their ears and dizziness. This suggests that other cranial nerves might also be involved.

Anticonvulsant medicines such as carbamazepine (Tegretol, Carbatrol) and oxcarbazepine (Trileptal) are usually effective at controlling geniculate neuralgia. Some patients also have been helped by methysergide (Sansert), a medicine that's usually used for migraines.

If medication doesn't help, microvascular decompression and many of the same other therapies used to treat TN often help this pain as well. A partial cutting of the nervus intermedius also usually brings relief.

Occipital neuralgia

Yet another pain in this same class is occipital neuralgia, which is an injury to or problem with the occipital nerve. This nerve serves the back of the head, so when a blood vessel or tumor impinges on it, people get an aching, throbbing sort of pain in the affected side of the back of the skull. (We have two occipital nerves – one that serves the back right of the head and one that serves the back left.)

Head trauma, "whiplash" neck injuries and arthritic changes in the upper spine also are believed to cause some cases of this neuralgia.

In many cases, the aching, continuous pain of occipital neuralgia is superimposed with the come-and-go sharper pains that are more character-istic of trigeminal neuralgia. Unlike TN, these stabs typically aren't trig-gered. They just seem to happen randomly.

Although many people get headaches in the back of the skull, this is a different type of pain from the common, dull-pain, muscle-tension headaches. Those are almost always caused by stress.

If occipital neuralgia isn't discerned from similar pains such as migraines, cluster headaches and muscle-tension headaches on the symptoms or examination alone, the type of medicine that works usually gives an answer. Over-the-counter pain-killers usually control tension headaches, but indomethacin (Indocin) or sumatriptan (Imitrex) might be needed to control a migraine. Local nerve blocks (done by injecting anesthetics) also can help sort out the problems.

The sharper jabs of occipital neuralgia are often relieved by the same anticonvulsant medicines used to treat TN (carbamazepine, oxcarbazepine, and the like). The more constant, burning pain, on the other hand, seems to respond better to gabapentin (Neurontin) or tricyclic antidepressants such as amitriptyline (Elavil), nortriptyline (Pamelor) or desipramine (Norpramin).

If a tumor is the suspected cause, removing it or treating it with radiation is likely to stop the pain. Tumors can be detected by X-ray, CAT scan or magnetic resonance imaging (MRI).

One other treatment that's been tried with some success is repeated anesthetic injections combined with a course of steroids. If those options fail and the pain persists, neurosurgeons can do a variety of procedures ranging from selectively injuring part of the occipital nerve to severing it altogether (which stops the pain but produces a numb scalp).

Vagal/ superior laryngeal neuralgia

When the vagus nerve is compressed by a blood vessel or tumor, pain occurs in the regions served by the nerve's auricular and superior laryngeal branches. Those areas include the side of the throat, beneath the jaw and under the ear.

The pain is much like TN – sharp, stabbing and fleeting. The most common trigger zone is the voice box or "larynx." Talking, swallowing, yawning and coughing are all apt to set off attacks of this neuralgia.

When other branches of the vagus nerve are affected, patients may experience hiccups, excessive salivation and coughing.

This pain usually responds to the same medicines that control TN pain. Anesthetic sprays and injections are temporary reliefs that also can help zero in on a diagnosis. Sometimes this pain goes away on its own.

If medicines don't help and the pain persists, microvascular decompression of the vagus nerve is usually effective.

Sphenopalatine neuralgia

Also known as *"Sluder's syndrome,"* this pain feels like a headache behind an eye with pain that radiates into the sinus area, the roof of the nose, the upper jaw and the palate on that side. The aching pain may even reach to the back of the nose, the teeth, the temple and maybe even the back of the head and neck on that side.

Nasal and sinus congestion almost always accompanies sphenopalatine neuralgia, and tearing of the eyes and redness in the face are common as well.

The pain is similar to cluster headaches, but the duration is longer. Many times this pain comes on following a sinus infection. It affects women twice as often as men.

Different medical texts offer differing explanations for the cause. One theory is that an infection irritates the cluster of nerves known as the *"sphenopalatine ganglion"* near the sinus. Another is that dilation of the nearby maxillary artery irritates or injures this ganglion. And a third is that inflammation or unfortunate anatomy results in painful contact between the septum (the cartilage that separates our two nasal cavities) and the mucous-covered turbinate bones at the base of the nose.

Nasal decongestants and other medicines that reduce inflammation may help relieve some of the pain. Anesthetic nasal sprays and anesthetic injections (sphenopalatine ganglion blocks) usually give quick pain relief.

Symptoms usually go away on their own over time. But in severe, chronic cases, surgery is sometimes done, usually to separate the septum and turbinate bones.

SUNCT

This pain is very similar to first-division (upper-branch) TN pain and, in fact, is often confused with that, although SUNCT is thought to be a separate condition more akin to a migraine in origin.

SUNCT stands for *"Short-lasting, Unilateral, Neuralgiform headaches with Conjunctival injection and Tearing."* The name describes the symptoms in a nutshell.

This pain comes on suddenly and strikes in bursts of 10 to 60 seconds, although some attacks may linger for up to 4 or 5 minutes. Then, like TN, the pain goes away. SUNCT sufferers may get only one attack a day, but others have reported up to 30 attacks an hour. Five to six attacks per hour are the norm, generally during the day.

Also as in TN, SUNCT pain tends to run in cycles that last anywhere from days to months. Then the attacks stop. Pain-free remissions may last for several months to a year. Occasionally the pain stays away for up to 7 years.

SUNCT pain is "unilateral," meaning it occurs on just one side, usually centered around the eye and sometimes radiating out into the forehead and temple. It's similar to a nerve pain or "neuralgia," usually described in such terms as "sharp," "stabbing" or "burning" with an electrical quality to it. When attacks occur, the pain is accompanied by tearing of the eyes, red eyes ("conjunctival injection" in medicalese), a runny nose and nasal congestion. Some people also get a sweaty forehead, swollen eyelids and a feeling of increased pressure in the affected eye.

Attacks sometimes are provoked by the same kinds of things that set off TN attacks – touching the face or hair, chewing, blowing the nose, brushing teeth, turning the neck. Other times, attacks occur at random with no trigger.

Because of these TN-like characteristics, it's easy to see why SUNCT pain is often confused with TN. Some medical literature even refers to it as a variant of TN.

The big difference, however, is the suspected underlying cause. SUNCT is thought to be related to an inflammation of the blood vessels in the affected region. What causes that is unclear, but one theory is that a malfunction in the hypothalamus portion of the brain may set up the inflammation – much like the suspected cause of migraines. Alcohol, stress and possibly estrogen levels also may play a role.

"This is a problem of the brain, not a problem of the trigeminal nerve," says Dr. Steven Graff-Radford of Cedars Sinai Medical Center in Los Angeles. "It's likely to be a neurovascular problem."

Others believe SUNCT may be caused by a problem with the nervus intermedius, that branch of the geniculate nerve that's involved with geniculate neuralgia.

In a few reported cases, people with SUNCT were found to have malformed blood vessels in the brain that were corrected by surgery.

Two medicines that have been most effective in treating SUNCT pain have been the anticonvulsants lamotrigine (Lamictal) and gabapentin (Neurontin.) Others have found relief from the anticonvulsant carbamazepine (Tegretol, Carbatrol) and from steroids. Dr. Graff-Radford says that sumatriptan (Imitrex) also is being investigated as a possible medical treatment.

In cases in which medicines didn't help, a few SUNCT sufferers have tried and got relief from glycerol injections (see Chapter 10).

First described in 1978, SUNCT is more common in men than women. The average age at diagnosis is 51.

Temporomandibular disorders

This group of disorders is high on the list of face pains, coming in somewhere just behind dental pain and headaches. An estimated 10 million Americans have some kind of temporomandibular disorder (TMD). Probably the best known of this group is temporomandibular joint pain (TMJ), which is pain in the jaw joint.

But TMD also includes pains involving the jaw muscles, nerves, and the tendons and ligaments supporting the jaw. The pain associated with

TMD can range from fairly minor, achy, localized jaw pain to severe, chronic pain. This pain can come on rather suddenly or work its way up from a minor irritant to a major problem over time.

One or more areas are usually tender to the touch. Chewing and talking are common aggravating factors. And many people have trouble opening their mouth wide. In many cases, the jaw makes clicking or popping sounds when moved, although that alone doesn't mean it's TMD.

Sometimes TMD pain radiates out into the face and can even cause deep ear pain, headaches in the temples and above the eyes, and even referred pain in the neck and shoulders.

Women are about six times more likely than men to get TMD, and the most common years it strikes is between the ages of 15 and 45.

A variety of causes may be behind TMD. Some are more speculative than others. But among the possibilities are sore jaw muscles from clenching or grinding teeth (*"bruxism"*), trauma to the mouth, arthritis, a poorly aligned bite, a displaced jaw disk and stress and other psychological factors.

TMD can become a secondary problem to trigeminal neuralgia if TN sufferers start clenching their jaws during pain attacks. This repeated stress on the jaw muscles can lead to soreness and tenderness.

Treatments vary depending on the nature of the problem. Muscle-related pains are very common and often respond well to simple rest, to heat or cold packs and/or to pain-killers such as ibuprofen (Advil), ketoprofen (Orudis), naproxen (Naprosyn, Aleve) and etodolac (Lodine).

Jaw exercises are often helpful for TMJ and muscle-related jaw pains. If it's too painful to start an exercise program, dentists and doctors may prescribe quick-numbing vapocoolant sprays, such as chloroethane or chlorofluorocarbon, right before exercising (the so-called "spray and stretch" plan).

In cases related to grinding or clenching teeth, acrylic plastic bite guards are often used to more evenly spread the force out over a wider area as well as protect the teeth.

Low doses of antidepressants such as amitriptyline (Elavil), nortriptyline (Pamelor), doxepin (Sinequan), imipramine (Norfranil, Tofranil) and clomipramine (Anafranil) also often help all kinds of TMD. Besides having pain-relieving and relaxation properties, these medicines boost the levels of serotonin in the brain, a chemical that's also thought to play a role in causing teeth-grinding.

TMD pain that isn't solved by any of those may respond to a series of anesthetic injections of lidocaine, bupivacaine or mepivicaine. And if that fails, some people are helped by taking muscle relaxants or trying steroid injections.

Other approaches that sometimes help include acupuncture (see Chapter 16), dental appliances or dental work to realign the bite, hot-pepper cream (Chapter 15), biofeedback (Chapter 20), TENS units (Chapter 15) and psychological counseling, particularly cognitive-behavioral therapy.

Surgery is rarely needed and is mainly directed at the relative few cases that involve an obviously misaligned jaw joint.

Conservative approaches are recommended first because TMD pain often improves with time and sometimes goes away on its own.

Myofascial pain

Muscles are the source of this condition, which is more of a dull, constant, aching pain than a sharp, stabbing one. It can occur in any of the body's skeletal muscles, but in the universe of face pain, the jaw is the main culprit.

Myofascial pain is more closely related to the TMD pains described above than TN, but one characteristic it does have in common with TN is trigger points. Myofascial pain sufferers almost always have one or more tender spots that set off pain when touched. The trigger points are usually less sensitive, though, than with TN. It takes more of a press than just a light touch to set them off.

People with this pain usually have trouble chewing and opening their mouths wide. The pain also often radiates into the teeth and ears. A hallmark that helps separate it from other pains is that there's generally a hard "knot" or taut area in one more spots of the muscle.

The cause of myofascial jaw pain isn't clear, but grinding or clenching of the teeth and similar overuses of the jaw muscle are suspected links. A jaw or mouth injury also may cause some cases. Other possible contributing factors include nutritional deficiencies (especially low levels of iron, calcium, potassium and Vitamins B-1, B-6, B-12 and C), chronic infections, sleep deprivation, poor posture and stress.

Treatments are similar to TMD. Jaw-muscle stretching and strengthening combined with anti-inflammatory pain-killers such as ibuprofen (Advil), naproxen (Aleve, Naprosyn) and ketoprofen (Orudis) often help new cases. Vapocoolant sprays or anesthetic injections can be used to help with exercise programs if the muscle is too painful at first. Tricyclic antidepressants such as amitriptyline (Elavil) also can help.

If that approach doesn't work, steroid injections have been used in cases in which inflammation seems to be a key factor. More recently, doctors are investigating the use of Botox injections as a possible help. (Botox is an acronym for the botulinum toxin, which has a mild muscle-paralyzing effect at low doses.)

Other therapies that sometimes help include acupuncture (Chapter 16), massage, TENS units (Chapter 15), biofeedback (Chapter 20) and ultrasound.

Temporal arteritis

Also known by the newer name of *"giant cell arteritis,"* this pain stems from an inflamed artery in the temple. The inflammation causes an intense, aching, throbbing and sometimes burning pain in the temple area, often radiating up into the head. It's primarily a constant pain, but sometimes it comes and goes.

Temporal arteritis usually occurs on one side of the head, but it can happen on both sides. It is most common in older persons, especially those who have polymalgia rheumatica.

The artery inflammation is thought to be an immune reaction, but what causes that is unknown. Arteritis also can affect other arteries, such as in the arms, legs and occasionally the heart.

When it strikes the temples, the area is very tender to the touch. Sometimes vision disturbances accompany it. Chewing often provokes the pain.

Besides evaluating the symptoms, doctors can diagnose this condition by blood test (an elevated erythrocite sedimentation rate is a clue) and more accurately by examining a biopsied section of the artery.

Oral steroids such as prednisone are the primary treatment. Relapses are common, though, so repeated courses of steroids may be needed to keep knocking down recurring bouts. It's important to treat temporal arteritis because chronic, untreated inflammation of the temporal arteries can lead to blindness.

Sinusitis

When infections, allergies and/or irritants strike the sinuses, inflammation and pain can result. That produces a fairly common condition known as sinusitis.

Sinusitis is most often an infection, caused either by a bacteria or virus. Cases are usually short-lived and often follow common colds. When the infection or irritation is resolved, the pain goes away.

The key symptom is nasal stuffiness with thick, discolored mucous. The cheeks usually become tender (and often turn red), and the dull, pressure ache that results may radiate into the upper teeth. Fever and tiredness also are the norm in sinusitis.

X-rays and CAT scans can be used to verify sinusitis if it's not obvious from the symptoms. If the cause is bacterial, antibiotics may clear it up in a few days. In viral cases, the symptoms are treated with antihistamines, nasal decongestants, pain-killers and/or pain-killers. Most patients recover in 7 to 10 days, although some cases can hang on for a few weeks.

In chronic or very severe cases, surgery can be done to clean out the sinuses.

Chronic paroxysmal hemicrania

This one's a rare upper-face pain that occurs in bursts, such as TN and SUNCT.

The nature of chronic paroxysmal hemicrania pain, though, feels much like that of cluster headaches – excruciating, throbbing, pulsating and "clawing." It's most common in the eye and temple regions but sometimes occurs in the cheek or forehead. The pain may radiate out into the neck or shoulder.

Attacks can happen anytime day or night. They come on suddenly, quickly build in intensity and throb away for anywhere from 2 to 30 minutes. An average attack is about 20 minutes. Then the pain is gone.

Pain occurs on one side at a time, but it has been known to switch sides. Tearing of the eyes, nasal congestion and a runny nose sometimes accompany attacks.

When the pain is active, sufferers typically have eight to 15 attacks a day. This can go on for years without treatment. But there is also an episodic version of paroxysmal hemicrania in which remissions may last for months, again much like TN.

The cause is unknown. It strikes women two to three times more often than men, and the first bout of it is often when people are in their 20s – earlier than most face pains.

Despite the unknown cause, chronic paroxysmal hemicrania responds very well in most cases to oral indomethacin (Indocin), a non-steroidal anti-inflammatory medicine that's often used for arthritis, bursitis and tendonitis.

Other medicines that have been used to successfully treat this pain include steroids, verapamil (Calan, Isoptin, Verelan), naproxen (Aleve, Naprosyn), acetazolamide (Diamox) and even ordinary aspirin.

Raeder's paratrigeminal syndrome

This condition, sometimes called just *"Raeder's syndrome"* or *"para-trigeminal neuralgia,"* is another rare, upper-face pain that affects the ophthalmic branch of the trigeminal nerve. It's a one-sided, headache-like face pain that strikes almost exclusively men.

The pain is mostly constant in the eye region and has a deep, boring, throbbing quality to it, although there may be occasional sharp pains as well. Attacks may last for a few days to a few weeks at a time.

Raeder's syndrome has a few other distinguishing characteristics that help set it apart from other pains. One is a drooping of the eyelid on the affected side. Another is constriction or contraction of the pupil. Some people also report an unpleasant taste in the mouth.

Most cases of Raeder's syndrome are thought to be caused by either an infection or inflammation of the nerve, but some cases are associated with usually benign tumors.

In the latter case, removing or treating the tumor can fix the problem. In the other cases, painkillers, steroids and megadoses of Vitamin B may help. Anti-inflammatory medications and some of the medicines used to treat TN – especially gabapentin (Neurontin) and carbamazepine (Tegretol, Carbatrol) – also sometimes help. Avoiding alcohol and other agents that dilate blood vessels may help as well.

The good news is that non-tumor-related cases of Raeder's usually resolve themselves in two to three months.

Orbital myositis

This is another pain around the eyes, caused by an inflammation of the tissues in the "orbit," or eye socket. Why the inflammation occurs is unknown.

The pain is an achy, pressure type of pain that's usually accompanied by swelling and drooping of the eyelids, red eyes and even swollen eye-balls, which makes the eyes look like they're protruding. Because of the swelling, the eye muscles may not work properly, leading to double vision or difficulty moving the eyes.

Orbital myositis is more common in people in their 30s and 40s, and it affects women twice as often as men.

The swelling is usually eased by steroid medications (e.g. prednisone) and other medications that suppress the immune system. In chronic cases, some people have been helped with Botox (botulinum toxin) injections.

Tolosa-Hunt syndrome

A third eye-area pain is Tolosa-Hunt syndrome, also known as *"painful ophthalmoplegia."* It's thought to be caused by an inflammation in the sinus and/or orbital cavities.

The pain is usually constant and boring around one eye, although it occasionally affects both sides. The pain is usually accompanied by a malfunction in the eye muscles, which can cause visual problems such as double vision. Depending on what nerves are affected, it also may lead to drooping and swollen eyelids, numbness of the surface of the eyeball (cornea) and even loss of vision in a severe case involving the optic nerve.

This one's hard to diagnose because it has no one, distinguishing feature that sets it obviously apart from other disorders that share some of the same symptoms.

One characteristic that stands out somewhat is its treatment – Tolosa-Hunt usually responds very well and very quickly to steroids, normally within 24 to 72 hours, according to Dr. Danette Taylor, a neurologist at the University of Michigan.

Most of the time this disorder goes away on its own, although malfunctioning eye muscles may take weeks to return to normal after the pain is gone. In rare cases, eye problems never do fully resolve.

If steroids don't work, Dr. Taylor reports that immune-suppressing medications such as azathioprine (Imuran) or methotrexate (Amethopterin) may help.

Lupus and Sjogren's syndrome

Lupus and Sjogren's are both immune-system disorders that, like multiple sclerosis, can result in nerve pain as a secondary symptom.

Lupus is a chronic, inflammatory disease that can affect various parts of the body, especially the skin, joints, blood and kidneys. It occurs when the body's immune system loses it ability to recognize the difference between foreign substances and its own cells, allowing antibodies to attack healthy, normal cells. This leads to inflammation, tissue injury and pain.

Sjogren's is similar in cause and affects the body's moisture-producing glands. Its main symptoms are dry eyes and dry mouth, but it can also affect other organs.

A condition called *"mixed connective tissue disorder"* – which has overlapping features of lupus, myositis and scleroderma (a hardening of the skin caused by overproduction of collagen) – is a third even less common but similar disorder that sometimes results in face pain.

When any of these problems involve the trigeminal nerve, injury to the nerve occurs and a chronic, neuropathic pain can result. "Chronic neuralgia from such an attack is rare," says Dr. Daniel Wallace, the chief of rheumatology at Cedars-Sinai Medical Center in Los Angeles. "In my practice of 2,000 active lupus patients, I can think of three or four with chronicity from trigeminal neuralgia."

Steroids and medications that suppress the immune system are usually used to treat the underlying causes. The pain usually responds to medications that work for neuropathic pain, such as the anticonvulsant gabapentin (Neurontin) and tricyclic antidepressants. Susan Urban, a TN support-group leader from Massachusetts who has face pain related to lupus, said nothing helped her, including steroids, until she began taking the antidepressant amitriptyline (Elavil). Sharper pains also may be helped by carbamazepine (Tegretol, Carbatrol) or oxcarbazepine (Trileptal).

Atypical odontalgia

This is a poorly understood condition in which the patient reports severe pain in a tooth – usually an upper molar – but nothing can be found wrong with the tooth. For that reason, sometimes it's suggested that the pain might be stemming from the middle branch of the trigeminal nerve.

However, atypical odontalgia is different from classic TN pain in that it's a constant, burning, aching and often throbbing pain rather than sharp and fleeting. The pain may radiate to other nearby teeth, and even when teeth are removed, the pain persists in or returns to the gum. Or the pain simply moves into the next tooth.

Many patients say this pain seemed to occur after a dental procedure or some sort of tooth or face trauma. While nerve damage might explain it, other clinicians believe the pain is related to a blood-vessel inflammation.

Sometimes patients are told this pain might by psychogenic in nature, but psychological tests generally turn out to be normal. Atypical odontalgia sufferers also are usually not depressed. However, antidepressant medications seem to be the most effective treatment – apparently because of its pain-relieving, brain-chemistry properties.

Pain relievers and sedatives are usually not effective for atypical odontalgia.

Burning mouth syndrome

A burning sensation in the mouth can be a symptom of several disorders, but when no obvious injury or cause can be determined, the name *"burning mouth syndrome"* and sometimes *"glossodynia"* is given to the symptoms.

A variety of causes have been suggested, including fungal infections, allergies to dental fillings, nerve damage, nutritional deficiencies (especially Vitamin B-12, iron and folic acid), stress and psychological disorders. None have been proven.

This pain has a burning quality to it and often affects the tongue. It may be continuous or may occur off and on. Most people say the pain is usually worst in the evening. About half of the people also complain of a dry mouth and many report altered taste in addition to the pain.

Burning mouth syndrome primarily affects post-menopausal women. The good news is that in about half of the cases, this condition goes away by itself within 6 or 7 years.

Some people get relief from low doses of the tranquilizer/anticonvulsant clonazepam (Klonopin), and others have been helped by antidepressants and/or cognitive-behavior psychological counseling.

CLUES TO POSSIBLE DIAGNOSES

The following characteristics may give some hints to the type of pain you may be experiencing. None of the following can supplant a careful history and exam by your physician, but they may point to conditions worth exploring further.

Pain in throat?	Glossopharyngeal or superior laryngeal neuralgia.
Pain in back of head?	Occipital neuralgia.
Pain in side of head, tender temple, blurred vision?	Temporal arteritis.
Throbbing pain in side of head, temple tender?	Migraine, paroxysmal hemicrania.
Dull, aching, constant pain on both sides of face?	Sinusitis.

...Continued from previous page

**Dull, aching, fleeting pain
on both sides of face?** Periodontal pain, vascular orofacial pain.

**Variable pain that
moves around face?** Atypical facial pain.

**One-sided pain affecting
teeth or mouth only?** Odontalgia, pulpitis, myofascial pain,
temporomandibular joint disorder,
neuralgia-inducing cavitational osteonecrosis
(NICO), cracked tooth.

**One-sided pain affecting
eye and forehead?** Tolosa-Hunt syndrome, orbital myositis,
Raeder's paratrigeminal syndrome.

**One-sided pain affecting eye
and forehead with facial
flushing and tearing?** SUNCT, cluster headaches.

**Sharp, stabbing,
one-sided pain?** Trigeminal neuralgia-1, Lyme disease.

**Aching, stabbing,
one-sided pain?** Trigeminal neuralgia-2, symptomatic TN.

**One-sided pain with
crusting lesions?** Post-herpetic neuralgia.

Stabbing, deep-ear pain? Nervus intermedius neuralgia,
geniculate neuralgia.

**Burning one-sided pain
with numbness?** Neuropathic pain, deafferentation pain,
trigeminal neuritis.

THE MANY FACES ...

CONDITION	WHERE IT HURTS	HOW IT HURTS	NATURE OF THE PAIN
Trigeminal neuralgia (TN-1)	1 side of face, anywhere from forehead to jaw	Sharp, stabbing, jolting	Fleeting; usually triggered by light touch; periods of remission
Atypical trigeminal neuralgia (TN-2)	1 side of face, anywhere from forehead to jaw	Burning, aching pain with sharp stabs	Mostly constant; stabs may or may not be triggered and/or go into remissions
Trigeminal neuropathic pain	1 side of face, anywhere from forehead to jaw	Dull, burning, boring; often tingling or numbness	Constant; occasional triggered stabs possible
Trigeminal deafferentation pain	1 side of face, anywhere from forehead to jaw	"Burning numbness" (burning pain with tingling, numbness)	Constant; occasional triggered stabs possible
Post-herpetic neuralgia	Usually eye/forehead region of 1 side	Deep, aching, boring, sometimes sharp, jabbing	Constant; skin hypersensitive
Symptomatic trigeminal neuralgia	1 side of face, anywhere from forehead to jaw	Sharp, jolting, stabbing, sometimes with burning, aching	Usually fleeting, triggered by light touch with emissions; burning ache may be constant
Atypical facial pain	Anywhere on face	Varies	Usually constant, may move around
Pulpitis	In or radiating out from a tooth	Throbbing, aching	Constant but hurts worse in waves
Cracked tooth	In or radiating out from a tooth	Sharp, aching	Triggered by pressure on tooth

... OF FACE PAIN

CAUSE/PRESUMED CAUSE	PRIMARY TREATMENTS
Blood vessel(s) compressing trigeminal nerve	Anticonvulsants, antidepressants, surgery, sometimes upper-cervical chiropractic, acupuncture, other CAM therapies
Possibly blood vessel(s) compressing trigeminal nerve	Antidepressants, anticonvulsants, steroids, surgery, sometimes upper-cervical chiropractic, acupuncture, other CAM therapies
Physical injury to trigeminal nerve	Antidepressants, anticonvulsants, hot-pepper/anesthetic cream, nerve/brain stimulation, neurectomy, CAM therapies
Physical injury to Trigeminal nerve	Antidepressants, anticonvulsants, hot-pepper/anesthetic cream, nerve/brain stimulation, neurectomy, CAM therapies
Herpes zoster viral attack following shingles	Antiviral medication early; non-steroidal painkillers, anticonvulsants, antidepressants, anesthetic cream, acupuncture
Pain secondary to multiple sclerosis (myelin loss), brain tumor or other condition	Shrink or remove tumor or address primary disorder. In MS, anticonvulsants, antidepressants or nerve-injuring surgery
Unknown, possibly psychogenic	Antidepressants, CAM therapies, psychological evaluation
Bacterial infection of tooth pulp	Root canal or tooth removal
Crack from force of physical injury	Adhesives, tooth crown early; root canal or tooth removal if opening leads to pulpitis

CONDITION	WHERE IT HURTS	HOW IT HURTS	NATURE OF THE PAIN
Periodontal pain	In and around teeth and gums	Severe, aching	Triggered by biting and chewing
Vascular orofacial pain	Anywhere in mouth	Throbbing	Fleeting
NICO	Upper or lower jaw	Ranges from sharp, stabbing to dull, aching	May be constant or fleeting; hurts when painful area is pressed
Cluster headache	Usually eye and temple and radiating from there	Searing, "like a red hot poker;" also red eyes, tearing	Pain runs in 30-60 minute episodes several times a day; remissions common
Cluster tic syndrome	1 side of face, anywhere from forehead to jaw	Sharp, stabbing and searing, boring	Sharper pains are fleeting, searing pain is more constant
Facial migraines	Nostrils, cheeks, gums, teeth	Severe, throbbing	Happens in episodes of a few hours to three days
Trigeminal neuritis	1 side of face, anywhere from forehead to jaw	Dull, burning; tingling also common	Usually constant
Lyme disease	Usually 1 side of face, anywhere from forehead to jaw	Sharp, stabbing, sometimes with burning, aching	May be fleeting or more constant
Glossopharyngeal neuralgia	Throat, base of tongue	Sharp, jolting, stabbing	Fleeting; usually triggered by swallowing, yawning, drinking
Geniculate neuralgia	Deep in ear	Like an "ice pick in ear," sharp, stabbing	Fleeting; triggered by light touch, chewing, swallowing, talking
Occipital neuralgia	1 side of back of head	Aching, throbbing	Constant ache with occasional sharper stabs; no triggers
Superior laryngeal neuralgia	Side of throat, beneath jaw, under the ear	Sharp, jolting, stabbing	Fleeting; usually triggered by talking, swallowing, yawning

CAUSE/PRESUMED CAUSE	PRIMARY TREATMENTS
Inflammation around receding gums	Cleansing, antibiotics early; removal of teeth if severe
Constricted blood vessels in mouth	Painkillers, antidepressants
Infection that erodes jawbone and nerves that traverse it	Jawbone surgery to scrape out bony cavities; antibiotics
Dilation of arteries in skull or possibly inflammation of blood vessels or nerves	"Triptan" medications, steroids, anesthetic nasal spray, CAM therapies
Thought to be a combination of trigeminal neuralgia and cluster headache	Same treatments as trigeminal neuralgia and cluster headache
Inflammation of blood vessels	"Triptan" medications, spray or injection of Imitrex; exercise, Indocin, Inderal or Sansert to prevent
Inflammation of trigeminal nerve, possibly from infection, toxin or allergen	Anti-inflammatory medications; antibiotics if bacterial infection suspected
Bacterial infection resulting from tick bite	Antibiotics, anti-inflammatory painkillers, antidepressants
Blood vessel or tumor compressing glossopharyngeal nerve; secondary effect of multiple sclerosis	Anesthetic spray to throat, anticonvulsants, surgery
Blood vessel or tumor compressing geniculate nerve	Anticonvulsants, Sansert, surgery
Injury to head or neck or blood vessel or tumor compressing occipital nerve	Anticonvulsants, antidepressants; shrink or remove tumor; upper-cervical chiropractic
Blood vessel or tumor compressing branch of vagus nerve	Anticonvulsants, surgery

Condition	Where it hurts	How it hurts	Nature of the pain
Sphenopalatine neuralgia	Behind eye, radiating into sinus, upper jaw, palate	Aching; nasal congestion, red eyes, tearing	Lasts in waves of several hours at a time
SUNCT	Eye on 1 side, radiating into forehead, temple	Sharp, stabbing with red eyes, tearing, nasal congestion	Short bursts of a minute or less; sometimes triggered, sometimes not
Temporomandibular disorders (TMD)	In and radiating out from jaw joint	Aching to severe	Constant but aggravated by pressing, chewing, talking
Myofascial pain	Jaw on 1 side, radiating into teeth and ears	Dull, aching	Constant; tender spots sensitive to pressure
Temporal arteritis	Temple on 1 side, radiating up into head	Intense aching, throbbing	Usually constant but flare-ups may be triggered by chewing or touch
Sinusitis	Upper cheeks, radiating into upper jaw	Dull, pressure ache; nasal stuffiness, discolored mucous	Constant; often follows cold but usually short-lived
Chronic paroxysmal hemicrania	Eye, temple, cheek or forehead on 1 side	Throbbing, pulsating, clawing; tearing of eyes	Sudden attacks of 15-30 minutes and then pain is gone; remissions sometimes
Raeder's paratrigeminal syndrome	Eye/forehead on 1 side	Deep, boring, throbbing; some stabs	Constant pain; also drooping eyelid, constricted pupil
Orbital myositis	Around eye on 1 side	Achy, pressure	Mostly constant; also red, swollen eyeball, swollen eyelids
Tolosa-Hunt syndrome	In and around eye, usually on 1 side	Boring	Constant; double vision may occur
Atypical odontalgia	In or around tooth, often an upper molar	Burning, throbbing	Constant
Burning mouth syndrome	Mouth or tongue	Burning	May be constant or fleeting; usually worst in evening; dry mouth common

Notes: For definitions of the first seven conditions, see Chapter 4. The next five are dental pains and are described in Chapter 5. "NICO" refers to "neuralgia-inducing cavitational osteonecrosis." "SUNCT" refers to "short-lasting, unilateral, neuralgiform headaches with conjunctival injection and tearing."

CAUSE/PRESUMED CAUSE	PRIMARY TREATMENTS
Sphenopalatine nerve infection; dilation of artery in cheek; inflammation	Anti-inflammatory medications; anesthetic nasal spray and injections; septum surgery
Inflammation of blood vessels in eye/forehead	Anticonvulsants, steroids, possibly Imitrex; glycerol injection, CAM therapies
Overworked jaw muscle from clenching or teeth-grinding; trauma; poorly aligned bite; arthritis	Rest; heat/cold packs; painkillers; jaw exercises; vapocoolant sprays; antidepressants; dental appliances; CAM therapies
Overworked jaw muscle from clenching or teeth-grinding; trauma	Jaw exercises, anti-inflammatory painkillers; antidepressants; CAM therapies
Inflamed artery in temple caused by unknown immune reaction	Steroids
Bacterial or viral infection of sinuses	Antibiotics, antihistamines, nasal decongestants, painkillers; sinus surgery in severe, chronic cases
Unknown	Indocin, steroids, verapamil painkillers; CAM therapies
Infection or inflammation of upper branch of trigeminal nerve; sometimes a benign tumor	Painkillers, steroids, anti-inflammatory medications, anticonvulsants for stabs; often goes away on own
Inflammation of tissues of the eye socket	Steroids, immune-suppressing drugs; Botox injections in chronic cases
Inflammation in the sinus and/or eye socket	Steroids, immune-suppressing drugs
Unknown	Antidepressants, CAM therapies
Unknown	Klonopin, antidepressants, CAM therapies

Notes: Under treatments, "CAM therapies" refer to a host of treatments described in Chapters 15-18 and some in Chapter 20. "Triptan" medications are those whose generic names end in "triptan," such as sumatriptan, rizatriptan, naratriptan, almotriptan and zolmitriptan.

CHAPTER 7

MEDICATIONS FOR FACE PAIN

"Most doctors agree that medical treatment is the best first step."
—Dr. Donald J. Dalessio, La Jolla, Calif., neurologist

There's at least one bright side of having trigeminal neuralgia today... it's better than having it in the 1600s or 1700s. Back in the pre-drugstore days, physicians didn't have very effective medicines.

They didn't even have a handle on what was causing this excruciating face pain. And so they tried all sorts of agents that they did have – purgatives to cleanse the bowels, bee and cobra venom, even hemlock to try and "poison" the pain away. "You must be pretty desperate if you try to use hemlock to get rid of TN," says Baltimore neurosurgeon Dr. Benjamin S. Carson Sr.

Colonial-era and early 19th-century physicians also tried the few pain-relieving medications available at the time, primarily opioids and herbal remedies.

As technology developed, doctors tried radiation and X-ray therapy, and in the late 1800s, the new "galvanic therapy," a system that involved hooking up patients to electrodes for steady, low-level doses of electric current.

A break-through, of sorts, came in the mid-1800s when the French physician Trousseau theorized that TN pain might have something to do with abnormal conduction of the nerves.

That prompted doctors in 1876 to use an antiepileptic (i.e. anticonvulsant) drug for the first time. The drug they used – potassium bromide – worked well enough that doctors began to think of TN as a variation of epilepsy. Some even began calling it "neuralgia epileptiform."

Anticonvulsants: Still the main type

Fast-forward more than a century, and we're still using anticonvulsant drugs as our front-line class of medicines to treat TN. Newer and better anticonvulsants have long replaced potassium bromide, but their action on the body is basically the same.

In TN, the problem is that an injured or compromised trigeminal nerve has become hypersensitive and is firing off errant pain signals at the slightest provocation. One way to deal with that is by giving medicine that alters these signals and calms down the whole system. That's exactly what anticonvulsants do. They throw a "wet blanket" over the neurological fire.

It's the same theory behind treating epilepsy. In that disorder, the nervous system is firing away too fast, and by slowing down the nervous system with anticonvulsants, the symptoms ease. That's why anticonvulsants work for both TN and epilepsy.

Although this approach works better than anything we've found so far, the down side is that it's not a very selective way to quell TN pain. Anticonvulsants not only slow down the pain-firing nerve signals, they also slow down everything else nerve-related – our reaction times, our memory cells, our coordination and so on. That's what leads to the unwanted side effects that often accompany anticonvulsants.

Research is under way to develop new medications that block pain signals without taking down everything else with it. (More on that research in Chapter 22, "Possibilities.") In the meantime, the aim is to find a medicine and a dose that knock out pain with as few side effects as possible.

What usually doesn't work

The normal arsenal of pain-killing medications is largely useless in treating TN pain.

Over-the-counter analgesics such as aspirin, acetaminophen, ibuprofen and naproxen generally have no effect on TN pain. Even narcotic painkillers such as Vicodin (hydrocodone and acetaminophen) and Darvocet (propoxyphene and acetaminophen) may do little more than take the edge off pain at standard doses.

Potent narcotics at high doses may work, but that makes most people feel significantly groggy or "out of it." Because of that and concerns about addiction, most doctors don't turn to heavy doses of narcotics unless other therapies have failed.

Pain-killers are much more effective at stopping soft-tissue pains – in muscles, tendons, joints, skin, ligaments and the like. But TN is a sharp, electrical pain originating in a nerve, and for that pain, anticonvulsants have been found to work best.

Finding better anticonvulsants

Another medical breakthrough came in 1942 when researchers developed a new anticonvulsant called phenytoin (Dilantin). It quickly became the leading epilepsy drug, and is still widely used today.

Phenytoin also worked fairly well for TN, and for about 20 years, it was the leading TN medicine.

Then in 1962, along came what is often called the "gold standard" of TN medication – carbamazepine (Tegretol). This was far more effective than phenytoin. Some early reports suggested that upwards of 80 to 90 percent of trigeminal neuralgians were being helped by this new anticonvulsant.

Although the effectiveness figures are more in the 65 percent to 80 percent range these days, carbamazepine is still the medication of first choice for many doctors.

Quickly gaining ground on carbamazepine is the new anticonvulsant oxcarbazepine (Trileptal). Very similar in makeup to carbamazepine, oxcarbazepine is often called a "cousin of Tegretol."

Neurologists are reporting that oxcarbazepine works as well as carbamazepine for TN pain, but it's often tolerated better with fewer side effects. It's also different enough from carbamazepine that many people who had an allergic reaction to carbamazepine are able to take oxcarbazepine.

Also becoming very popular in TN medication are two recent timed-release versions of carbamazepine – Tegretol XR and Carbatrol. Both of these last up to twice as long as regular carbamazepine tablets, cutting down on how often neuralgians have to take their medication.

Gabapentin (Neurontin) is yet another anticonvulsant that came along in the 1990s, offering one more alternative that also seems to be particularly effective in helping burning, aching pains.

Several other anticonvulsants were approved in the late 1990s, including topiramate (Topamax), lamotrigine (Lamictal) and levetiracetam (Keppra). Each of these has shown early signs of helping face pain, offering more alternatives for those who either can't take or weren't helped by other anticonvulsants. If nothing else, these three may be helpful as "add-on" medicines when one drug alone isn't doing the job.

Two other new anticonvulsants – tiagabine (Gabitril) and zonisamide (Zonegran) – also may help some people, although they haven't been used enough to tell what role they might play in face pain.

Finally, there's another anticonvulsant from the 1980s – valproate (Depakote) – that helps about half of those with nerve-related face pain. It can be used either as a stand-alone TN drug or as an add-on drug.

Beyond anticonvulsants

While anticonvulsants are the most effective class of drugs in treating TN and related face pain, it isn't the only kind of drug that helps.

In the 1980s, a pair of muscle-relaxants – baclofen (Lioresal) and tizanidine (Zanaflex) – were found to be helpful to some neuralgians. Baclofen is by far the more commonly used (and more effective) of the two, but it's been much more helpful as an add-on medication to anti-convulsants than as a stand-alone pain-fighter.

Tricyclic antidepressants such as amitriptyline (Elavil), imipramine (Norfranil, Tofranil) and nortriptyline (Pamelor) also have been used in a variety of face pains, especially the more constant, burning types. These medicines affect brain chemicals that play a role in chronic pain as well as depression.

"A wide range of chronic pains in addition to facial pain are responsive to antidepressant drugs," says London oral-medicine specialist Dr. Joanna Zakrzewska. "There is much evidence to suggest that treatment of pain with antidepressant drugs is independent of its antidepressant activity."

As with the muscle-relaxants, tricyclic antidepressants also may be useful as add-on medicines to some anticonvulsants. They are often used in patients who have mixed symptoms – a combination of sharp, stabbing pain but also a more constant, burning pain. An anticonvulsant may knock out the stabs while the antidepressant eases the burning ache.

Clonazepam (Klonopin), a tranquilizer that also has anti-seizure properties, has been used occasionally for TN treatment since 1975. Four studies totaling 64 people found it helped about two-thirds of the people, although it's one of the more sedating face-pain drugs.

One other medicine – pimozide (Orap) – is an antipsychotic drug that's primarily used to reduce the tics of Tourette's syndrome, but it was found to be effective against TN as well. Because it has more potentially serious side effects than most other TN drugs, it's used sparingly.

If all else fails, opioids such as morphine sulfate (MS Contin), oxycodone hydrochloride (OxyContin) and fentanyl are options for intractable pain.

No "just-for-TN" drug

One thing all of those medications have in common is that they were all developed for conditions other than TN. In fact, no drug that's used to treat TN was developed specifically for TN. Few studies have ever even been done to examine how well existing drugs control TN pain.

For one thing, it's difficult to find enough people to conduct an efficient drug trial. Plus the come-and-go nature of TN makes it tough to evaluate a test drug's true efficacy. But the main reason there's no just-for-TN medicine is that it's just not a very good investment for drug companies.

Developing and bringing a new drug to the U.S. market is a very expensive proposition – somewhere along the order of $70 million to $100 million. The U.S. Food and Drug Administration requires three different phases and years worth of testing on thousands of people before a new drug can be approved. The majority of new-drug proposals do not make it.

When a prospective new drug would treat something common such as diabetes, high blood pressure or heart disease, investing in the idea makes more sense. Millions of potential customers make that potential payoff worth the considerable risk and investment.

In uncommon disorders such as TN, the customer base is more in the thousands than millions. And that payoff-vs.-risk outlook doesn't look as rosy when a drug company decides where to invest its research dollars.

Due in part to requests by the Florida-based Trigeminal Neuralgia Association, the U.S. government's National Institutes for Health in the late 1990s funded two different drug studies. One involved dextromethorphan, a common ingredient in cough suppressants that was thought to have face-pain-fighting properties at higher doses. The other involved a different version of baclofen called "L-baclofen." The dextromethorphan study turned up no benefit, and the L-baclofen study has not been completed.

Even more promising, the National Institute of Neurological Disorders and Stroke and the National Institute of Dental and Craniofacial Research in 2003 announced that more than $5 million would be awarded in grants for TN and other face-pain research through 2006. Some of that money could end up leading researchers to improved and more selective TN medication.

The path to medication

Once TN is suspected, most patients end up going to a neurologist – the specialist most versed in medications involving the nervous system. This is often the first person neuralgians encounter who seems to know much about this condition at all.

This is where most people learn the first few key details about this disease with the big name. This is usually where they learn, first, that it's not a fatal problem, and then that the pain is most likely being caused by a blood vessel compressing the nerve.

One of the most important things the physician – whether it's a neurologist, neurosurgeon, family doctor or some other specialist – will do at this point is some detailed investigating to figure out exactly what you've got. Is it a case of classic TN? A mixed case of classic and so-called "atypical" TN (or TN-2, under the proposed new classification scheme discussed in Chapter 4)? Or is it really one of the other face pains discussed in Chapter 6 masquerading as TN?

Accurately nailing that down gives the best chance of going to the best medicine right off the bat.

"Before we start giving a lot of medicines, we ought to be sure of the diagnosis," says Dr. Zakrzewska.

Depending on which pain you have and even which variation of TN you have, different medications might be indicated. The sharp, stabbing pain of TN, for example, generally responds best to anticonvulsants such as carbamazepine (Tegretol, Carbatrol) or oxcarbazepine (Trileptal), while a more constant, burning, aching pain might respond better to gabapentin (Neurontin) or amitriptyline (Elavil). On the other hand, pain from a cluster headache isn't likely to respond to any of those medicines.

Neurologists usually do several types of tests to help nail down the diagnosis. This may include pin-prick and light-touch tests of the nerve endings, checks to see if muscles are working properly and balance and coordination tests.

They also may order a CT or MRI scan of the brain to rule out a tumor or multiple sclerosis. But the most helpful diagnostic aid is the patient history – especially the answers to such questions as where it hurts, how it hurts, what makes it hurt more or less, and so on.

Your description of these kinds of things is hugely important because as we saw in Chapter 6, a lot of conditions share similar symptoms. Sometimes it's just one key characteristic that sets one condition apart from another. The more accurate and detailed information you can give the doctor, the better your chance of getting an accurate diagnosis and therefore therapy that's most likely to help. It may help to jot down notes ahead of time and take them along to help you remember details.

Dr. Zakrzewska highly recommends a "pain diary" to help keep track of changes in the frequency and severity of the pain – both before and after medication.

"I think diaries help give patients some control over their situation," she says. "It also helps me note changes in their pain over time, side effects and other stress factors involved."

She says a continuing diary helps doctors adjust dosage levels and determine if or when a different medicine altogether should be tried.

Medication's role in TN

Assuming you've got TN or a variation of it, the neurologist or other diagnosing physician most likely is going to recommend treating the pain with medication. Even the most ardent proponents of surgery suggest medicine as the best first step – if for no other reason than to get patients out of pain quickly and allow them to "buy time" to consider longer-term options.

Medications also might help to confirm the diagnosis. If a sharp pain responds to carbamazepine (Tegretol, Carbatrol), for example, that's a good clue that the problem really is TN or a variation of it. Just because it *doesn't* work, though, doesn't mean it's *not* TN. No medication works 100 percent of the time, and up to 20 percent of neuralgians never do respond to any single medication.

The diagnosing doctor should make clear early on that this isn't a case where any medication will "cure" or "fix" TN. It's not like an infection in which a 10-day course of antibiotics gets rid of the symptoms and the cause behind them.

Rather, TN medications control the symptoms of pain. They don't affect the presumed causes. For that reason, medications are likely to be needed for as long as the underlying causes at are work – at least during active pain cycles. In other words, medications may be needed long-term.

If the pain stays under control and the side effects remain acceptable, lifelong control with medication is possible. For about half of neuralgians, medication is the only therapy they ever use. People who are prone to seizures also are on lifelong courses of the same anticonvulsants, so there are no maximum time frames on how long these medications can be used.

With the possible exception of opioids (used only after most everything else has failed), none of the TN medications are addicting. When pain goes into remission or is addressed by other therapies, neuralgians are generally happy to stop taking medication.

Picking the "right" medicine

The good news is that there are far more medications in the TN arsenal today than ever before. This gives both the doctor and the neuralgian many more choices than they had just a few years ago. Ideally, this decision will be a team effort since each has key facts the other needs to come up with the best choice.

In the past, the doctor/patient relationship often was more of an authoritarian one in which the doctor decided what was best and told the patient what to do. These days, patients tend more toward being "medical consumers" who want a greater role in the treatment decisions.

Some research suggests that treatment outcomes are better when patients have a role in the decision. For instance, patients are more likely to stick with a treatment and have more positive expectations when they helped make the treatment decision.

Given the new drug choices, doctors have more leeway to tailor a treatment program to individual patients' goals, priorities and concerns.

Some people, for example, are mainly interested in the best pain relief and are willing to tolerate potential side effects to get it. Others are less willing to make that trade, such as someone who operates heavy machinery for a living and can't afford to have any loss of coordination. Some people don't like the prospect of taking medications at all. Rather than even start on a medicine, they may rather try some of the complementary and alternative therapies discussed in Chapters 15-19, such as acupuncture, chiropractic care, hot-pepper creams, nutrition therapy and the like.

Sorting out customized treatment programs like this takes time and good communication – both tough to achieve in today's fast-paced medical environment.

Conflicts with other medicines, conditions

Before starting any medication, you should inform your doctor about any other conditions you have and any other medicines you're taking – including herbal ones and seemingly innocuous over-the-counter ones such as antacids and acetaminophen (Tylenol).

In some cases, other medications can interfere with how well your TN medication will work. Antacids, for example, can prevent anticonvulsants from working as well as they should.

Other times, a TN medication may interfere with the workings of another drug. Many anticonvulsants, for example, can reduce the effectiveness of birth-control pills.

And sometimes one drug will magnify another drug's effect, possibly leading to toxic situations. When carbamazepine (Tegretol, Carbatrol) and MAO-inhibiting antidepressants are taken together, for example, reactions including sudden high body temperature, dangerously high blood pressure and even seizures can result.

Many anticonvulsants can affect liver or kidney function, depending on how the body processes and excretes them. So someone with a pre-existing liver problem might be better suited taking an anticonvulsant that's processed by the kidney, and vice versa.

A few other medications can pose potential problems for those with diabetes, high blood pressure, heart disease, lung disease and stomach disorders. This doesn't mean you can't take anticonvulsants and other TN medications if you have any of these conditions. It just means your doctor needs to know this information to help choose the best medication and to determine what precautions, if any, ought to be taken.

"Tegretol and Dilantin have been around for ages, and we know what the problems are," says Dr. Steven Graff-Radford, a face-pain specialist at Cedars-Sinai Medical Center in Los Angeles. "We can watch for them and weigh the pros and cons."

He adds that better research has led to newer medications that have fewer known side effects.

All of these are considerations that should go into deciding which medication is right for you.

Pharmacists also can be invaluable in heading off drug interactions. That's one of the drawbacks of jumping around from pharmacy to pharmacy for different medicines. If you pick one pharmacy and go there for all your medications, the pharmacy will have a record of everything you take and should be able to catch conflicts. If you do decide to use more than one pharmacy, make sure each has a complete and current record of all of your medications.

How to take TN medications

Most TN medications – and anticonvulsants in particular – aren't taken like pain-killers. You can't take them when you're having pain and skip them when you're not. Medication levels must build up in the bloodstream until they reach a point where they calm the nervous system enough to stop those errant pain signals from getting through.

Anticonvulsants need to be both increased gradually and decreased gradually. Going up too quickly can magnify the side effects, giving people a feeling similar to marked drunkenness. Suddenly stopping anticonvulsants and baclofen can lead to mood changes, anxiety, hallucinations or seizures. For these reasons, it's important to follow the doctor's dose schedules. These schedules may spell out a starter dose, then call for increases every few days until either the pain is relieved or a maximum dose is reached.

A DOSING SCHEDULE

Dr. Joanna Zakrzewska tries to make it easy for her patients to start new TN medications gradually. She gives them a dosing schedule that lists how much medicine to take each day, at what time and how to increase it.

Here's a sample of a schedule she typically gives
for starting carbamazepine (Tegretol):

Daily dose	Day	Morning	Lunch	Afternoon	Night
200 mg	1-3	100	—	—	100
300 mg	4-6	100	100	—	100
400 mg	7-9	100	100	100	100
500 mg	10-12	200	100	100	100
600 mg	13-15	200	100	100	200
700 mg	16-18	200	200	100	200
800 mg	19-21	200	200	200	200

Note: You can do the changes more slowly, if you'd like. The amount of drug you need is related to your body weight and age, so you may start at a different point in the scale. Stop at the point at which you get good control of pain and few side effects. After three to four weeks, you may need further adjustment as your liver gets used to handling the drug. When stopping the drug, you need to go down in the same way.

— *Source: Pain Research and Clinical Management: Assessment and Management of Orofacial Pain*
(Elsevier, 2002)

Once an effective level is reached, doses need to be taken regularly.

"Believe me, Tegretol sitting in a bottle on the bathroom or kitchen shelf is not going to help your pain," San Diego neurologist Dr. James Nelson told the Trigeminal Neuralgia Association's San Diego support group. "You have to remember to take it on time."

Depending on how much medicine is needed to control pain and how long the medication works, the doses may be spread out over three or four times during the day. That's done to keep consistent levels of the medicine in the blood. If a dose or two is missed, blood levels may drop to the point where the pain breaks through.

Some neuralgians say this happens to them first thing in the morning. They take a dose of medicine before bed and then go 8 hours without a new dose. What can happen is that the blood level of the medicine wanes enough overnight that there's no longer enough to prevent that first rub of the lip in the morning from setting off a pain attack.

Drug companies are addressing that by coming up with new formulations of "time-release" medicines that spread out doses over longer periods of time. Tegretol XR and Carbatrol, for example, are two recently developed brands of carbamazepine that allow neuralgians to take doses twice a day instead of three or four times a day.

Taking fewer doses also means fewer missed doses. Studies have found that the more doses of medicine people have to take each day, the less likely they are to stick with the schedule. One study found that 70 percent of people follow a medication program when they must take pills only once or twice per day, but the number drops to 52 percent when they have to take three pills a day and goes down to 42 percent when they have to take pills four times a day.

"This is why the pharmaceutical industry is looking at developing pills that work for 24 hours, or at least for 12 hours," says Dr. Nelson.

Before starting some TN medications, doctors may want to order blood tests and/or liver or kidney function tests. These give pre-medication or "baseline" readings to help doctors later compare changes that might indicate an adverse reaction to the medication.

Allergic reactions

One other thing to watch for when starting a new TN medication is the possibility of an allergic reaction. These are usually rare and not serious, but one exception is a skin rash that develops after starting carbamazepine and a few other TN medications. This is a symptom of a serious and potentially life-threatening disorder called Stevens Johnson Syndrome. If a rash develops that indicates this disorder, the medicine should be stopped as soon as possible.

Dr. Nelson says he sometimes finds that people have less-threatening allergic reactions to the dye used in pills as opposed to the medicine itself. He says switching from one company's version of a medicine to another company's version (i.e. switching from a generic carbamazepine to brand-name Tegretol) may solve the reaction.

For people concerned about allergic reactions, Dr. Graff-Radford says allergists can do a skin test of the medicine ahead of time before a patient starts ingesting pills.

Besides that alert and any other important precautions, the doctor or pharmacist should give instructions on whether to take the medication with or without food. Some should be taken with food to lessen the chance of nausea. Others seldom cause nausea and work best when taken on an empty stomach.

And details should be given on anything else that should or shouldn't be done in order to take the medication safely and effectively. For instance, alcohol and other sedatives should be avoided with almost all TN medicines because they can magnify drowsiness.

All of this is listed on detailed handouts that pharmacies must make available for all medications they dispense by prescription. Pharmacists also are required by law to offer counseling and to answer questions that consumers have about medications they're about to take.

The right dose

After deciding which medication is likely to give the best results, the next step is to find the right dose. What's tricky here is that not everyone reacts the same way to the same medicine.

A medication that works wonderfully for one patient may do nothing for another, no matter what the dose. Or one patient may function fine on 1,200 mg of carbamazepine per day while another falls asleep on 200 mg. "Everybody responds to drugs very differently," says Dr. Zakrzewska.

Coming up with the "right" medicine at the right dose is therefore a matter of trial and adjustment. You basically try what *should* work and see if it *does* work. You see which, if any, side effects occur. You judge how well the pain is controlled and whether that outweighs the side effects.

QUESTIONS TO ASK WHEN TAKING A NEW DRUG

- What kind of medicine is this, and how does it work?

- How long should I expect it to take before it gives pain relief?

- Is there a schedule for gradually increasing the dose?

- Do I need any blood tests or other tests before starting? Will I need regular retests?

- Might this medication affect any other conditions I have?

- Does it conflict with any other medications I'm taking? Are there medicines (including prescription, over-the-counter and herbal) that I shouldn't take with this?

- Should I take the medicine with food or on an empty stomach? And are there foods or drinks I should avoid while on this medicine?

- Are there any allergic reactions to watch for?

- What are possible side effects, both common ones and more serious ones that I should report immediately?

- What if the medicine isn't helping or if a flare-up or break-through pain occurs? Should I call or can I increase the dose gradually to a certain level?

- When should I come back for a follow-up visit?

The strategy of most doctors is to start low on a medication of choice and gradually increase the dose until either the pain is relieved or the patient develops intolerable side effects. With experience, doctors have been able to come up with average doses that usually work for TN. But you may need more or less. Either way, never take any dosage other than what the prescribing doctor says.

Pain relief doesn't usually happen gradually as the doses go up. It's usually an "all-or-nothing" thing, says Dr. Nelson. "The blood level must get up to the level of pain, and then the pain can go to zero," he says.

Just because 800 mg a day of carbamazepine controls your pain doesn't mean 600 mg will control most of it and 400 mg will control some of it. You may get no relief at all until you're up to 800 mg consistently.

Because most anticonvulsants should be built up gradually to avoid sudden side effects, it may take at least a few days and maybe even a few weeks to reach complete relief. In the meantime, if the pain is unbearable, there are a host of temporary, short-term treatments to knock down attacks until the longer-term medications kick in. These include topical anesthetics, anesthetic injections and eyedrops, temporary doses of phenytoin (an anticonvulsant that can be taken at relatively high doses quickly, including intravenously) or a few days worth of an opioid medication such as morphine.

Ideally, the selected medicine will work, and you'll get out of pain at a dose that doesn't cause side effects – or only side effects that are tolerable and worth the tradeoff for pain relief. In that case, keep taking the effective dose, report back to the doctor at the suggested intervals, and make sure you have plenty of medicine on hand. Refill early. Don't run out.

What if the pain is gone?

Once the pain is under control for awhile, some neuralgians start to question whether they still need medicine. They wonder: How do I know whether it's the medicine stopping the pain or one of those remissions taking place?

The answer is you *don't* know. "The only way to determine whether there has been a remission is to withdraw the drug," says Dr. Zakrzewska, who suggests at least one month of pain control before trying a dose reduction.

Some people are very reluctant to mess around with success and would rather keep the "protection" of the medicine whether there's a remission in progress or not. Others prefer to take no more medicine than absolutely necessary and to get off medication altogether whenever possible – even if it's for a brief period.

Neither way is right or wrong. It's another one of those individual decisions. There may even be times when you want to *increase* dosage rather than decrease it, such as before major dental work or before a wedding or other important event that you don't want to risk missing because of a pain flare-up. Either way, never fool around with doses without the guidance of the prescribing doctor. He or she can give you advice on how to gradually increase or lower doses. Some may even give experienced patients schedules ahead of time with instructions on how and when to make changes.

Overdoing it with medicine can lead to unnecessary reactions and toxic side effects. But getting off the medication has its potential down side, too. You may not get much, if any, warning that you're about to "bottom out." Example: You may cut back a little and still have no pain, cut back a little more and still have no pain, then cut back a little more and suddenly get huge waves of pain for days until you're able to build the blood levels back up.

Or you may get off the medication altogether and do fine for days or weeks or even months. Then instead of coming back gradually, the pain fires back up suddenly and at full intensity. Once again, it may be days until you can get enough medication back into the bloodstream to control the pain again.

Veteran neuralgians who have been through this medication game of cat and mouse say they sometimes get "early rumblings" and other signs that the pain is coming back. Other times not.

To prepare in case you ever find yourself in an emergency or breakthrough pain situation, see the sidebar in Chapter 8 for a list of tips on how to quickly knock back these "sneak attacks."

What if the medicine "wears off?"

Sometimes medicines that were working quite well start to go downhill for no apparent reason – even if you weren't changing doses. Pain may start to break through even at a dose that has long controlled the pain.

Dr. Zakrzewska says there are two reasons for this. One is that the body has adjusted to the medication and has become more adept at breaking it down and getting rid of it. The other explanation is that the nerve injury has continued to worsen, and the resulting pain is just becoming more severe or chronic.

Increasing the dose is one option to regain pain control in both of these scenarios – assuming the new drug level doesn't create intolerable side effects.

Another option is to switch medications. Different TN medications work in different ways. Even the different anticonvulsants have different mechanisms for preventing seizures and stopping pain. So switching medicines is like starting anew with a fresh approach. Ideally, this alternate approach will work as well as the first one.

Even temporarily switching away from an effective medicine for 6 to 8 weeks is usually enough time for the drug to work well again when it's reintroduced. This is called a "drug holiday."

Doctors often take advantage of this phenomenon when treating epilepsy and Parkinson's disease, which require long-term and usually lifelong medication. On average, anticonvulsants tend to become less effective in epilepsy after 4 to 6 years, and Parkinson's drugs tend to wane after about 2 to 3 years. So by rotating in alternate drugs for a 6 to 8 weeks at some point within those time frames, the most effective medication can be maximized.

If a single drug isn't doing the job alone for TN pain, two or more drugs can be tried together. Some medications enhance one another, and some work much better as add-ons to other drugs as opposed to being used alone.

For example, the muscle relaxant baclofen (Lioresal) may not stop TN pain by itself, but it may be very helpful when added to an anticonvulsant. Or a combination of carbamazepine (Tegretol, Carbatrol) and gabapentin (Neurontin) – both anticonvulsants – may together control pain that neither of them alone was helping.

In the case of multiple drugs, it doesn't matter which drug was started first and which was added later. It's the combination of them working together that makes the difference.

Taking more than one medication doesn't always mean more side effects. It's possible for a neuralgian to have better pain relief and fewer side effects by taking lower doses of two medications than a high dose of a single medication.

Dealing with side effects

The most common side effects of TN medications are what you'd expect from drugs that slow the nervous system – things like drowsiness, lethargy, slowed reaction times, less sharp thinking and impaired coordination. Also somewhat common are headaches, dizziness and nausea, at least in the early stages.

Few people experience all of these. A few don't notice any of them, but the majority experience at least a few side effects. As Dr. Zakrzewska puts it, "There is no single drug that doesn't give side effects."

How annoying the effects are varies from person to person. Some people just have more severe reactions to certain chemicals than others. In
other cases, it's a difference in perception. Two people may have the exact
same amount of acid churning around in their stomachs, for example,
but one may complain of nausea and the other doesn't.

Fortunately, side effects tend to ease as the body adapts to the medicine. That's why most doctors advise their patients to give a new medicine at least a few weeks' trial. That's usually enough time to tell if: 1.)
the medicine is going to do a good job against the pain, and 2.) not cause
lingering side effects that the patient finds intolerable.

Until you see how you're going to react to a new medication, it's a
good idea to avoid driving, operating machinery and anything else that
could be dangerous to do in an impaired state. You don't want to solve
your face pain but fracture your spine (or worse) in a car accident.

If intolerable side effects persist after a few weeks or if pain is breaking through, it's time to call your doctor. Don't try to adjust the medication yourself or suddenly stop taking it. There are plenty of other medications that may help. But you'll probably need to gradually decrease
the dose of Medicine No. 1 as you gradually build up on Medicine No.
2. Remember, anticonvulsants in particular should be adjusted slowly.

Unpleasant side effects almost always go away within a few days of
stopping a medication, although some neuralgians say they've had lingering effects for several weeks.

If you keep trying one medicine after the other and none of them give
relief or have tolerable side effects, at some point it's time to move on to
another option. Some people are ready to move on after a couple of failures; others are willing to try every last medicine in the book before giving up. It's up to you to decide when you've given fair trial.

The important thing to remember is that even if medicines don't help,
that's just one method of dealing with this pain. The rest of this book
will discuss the many other treatment options available. But first, let's
take a closer look at the main medications currently being used to treat
TN and related face pains.

A drug-by-drug rundown

Please keep in mind that the following drug information is by no means exhaustive. Not every possible side effect, interaction or precaution is listed, and our intention is not to suggest one medication over another. What we are suggesting is that it's best to develop your own personal medication game plan with the help of a trusted doctor.

For more detailed drug information, there are numerous drug reference books as well as a variety of web sites that give in-depth drug-by-drug rundowns.

Some worthy printed references to consider:

- *"Physicians Desk Reference"* (Thomson Healthcare, $92.95 hardcover)
- *"The PDR Pocket Guide to Prescription Drugs"* (Pocket Books, $6.99 paperback)
- *"Mosby's Medical Drug Reference"* (Mosby, $39.95 hardcover)
- *"Nursing Drug Handbook"* (Springhouse Publishing, $37.95 paper back)
- *"Consumer Reports Consumer Drug Reference"* (Consumer Reports, $44.95 hardcover)
- *"Complete Guide to Prescription and Non-Prescription Drugs"* (Perigee, $17.95 paperback)
- *"The Essential Guide to Prescription Drugs"* (HarperResource, $20.95 paperback)
- *"The Pill Book"* (Bantam Books, $19.95 paperback)

And some web sites worth checking out:

- The U.S. National Library of Medicine and National Institutes of Health's Medline Plus site at
  www.nlm.nih.gov/medlineplus/druginformation.html
- Web site of *"Physicians Desk Reference"* publisher Thomson Healthcare at www.pdrhealth.com/drug_info/index.html
- WebMD at
  http://my.webmd.com/medical_information/drug_and_herbs/default.htm
- Medscape, which offers drug articles, drug studies and other information at www.medscape.com
- Center Watch, a clinical trials listing service, which publishes drug-trial results, trials in progress and new drugs recently approved by the U.S. Food and Drug Administration at www.centerwatch.com

Let's now take a look at the main medicines used in treating TN and related face pain along with how they're used, how they're taken and the key things you should know about them. Refer to the charts at the end of the listing for additional details.

• ANTICONVULSANTS •

CARBAMAZEPINE (Tegretol, Carbatrol)

How it's used in face pain. From the time it was first tried on Scandinavian TN patients in 1962, carbamazepine has been *the* TN drug of choice. It's still the leading TN drug worldwide, although the similar and newer oxcarbazepine (Trileptal) is beginning to rival its popularity.

It's also still the only medicine officially approved by the U.S. Food and Drug Administration for use in TN. All other medicines are considered "off-label" uses when prescribed for TN.

Carbamazepine's strong suit is dealing with the sharp, electrical stabbing nature of nerve pains. It's a bit less helpful with the more constant, burning types of nerve pain, but often alleviates that as well.

Besides sometimes being called the "gold standard" for treating classic TN, carbamazepine also is often effective in treating TN variants (i.e. post-herpetic neuralgia, trigeminal neuropathic pain related to injuries, cases caused by multiple sclerosis, etc.) And it's often effective in helping other sharp, nerve-related pains such as that caused by glossopharyngeal neuralgia, geniculate neuralgia, occipital neuralgia, SUNCT and Raeder's paratrigeminal syndrome. (See Chapter 6 for more on these.)

How it's taken. Carbamazepine comes in 100 mg chewable tablets, in scored 200 mg pills and in liquid form. It's usually started at a level of 200 mg a day (split over two doses) and increased every few days until the pain is gone. An average maintenance dose is 800 mg a day (split over three or four doses). The usual maximum is 1,200 mg a day, although some people have taken even more with careful monitoring.

Carbamazepine is most effective when taken with food (with the exception of grapefruit juice, which interferes with the drug's absorption rate.) Doses last about 6 to 8 hours. Sometimes the liver adjusts to processing it after four weeks or so, and dose adjustments are often needed around that time.

Two controlled-release versions of carbamazepine also are available – Tegretol XR and Carbatrol. The advantage of both of these is that they break down gradually and allow patients to take doses only twice a day instead of three or four times.

The gradual breakdown of these controlled-release versions also evens out the drug levels in the blood, reducing side effects that can result from the ebb and flo of regular pills.

Tegretol XR comes in 100 mg, 200 mg and 400 mg tablets. These remain active for about 12 hours per dose and should be taken with food.

Carbatrol comes in 100 mg, 200 mg and 300 mg capsules. These also remain active for about 12 hours per dose but need not be taken with food. Carbatrol capsules have the added advantage of allowing patients to open the capsules and sprinkle the tiny medicated "beads" on food – a benefit to those who have trouble swallowing pills.

Both of these versions contain the same active ingredient – carbamazepine – and so both carry the same precautions and potential types of side effects as the original Tegretol.

Key points. Sometimes carbamazepine goes to work rather quickly. Some people notice improvement within the first one to three days on doses as low as 100 mg.

Within two to three weeks, anywhere from 60 to 85 percent of patients respond to carbamazepine, depending on whose studies you believe. About 7 percent of patients find they are allergic to the drug (a severe skin rash is a key symptom) and stop taking it early on.

Over time, others find the side effects to be intolerable, and over more time, the pain can begin to break through even at higher and higher doses. In the long run, one study found that after 10 years, only about 40 to 56 percent of all patients are still getting adequate relief from carbamazepine.

Carbamazepine is metabolized by the liver. (Metabolism refers to how the body processes a drug in order to eliminate it from the body. This is done in either the liver or kidneys. Problems with these organs can impair the body's ability to get rid of drugs, allowing toxicity to occur.)

Even in its brand-name Tegretol version, carbamazepine is one of the least expensive anticonvulsants. And generic carbamazepine is often only a third of that cost.

Precautions. Besides that potentially life-threatening allergic reaction (signaled by the skin rash, fever and mouth sores), carbamazepine can cause a few serious blood disorders.

The most serious is *aplastic anemia*, a rare but potentially fatal disorder caused by damage to the bone marrow. Four other conditions also can occur: 1.) *leukopenia,* a deficiency in white blood cells, which protect the body against disease-causing microorganisms; 2.) *neutropenia,* a diminished number of neutrophils, which is a type of white blood cell; 3.) *thrombocytopenia,* a decrease in platelets, which is the component of blood needed for clotting, and 4.) *hyponatremia,* abnormally low levels of blood sodium.

All of these disorders can be headed off by keeping tabs on the patient's blood, which is one reason why doctors routinely order periodic blood tests for those on carbamazepine therapy. Blood tests will show if any of these side effects is developing so the medicine can be decreased or stopped before problems develop.

Blood tests also can tell doctors how much carbamazepine is being absorbed and carried in the blood.

Usually if there's going to be a problem taking the drug, it'll show up within the first month. Some of the potential side effects may sound scary, but it's important to remember that the serious ones are very rare.

"In 35 years as a neurologist, I have never seen one case of bone-marrow depression with this medicine," say Dr. Nelson.

"I've never seen (carbamazepine) cause a life-threatening situation," adds University of Cincinnati neurologist Dr. John H. Feibel. "Many people are afraid of this drug, and they shouldn't be."

The most common side effects of carbamazepine are drowsiness, sluggishness, dizziness, impaired coordination, impaired memory, nausea, blurred vision and occasionally headaches, a sensitivity to sunlight and loss of appetite. It also sometimes causes noticeable water retention.

Long-term use may cause a folate vitamin deficiency, so some doctors advise patients to take a daily supplement of folic acid.

Carbamazepine does have an effect on several other medications that patients may be taking for other conditions. For example, it decreases the effectiveness of some oral contraceptives. It also can lessen the effectiveness of blood-thinners, such as warfarin (Coumadin) and aspirin. And it can lead to sudden rises in body temperatures, dangerously high blood pressure and even convulsions when taken with MAO-inhibiting antidepressants.

Carbamazepine should be used with caution by pregnant women, people who are allergic to tricyclic antidepressants, people who have glaucoma, and people with a history of liver, kidney, heart or bone-marrow problems.

OXCARBAZEPINE (Trileptal)

How it's used in face pain. Think of this as carbamazepine with fewer side effects. It is closely related to carbamazepine (it's even sometimes called a "cousin" or "sister" drug to carbamazepine), and so it works for most of the same kinds of pains – especially the sharp, stabbing attacks of classic TN.

It was approved for use in the United States in 2000 after being used for about a decade in Canada and some European countries.

However, the makeup of this new anticonvulsant is different enough that most people tolerate it better than carbamazepine. Most of the potentially serious side effects and drug interactions have been eliminated, and even some of oxcarbazepine's more common side effects are milder than carbamazepine's.

Oxcarbazepine also is used to treat burning nerve pains as well as glossopharyngeal neuralgia, geniculate neuralgia and Raeder's paratrigeminal syndrome. Essentially, any condition that responds to carbamazepine also is likely to respond to oxcarbazepine.

How it's taken. Oxcarbazepine comes in 150 mg, 300 mg and 600 mg tablets as well as in liquid form.

Dr. Graff-Radford says this drug is a bit less "potent" than carbamazepine and so the doses are slightly higher – about 300 mg of oxcarbazepine for every 200 mg of carbamazepine. He starts the drug with a 150 mg dose at bedtime and then adds 150 mg every 4 to 7 days, splitting it over two or three doses. Others start with 300 mg a day over two doses and bump it up a little faster.

As with carbamazepine, sometimes pain relief from this medication is pretty quick at low doses – anywhere from 400 mg to 1,000 mg per day. But most people need somewhere between 1,200 and 2,000 mg a day for good, consistent, long-term pain control. The usual maximum is 2,400 mg.

Oxcarbazepine can be taken with or without food.

Key points. At least four different studies in Canada and Europe have found oxcarbazepine is just as effective as carbamazepine in treating TN. In his first three years using it, Dr. Nelson says that 70 to 80 percent of his patients got pain relief from oxcarbazepine – about the same as carbamazepine.

But because of the improved side-effect and drug-interaction pro-file of this newcomer, it's become a drug many doctors are now pre-scribing first. Dr. Nelson says oxcarbazepine breaks down into a sim-pler form in the body. "That leads to much more stable blood levels, and that converts into much better tolerability," he says. "Head-to-head recent reports show the side-effect profile of this is seemingly superior (to carbamazepine)."

One other important factor is that allergic reactions to this drug are much less common than with carbamazepine. That means that some people who couldn't take carbamazepine because of an allergy may be able to safely take oxcarbazepine.

A possible drawback of oxcarbazepine is its cost. As a new intro-duction, it's significantly more expensive than older anticonvulsants, including carbamazepine.

Oxcarbazepine is metabolized by the kidneys. Some doctors order an electrolyte test after the first month, but after that, regular testing is usually not done.

Precautions. Though the early experience is promising, oxcar-bazepine is not free from all side effects. Hyponatremia, one of the blood disorders that can occur with carbamazepine use, also can occur with oxcarbazepine. (This is the one that involves abnormally low blood sodium levels.) Periodic monitoring of blood sodium lev-els can head off this possibility.

Aside from a drop in blood-platelet count that about 1 percent of people experience, no other blood problems have been seen, includ-ing the potentially life-threatening aplastic anemia that's a rare com-plication of carbamazepine use.

Among the most common side effects of oxcarbazepine are dizzi-ness, drowsiness, double vision and lethargy. Nausea, tremors and coordination problems also are occasionally seen. These usually lessen after a few weeks, and most of the time they're milder than with car-bamazepine.

The main side effect to watch for early is an allergic reaction, which is marked by a severe skin rash and sometimes a sore throat and/or mouth sores.

There are no known serious drug interactions, but oxcarbazepine may lessen the effectiveness of some oral contraceptives.

GABAPENTIN (Neurontin)

How it's used in face pain. Gabapentin was approved by the U.S. Food and Drug Administration in 1993 as an add-on medication to help control epilepsy cases that were only partly controlled by other medications.

Since then, it's also been proven to work well enough for post-herpetic neuralgia that the FDA approved it for that labeled use in 2002. Doctors also have used gabapentin with success for various neuropathies, for the more burning, constant type of face pain, for SUNCT and for Raeder's paratrigeminal syndrome.

In TN, it's sometimes used as a stand-alone, front-line drug, but it's also often used in conjunction with carbamazepine or oxcarbazepine. As an add-on drug, it often helps when one drug isn't doing a complete pain-relief job. And it's especially useful as an add-on for mixed or TN-2 types of face pain – the carbamazepine or oxcarbazepine helps the sharp pain while the gabapentin helps the more burning, constant pain component.

Gabapentin pairs well with other anticonvulsants because it has a different mechanism of action than older medications. Gabapentin is thought to help nerve pain by increasing the body's production of gamma-aminobutyric acid (GABA), a body chemical that "tones down" or shuts off the firing of nerves. It also has no apparent adverse interactions with other anticonvulsants – or any other medications, for that matter.

How it's taken. Gabapentin comes in 100 mg, 300 mg and 400 mg capsules.

It can be increased to helpful levels fairly quickly. Gabapentin is usually started with one 300 mg capsule at bedtime on the first day, then increased to two 300 mg capsules in two doses the second day, and then to three 300 mg capsules in three doses the third day.

Some people get pain relief at that level, but if more is needed, additions should be in 300 mg increments every few days. Dr. Miroslav Backonja, associate professor of neurology and anesthesiology at the University of Wisconsin, analyzed four studies of 1,033 gabapentin patients and concluded that patients should go up to a dose of at least 1,800 mg total per day before judging whether the medicine will work.

The usual maximum is 3,600 mg per day, but some patients have tolerated as much as 4,800 mg per day. Gabapentin's effects last for 5 to 7 hours, so it's a medication best taken either three or four times a day.

Gabapentin can be taken with or without food, but it should not be used with antacids, which reduce gabapentin's absorption when taken within two hours before a gabapentin capsule.

Key points. The main reason gabapentin has become an extremely popular new medication for all sorts of nerve pain is its low side-effect rate. It gives good pain relief with no serious side effects, relatively few annoying side effects and no known drug interactions (other than the antacids mentioned above).

For those reasons, blood testing is normally not needed. Neither are kidney or liver function tests, although gabapentin is eliminated through the kidneys. (Dr. Nelson says testing is seldom needed because the body doesn't break down gabapentin; it uses it as is and passes it out whole in the urine.)

Since gabapentin has no apparent adverse drug interactions, it's a good choice for patients on a lot of other medicines, including other anticonvulsants and central nervous system depressants (i.e. antidepressants, antihistamines, sleep aids, anxiety medicines and some pain-relievers and muscle-relaxants). Many other anticonvulsants must be paired cautiously with other sedating drugs so the combined effects aren't intolerable or toxic.

Studies of 33 people who used gabapentin for pain relief found that it helped 82 percent of the time.

The main downside of gabapentin is cost. Like oxcarbazepine, it's a relatively new introduction and about as expensive as oxcarbazepine. Both of these can cost more than three times as much as carbamazepine – a potential problem for those with poor or no prescription drug coverage.

Precautions. There's not a lot to worry about here. An allergic rash can happen, but it's not common. The most serious possibility is leukopenia – a lack of white blood cells – but it's not likely enough that most doctors believe blood monitoring is necessary.

The most common side effects of gabapentin are drowsiness, dizziness and sedation. Occasional other side effects include nervousness or sadness, tremors, involuntary arm or leg movements and twitching eyes. The level of these problems are usually milder than with most anticonvulsants, and as is usually the case, side effects often ease in a few weeks as the patient adjusts to the medicine.

In clinical trials, only about 7 percent of the 1,748 test subjects opted to stop using gabapentin because of side effects.

LAMOTRIGINE (Lamictal)

How it's used in face pain. Lamotrigine was approved by the FDA in 1994, also primarily as an add-on medication for epilepsy. It is believed to work by blocking the passage of sodium in nerve cells and by slowing the release of glutamate, an amino acid that's important in transmitting pain signals to the brain. This was the first medication to attack pain and seizures in this way.

In TN, it seems to be much more effective as an add-on to other anticonvulsants such as carbamazepine or oxcarbazepine than as a stand-alone, front-line pain-killer. However, it sometimes works by itself, at least giving one more option to those who can't take carbamazepine or oxcarbazepine.

It's also been used with some success to treat SUNCT, post-herpetic neuralgia and some neuropathies, especially those related to diabetes.

How it's taken. Lamotrigine comes in 25 mg, 100 mg, 150 mg and 200 mg pills and in 5 mg and 25 mg chewable tablets.

When used as an add-on medication, the usual starting dose is 50 mg once a day for two weeks, then 100 mg per day in two divided doses for two more weeks. The medication can be increased at that rate up to the usual maintenance dose of 300 to 500 mg per day, taken in two divided doses.

Lamotrigine can be taken with or without food.

Key points. Little research has been done on lamotrigine's use as a nerve pain-killer. In one small 1997 study, though, 10 of 13 patients reported that lamotrigine gave them good or excellent relief when used as an add-on medication for face pain.

Since it has no serious adverse interactions with other drugs (and few interactions of any sort), it's a good drug to add when one drug isn't doing the job alone.

Blood tests and other monitoring are usually not needed because of the low likelihood of problems. Lamotrigine is metabolized by the liver.

As a relatively new medication, lamotrigine is about twice as expensive as carbamazepine, but not quite as expensive as oxcarbazepine, gabapentin and topiramate.

Precautions. The main problem to watch for with this drug is a potentially severe skin rash. In clinical testing, 5 to 10 percent of lamotrigine users developed a rash. Most of these cases were benign, but the problem is that it's difficult to tell the non-threatening rashes from the ones associated with the potentially life-threatening Stevens-Johnson syndrome. Rashes were even more common in children, affecting as many as one in 50 of the test subjects.

Dr. Nelson says a rash isn't always a sign of an allergic reaction and may occur when too much lamotrigine is taken too quickly. If a rash is going to occur, it normally will appear in the first two to eight weeks of starting lamotrigine, although rashes have been reported as long as six months later.

Other than that, lamotrigine seems to have relatively few and generally mild, tolerable side effects. Most common is the usual lineup for anticonvulsants – drowsiness, dizziness, tiredness, double or blurred vision, impaired coordination and nausea. A headache, insomnia and/or runny nose are other occasional side effects.

Lamotrigine also has only a few drug interactions, and none of them are serious ones. Valproate (Depakote) is the main one to watch because this drug may hinder the body from eliminating lamotrigine as quickly as normal. That can lead to toxic levels. If these two drugs are used together, the lamotrigine dose should be reduced from normal levels.

On the other hand, lamotrigine's effectiveness can be reduced by carbamazepine, phenytoin and the epilepsy drugs phenobarbital (Luminal) and primidone (Mysoline).

Lamotrigine also may cause increased skin sensitivity to sunlight.

TOPIRAMATE (Topamax)

How it's used in face pain. Similar in workings to lamotrigine, this anticonvulsant joined the TN arsenal at the end of 1996. Again, it was developed primarily as an add-on medication for epilepsy and other seizure conditions.

In clinical testing, topiramate proved to be a more effective seizure-controller than either gabapentin or lamotrigine. However, the early feedback from doctors on its effectiveness in treating face pain hasn't been as promising. Initial reports are that it seems to be a notch less effective for pain than carbamazepine and oxcarbazepine.

Dr. Graff-Radford, for example, says he's seen an effectiveness rate of about 60 to 70 percent. "I think it's good as an add-on drug, not a first-line drug," he says.

It also gives another option for those who can't take carbamazepine or oxcarbazepine.

Topiramate has been used with some success in treating migraines,

SUNCT, cluster headaches, post-herpetic neuralgia and the more burning, constant pains of neuropathies.

It is thought to enhance the body's ability to use GABA (the body chemical that inhibits nerve firing) as well block glutamate, one of the body's chemicals that is responsible for firing off nerve signals. (Lamotrigine also blocks glutamate.)

How it's taken. Topiramate comes in 25 mg, 100 mg and 200 mg tablets and in 15 mg, 25 mg and 50 mg capsules. The tablets should be swallowed whole (they have a bitter taste if chewed), but the capsules can be opened and the "sprinkles" taken with soft food (again without being chewed).

For seizures, topiramate is usually started at either 25 mg or 50 mg once a day before bed, then increased by 25 mg or 50 mg each week up to a maximum of 400 mg a day taken over two doses.

Dr. Graff-Radford said he starts his pain patients at a lower level – usually 15 mg a day right before bedtime – and adds 15 mg every 4 to 7 days until the pain is controlled. He says this more gradual increase helps limit some of the drug's sedating effects. He says he usually starts to see pain relief at about 45 mg per day. If more than 100 mg a day is needed, that's when he splits the medication over two daily doses, up to 400 mg maximum. "Getting to the first 100 mg is the biggest challenge," he says. "If you can get to that, you can tolerate it pretty well."

Topiramate can be taken with or without food, but unless directed otherwise, it's best to take each dose with a full glass of water.

Key points. While some people tolerate topiramate very well, others say it's one of the most sedating of the anticonvulsants. Try it for awhile before driving or operating equipment to see which way you'll react. Taking it at night (to the degree possible) also can help overcome this potential problem.

Serious side effects such as blood disorders and kidney or liver problems are very unlikely, and so regular blood testing normally is not needed. Topiramate is metabolized by the kidneys.

As a new drug, it's about three times more expensive than carbamazepine, or about the same cost as oxcarbazepine and gabapentin.

Precautions. Two main problems to watch for are a form of glaucoma and an increased incidence of kidney stones. Neither is common, but symptoms of either should be reported immediately. (1.5 percent of clinical test subjects developed kidney stones.)

Glaucoma can be blinding, so tell your doctor if you notice blurred vision, vision changes or pain around the eyes while taking topiramate. This usually resolves itself when the problem is recognized early and the drug stopped.

Low back pain and difficulty urinating are two key signs of possible kidney stones. Drinking several extra glasses of water a day can help counteract this potential problem. (That's especially important in hot weather or if you notice a rise in body temperature or decreased sweating.) Eating a high-protein, very low-carbohydrate diet can increase the risk of kidney stones while on topiramate.

Allergic reactions to this medicine are uncommon, but the symptoms are: difficulty breathing; hives, and swelling of the lips, tongue, face and throat. These also should be reported immediately.

A variety of less serious side effects are fairly common. Besides sleepiness, some of the most common ones are dizziness, impaired coordination, impaired memory, sluggishness, twitching eyes, tremors, nervousness, sadness, double vision, speech problems and nausea. Some people also have reported weight loss while on this medicine. Most side effects ease as the body adjusts to the medication.

Topiramate also conflicts with several other medications. For example, topiramate's effectiveness is decreased by carbamazepine, phenytoin and valproate. On the other hand, topiramate may decrease the effectiveness of valproate and some oral contraceptives, and it may increase the blood levels of phenytoin.

Topiramate also can be excessively sedating if taken along with other medications that depress the central nervous system, including antidepressants, antihistamines, sleep aids, anxiety medicines, narcotic pain-relievers and muscle-relaxants.

PHENYTOIN (Dilantin)

How it's used in face. This is the "granddaddy" of modern anticonvulsants. Originally developed as a hypnotic drug in 1908, phenytoin began to be used for treating epilepsy and other seizure disorders in 1938. Soon after, doctors began prescribing it for TN, and it quickly became the No. 1 TN drug until carbamazepine came along in the early 1960s.

Today it's seldom used as the first TN choice anymore because many other anticonvulsants have proven more effective. It's now mostly a fallback choice for patients who can't take carbamazepine or oxcarbazepine because of allergic reaction. Phenytoin also is sometimes used as an add-on drug when one medication alone isn't doing the job.

Because it's one of the few anticonvulsants that can be given in rather large doses quickly (including intravenously), phenytoin also is useful in treating sudden break-through attacks. This can be a godsend in new cases or in cases where a neuralgian has gone off medicine and experienced a sharp and sudden recurrence. A quick "loading dose" of phenytoin can knock back pain quickly while more effective, long-term anticonvulsants have a chance to build back up in the bloodstream.

How it's taken. Phenytoin comes in liquid form, in 50 mg chewable tablets, in 100 mg capsules and in 30 mg and 100 mg extended-release capsules. It and a closely related product – fosphenytoin (Cerebyx) – is available in IV form for those quick pain knock-backs described above.

When taken orally, phenytoin is usually started at 300 mg a day taken over three doses. It's then increased in increments of 100 mg every two to four weeks until symptoms are gone, which is usually in the 300 mg to 600 mg range. Some people are able to take up to 300 mg in a single dose of extended-release phenytoin (Dilantin Kapseals).

Phenytoin is best taken with food to minimize upset stomach, but antacids should be avoided within an hour or two before and after the medication is taken. Antacids can prevent the medication from being absorbed.

Key points. The main reason phenytoin isn't used more often these days for face pain is that it's just not as effective as most of the newer anticonvulsants. At best, studies have shown it gives either full or partial relief to 54 to 70 percent of patients. However, three more recent studies put its effectiveness at 42 percent, and others have reported rates as low as 25 to 30 percent.

Even when it works initially, phenytoin doesn't seem to be a reliable, long-term solution. One study found that the average duration of relief is about 18 months – significantly shorter than carbamazepine.

Most doctors advise at least one early blood test to make sure the medicine isn't affecting liver function. Phenytoin is metabolized by the liver. It sometimes turns urine pink, red or reddish-brown, which can be alarming to people but isn't a serious threat (unless it masks true bleeding from another problem).

On the plus side, though, phenytoin is one of the two most inexpensive anticonvulsants – rivaling generic carbamazepine in cost. That can be a big factor for those whose insurance plans won't pay for some of the more expensive newcomers.

Precautions. Phenytoin certainly isn't without its share of side effects and drug interactions. But the advantage of such a "veteran" drug is that it has a long track record of very few serious problems, and its precautions and potential problems are well known. Despite the detailed pre-market testing that's required, sometimes side effects of new medications don't become apparent until millions of people are taking it years after they've been approved.

About 10 percent of TN patients are unable to take phenytoin because of allergic reactions (i.e. a potentially serious skin rash), intolerable side effects or conflicts with other medications.

The most serious possible problems are blood disorders: thrombocytopenia (clotting problems), leukopenia (too few white blood cells), agranulocytosis (decrease in leukocyte cells need to fight infections), and pancytopenia (decrease in all types of blood cells). Some doctors order periodic blood tests to make sure there are no signs of any of these.

Long-term phenytoin use also can deplete the body of calcium and folate, so calcium and folic acid supplements are often advised in patients taking phenytoin.

The most common side effects are drowsiness, dizziness, sluggishness, impaired coordination and sore, thickened gums (*gingival hyperplasia*). Some patients also may develop tremors, twitching eyes, double vision, slurred speech, constipation, mood changes, confusion, nervousness, impaired memory and unwanted hair growth.

A variety of drugs interact with phenytoin. For example, phenytoin can decrease the effectiveness of such medications as valproate, some oral contraceptives, estrogens, carbamazepine, lamotrigine, the bronchodilator theophylline (Theo-Dur), the heart drugs quinidine (Quinalan) and digitoxin (Crystodigin), the transplant drug cyclosporin, and the anti-swelling drug furosemide (Lasix).

On the other hand, some medications can increase phenytoin levels in the blood, such as the sedative diazepam (Valium), valproate, the heart drug amiodarone, the blood-pressure drug diltiazem (Cardizem), the tuberculosis drug isoniazid (Laniazid, Nydrazid), the antifungal drug fluconazole (Diflucan), the arthritis drug phenylbutazone (Cotylbutazone) and the stomach drug cimetidine (Tagamet).

Phenytoin levels can be decreased by carbamazepine.

LEVETIRACETAM (Keppra)

How it's used in face pain. This is one of the newest of the new anticonvulsants, being approved by the FDA in 1999 as an add-on drug for seizures. It apparently works by preventing nerve cells from firing – a slightly different mode of action than older anticonvulsants.

It's also been tried for a variety of pains, but levetiracetam is so new that there's very little data so far on how likely it is to help. One study of 400 patients experiencing all sorts of pain (not just TN) reported some relief in 93 percent of the case, while another of 24 patients with neuropathic pain reported excellent or good pain relief 67 percent of the time.

For now at least, it's most likely to be used in TN as an add-on drug or as another fall-back option in case of failure or allergic reactions in other more proven anticonvulsants.

There's also some early evidence that it might be useful in treating migraines.

How it's taken. Levetiracetam comes in 250 mg, 500 mg and 750 mg tablets. One advantage is that it can be started at fairly high, effective doses, which is good for those in severe pain and anxious to get relief.

Levetiracetam is usually started at 500 mg a day, taken in two doses. An additional 500 mg can be added every two weeks up to a maximum of 1,500 mg.

It can be taken with or without food.

Key points. Although it's largely unproven as a pain-killer so far, some doctors are willing to try it because it has relatively few side effects and practically no drug interactions or serious side effects.

It's metabolized by the kidneys, and blood tests are not needed in most cases.

It's also a fairly long-acting medication – lasting up to 12 hours per dose. So it can be taken in just two doses per day instead of the three or four doses that some other TN medications require.

As a new drug, it's relatively expensive, although not quite as costly as oxcarbazepine, topiramate and gabapentin. It's been approved only for use in those over age 16.

Precautions. There's very little to worry about here – at least so far. The only known potentially serious side effects are the blood disorders leukopenia (too low white blood cells) and neutropenia (decrease in the neutrophil cells needed to fight infection). But both of these are very rare possibilities.

In the first few weeks of treatment, levetiracetam sometimes triggers psychological reactions, such as agitation, hostility, anxiety, depression and possible hallucinations. These also are uncommon and usually ease as the patient adjusts, but they should be reported nonetheless.

Allergic reactions can happen but also are rare.

Other than that, the side effects are the usual: dizziness, drowsiness, headache, impaired coordination, nausea and sometimes dry eyes and weakness.

Using levetiracetam with other sedating drugs (i.e. antidepressants, antihistamines and narcotics) can sometimes cause excessive sedation. There are no other known drug interactions

TIAGABINE (Gabitril)

How it's used in face pain. This anticonvulsant was approved by the FDA in 1997 as an add-on drug for partial-onset seizures in adults and children over age 12. It's thought to work by enhancing the body's ability to use GABA (the body chemical that inhibits nerve firing). That's one of the ways topiramate also is believed to work.

Because it's such a new drug, there's little feedback so far on how well it's likely to work for TN and related face pains. For now, it's mainly used as an occasional add-on drug when one drug alone isn't doing the job or as an alternative when other more proven anticonvulsants have failed or can't be taken.

How it's taken. Tiagabine comes in 4 mg, 12 mg, 16 mg and 20 mg tablets. The usual starting dose is 4 mg once a day, increased by 4 to 8 mg each week up to a maximum of 56 mg per day. The suggested usual maintenance dose is 32 to 56 mg per day.

Tiagabine works for about 7 to 9 hours, so it's a medicine usually taken three times a day.

It should be taken with food to minimize possible upset stomach.

Key points. One of the main advantages tiagabine has going for it is relatively few side effects and no known serious side effects or drug interactions. That makes it particularly useful as an add-on drug or one for people who are on a lot of other medications.

Blood testing is normally not needed because this drug has not been linked to the blood disorders that are occasionally seen in some other anticonvulsants. It's metabolized by the liver.

As a new drug, it's fairly expensive, so the main question to be answered is whether it's going to perform better than other less-expensive and proven anticonvulsants.

Precautions. The only somewhat troubling symptom some patients have seen so far is marked weakness when tiagabine is taken at high doses. That effect normally clears quickly once the drug is stopped or the dose is reduced.

Other than that, side effects are few and usually mild. The most common are dizziness, drowsiness, nervousness and nausea. Tremors, difficulty concentrating and stomach pain also are occasionally seen.

Tiagabine may slightly reduce the effectiveness of valproate, but it does not appear to effect levels of other anticonvulsants. The effectiveness of tiagabine, however, may be reduced by carbamazepine, phenytoin, phenobarbital and primidone (Mysoline).

Using tiagabine with other sedating drugs (i.e. antidepressants, antihistamines and narcotics) can sometimes cause excessive sedation.

VALPROATE (Depakote, Depakene)

How it's used in face pain. Valproate is one of the older anticonvulsants. Also known as valproic acid and divalproex sodium, it's been used since 1980, mainly to control both petit mal and grand mal seizures.

It seems to work much better in face pain as an add-on to other drugs than used by itself. However, because of the many interactions it has with other drugs, it must be paired carefully. Sometimes dose adjustments are required either in valproate or the other drugs already being taken.

Before some of the newer anticonvulsants came along, valproate was often paired with the muscle relaxant baclofen (Lioresal) for TN pain when carbamazepine failed or couldn't be taken.

It's also been used with some success in neuropathic pains, for preventing migraines and in the treatment of bipolar disorder.

How it's taken. Depakene brand of valproate comes in syrup form and in 250 mg capsules. Depakote comes in 125 mg capsules and 125 mg, 250 mg and 500 mg delayed-release tablets.

It also can be injected or given intravenously, which makes it an option for someone who needs immediate pain relief (such as in the case of a sudden pain break-through).

The dose levels vary by body weight, but the usual adult ranges are 600 mg to 2,000 mg a day.

Depakote capsules can be taken whole or opened and the coated beads sprinkled on food. (The beads should not be chewed.)

Valproate should be taken with food or milk to prevent upset stomach.

Key points. Valproate isn't widely used in face pain because there are many other drugs now that give much better relief with fewer side effects.

A pair of limited studies on valproate's effectiveness for TN found that about 80 percent get some relief but less than half get 50 percent or better relief. Bottom line: it's likely to be only marginally helpful.

Valproate is metabolized by the kidneys and has been known to cause liver problems in some people. Severe fatigue and malaise are possible signs of liver toxicity. For this reason, liver function tests are usually ordered for those on valproate. This medicine is not recommended at all for those with pre-existing liver conditions.

Blood tests also are often needed to guard against several other blood disorders (see below).

Precautions. In addition to liver disorders, valproate can cause a few potentially serious side effects, including: pancreatitis (a possibly life-threatening inflammation of the pancreas); bone marrow suppression; thrombocytopenia (a blood-clotting disorder), and leukopenia (too low white blood cells).

Some of the more common but less serious side effects are sedation, headache, dizziness, double vision, nausea, irritability, restlessness and impaired coordination. Tremors, weight gain and hair loss also are occasional side effects.

Valproate also interacts with a variety of other drugs in a variety of ways. The stomach drug cimetidine (Tagamet) and antibiotic erythromycin can increase valproate blood levels. On the other hand, valproate can lessen the effectiveness of the blood-thinner warfarin (Coumadin) and increase the blood levels of lamotrigine.

When used with other sedating drugs such as tranquilizers, antidepressants, antihistamines and narcotics, valproate can become excessively sedating.

ZONISAMIDE (Zonegran)

How it's used in face pain. Zonisamide was approved by the FDA in 2000 as an anticonvulsant for use as an add-on drug in the treatment of partial-onset seizures in adults and children over the age of 16. Its action is unknown but thought to be similar to some of the older anticonvulsants.

It's also unknown so far how useful or successful zonisamide will be in the treatment of TN and related face pains.

For now, it's used as an occasional add-on drug to other medications or another alternative when other more proven anticonvulsants fail or can't be taken.

How it's taken. Zonisamide comes in 100 mg capsules. It's usually started at 100 mg a day in a single dose and then increased after two weeks to 200 mg a day, taken either in one or two doses.

The medication can be increased every two weeks in 100 mg increments up to a maximum of 600 mg. It's usually taken in two doses.

Capsules should be swallowed whole and not chewed or broken apart.

Zonisamide can be taken with or without food, but patients on it should drink at least 6 to 8 glasses of water a day to limit the risk of kidney stones, which is a possible although uncommon side effect.

Key points. Time will tell what role it will play in TN and face pain. Other than a few problems from possible allergic reactions, zonisamide has relatively few side effects and hardly any drug interactions.

It's metabolized by the liver and eliminated through the kidneys, so it should be used with caution in people with pre-existing liver or kidney problems. Periodic blood tests may be ordered to make sure the drug is not causing liver, kidney or blood disorders.

As a new drug, it's fairly expensive.

Precautions. Initially, watch for an allergic reaction, especially a severe skin rash that might indicate a case of potentially life-threatening Stevens-Johnson syndrome. Two potentially serious blood disorders (agranulocytosis and aplastic anemia) also can occur rarely in people who are unusually sensitive to zonisamide.

Longer term, there is a slight increase in the incidence of kidney stones. Signs of that include sudden back or abdominal pain, difficulty urinating and/or blood in the urine.

More common but less serious side effects include drowsiness, sluggishness, fatigue, dizziness, headache, nausea and occasionally loss of appetite, weight loss, agitation, irritability and difficulty concentrating.

Carbamazepine, phenytoin and valproate have been found to make zonisamide less effective, so dose adjustments might be needed when these drugs are paired. Other than that, no other drug interactions have been found.

• ANTIDEPRESSANTS •
AMITRIPTYLINE (Elavil)
IMIPRAMINE (Norfranil, Tofranil)
NORTRIPTYLINE (Pamelor)

How they're used in face pain. All three of these are tricyclic anti-depressants that work in very similar, if not identical, ways – namely by increasing the amount of norepinephrine and serotonin in the central nervous system. The levels of these biochemicals are a key factor in depression, but they're also both used in nerve transmission.

Amitriptyline, imipramine and nortriptyline have long been used to treat depression. But they've also been found to have pain-relieving properties, particularly in relieving the more constant, aching pains that anticonvulsants often don't help. Desipramine (Norpramin) is another very similar medication in this class, but it's not used quite as often for pain as the above three.

The pain-relieving properties of these tricyclic antidepressants are separate from the antidepressive properties. Just because a doctor prescribes a tricyclic antidepressant for face pain doesn't mean he/she thinks you're depressed, anxious or "imagining" the pain for psychological reasons.

On the other hand, chronic pain can often lead to or occur along with depression, so antidepressants can be an effective way to deal with two problems by using just one medicine.

In TN, antidepressants are used most often for so-called "atypical" TN or TN-2 or for related face pains that are more constant, burning and/or aching as opposed to sharp and stabbing. In mixed cases, they can be taken along with an anticonvulsant. The aim is for the anticonvulsant to knock out the sharp pains while the antidepressant addresses the underlying, constant pain.

These antidepressants also have been used with good success on a variety of other face pains, including various neuropathies, temporomandibular disorders, myofascial pain, atypical odontalgia and burning mouth syndrome.

Dr. Graff-Radford says he normally sees an average 70 to 80 pain reduction when using antidepressants in continuous-pain cases.

Amitriptyline, imipramine, nortriptyline and desipramine also have all been used for treating post-herpetic neuralgia. Dr. David Bowsher, a research scientist at the Pain Research Institute in Liverpool, England, found that amitriptyline was very effective when given early in the course of post-herpetic neuralgia. In his study of 262 post-herpetic neuralgians, he found that 75 percent reported at least a 50 percent improvement in their pain when amitriptyline was given within the first six months of pain onset. The success rate dropped to only 25 percent when the medicine was given two or more years afterward.

How they're taken. Amitriptyline comes in 10 mg, 25 mg, 50 mg, 75 mg, 100 mg and 150 mg tablets. It's also an injectable medication. It's normally started at 50 to 100 mg at bedtime and then gradually increased to 150 mg daily – or up to a maximum of 300 mg per day, if needed. At higher doses, amitriptyline is usually taken three or four times a day.

Imipramine comes in 10 mg, 25 mg and 50 mg tablets. It's also injectable. It's normally started at 75 to 100 mg a day over two doses, then increased in 25 to 50 mg increments until pain is relieved. The usual maximum is 200 mg a day, taken in two or three doses (although it can be taken in one dose at bedtime).

Nortriptyline comes in 10 mg, 25 mg, 50 mg and 75 mg capsules and in liquid form. It's normally started at 75 to 100 mg a day over three or four doses, then increased gradually until the pain is gone, up to a maximum of 150 mg a day.

Each of these can be taken with or without food.

Key points. These drugs aren't without side effects, but as a group they're usually tolerated better than older anticonvulsants. They've been around a long time, and so they've got a known track record.

Dizziness and drowsiness are the two most likely side effects, although these usually subside within two weeks. Amitriptyline is the most sedating of the lot, so much so that it's sometimes prescribed as a sleep aid. Imipramine is the least sedating of the three. If drowsiness is a problem, the medicine should be taken at night (to the extent possible) to limit daytime doses.

Regular blood testing is normally not needed, except that plasma levels are sometimes recommended in patients who are taking more than 100 mg a day of nortriptyline.

As with anticonvulsants, patients should increase and decrease doses gradually. Antidepressants should never be stopped suddenly.

All three of these drugs are metabolized by the liver.

Cost-wise, these are relatively inexpensive drugs.

Precautions. Serious side effects are very rare, but an increased incidence of strokes, heart attacks and heart rhythm problems have been linked to tricyclic antidepressants. Nortriptyline also may cause blood disorders (agranulocytosis and thrombocytopenia), and amitriptyline may cause those two disorders or leukopenia.

Besides drowsiness and dizziness, more common side effects of amitriptyline are a dry mouth, increased appetite, urine retention, blurred vision, rapid heart beat and orthostatic hypotension – a feeling of blacking out when standing up due to gravity's effect on blood pressure.

Common side effects of imipramine are dry mouth, orthostatic hypotension, rapid heart beat, blurred vision, constipation, nausea and urine retention.

Common side effects of nortriptyline are blurred vision, headache, dry mouth, rapid heart beat, constipation and urine retention.

All three drugs can be especially sedating when taken with other central nervous system depressants, such as antihistamines, narcotics, anticonvulsants, tranquilizers and some muscle relaxants.

Tricyclic antidepressants interact with a few other drugs as well. Using them with MAO-inhibiting antidepressants can lead to excitability and a sudden rise in body temperature and blood temperature. They can reduce the effectiveness of the blood-pressure drug clonidine (Catapres). And the stomach drug cimetidine (Tagamet) can increase antidepressant blood levels to potentially toxic levels.

Tricyclic antidepressants also can increase skin sensitivity to sunlight, so excessive sun exposure should be avoided.

VENLAFAXINE (Effexor)

How it's used in face pain. This is also an antidepressant but not a tricyclic type. However, like the tricyclics, venlafaxine increases norepinephrine and serotonin levels in the central nervous system and therefore seems to help pain much like the tricyclics.

It's most commonly used to treat depression but also helps anxiety disorders as well as various chronic pains, especially neuropathic pains and other more constant, burning types of pain.

How it's taken. Venlafaxine comes in 25 mg, 37.5 mg, 50 mg, 75 mg and 100 mg tablets and in 37.5 mg, 75 mg and 150 mg extended-release capsules.

It's normally started at 75 mg a day taken over two or three doses, then increased by 75 mg a day every 4 to 7 days until the pain is gone. The usual maximum is 225 to 375 mg a day.

It's best taken with food to avoid upset stomach.

Key points. The main advantage venlafaxine has over amitriptyline, imipramine and nortriptyline is that most people don't experience quite as much drowsiness or impaired concentration.

This drug also hasn't had any of the rare serious side effects such as strokes and heart problems that have been linked to the tricyclics.

It's metabolized by the liver.

Precautions. Venlafaxine has many of the same less-serious side effects as tricyclic antidepressants, but they're generally mild and transient. Common side effects include headache, drowsiness, dizziness, nervousness, insomnia, nausea, constipation, dry eyes and loss of appetite.

At high doses, this medicine may cause a rise in blood pressure. It's also not recommended for those with pre-existing kidney problems.

Venlafaxine should not be taken with MAO-inhibiting antidepressants because it can cause agitation and a sudden rise in body temperature and blood pressure. Other than that, it has no other known drug interactions.

• MUSCLE RELAXANTS •
BACLOFEN (Lioresal)

How it's used in face pain. Baclofen was introduced in 1972 as a medicine to treat spastic muscles, primarily in people with multiple sclerosis or spinal cord injuries.

Pittsburgh neurologist Dr. Gerhard Fromm began trying it on TN patients in the early 1980s because it mimics the effect of a brain chemical that slows the activity of nerve cells. In 1984, Dr. Fromm produced the first study showing that baclofen was effective in treating TN.

His and two subsequent studies found that about 67 percent of neuralgians can expect to get good to excellent relief from baclofen. That's a little less effective than carbamazepine. But more importantly, Dr. Fromm and others found that baclofen paired very well with anticonvulsants and actually enhanced the effectiveness of medications such as carbamazepine and phenytoin.

Through most of the 1990s, baclofen was one of the "big three" TN medications. Some doctors prescribed it first – preferring the better patient tolerability of the drug over the possibility that it might not work as well as carbamazepine. Other doctors used baclofen as a back-up in case carbamazepine didn't work or patients couldn't tolerate it. Most, however, viewed it as the top add-on choice when carbamazepine or phenytoin alone weren't doing the trick.

The arrival in the late 1990s of a glut of new anticonvulsants with fewer side effects gave doctors many more alternatives, and so baclofen's use in TN has waned. However, it's still used fairly often, usually as an add-on to one of the many anticonvulsants.

Baclofen also is often a top choice for those who have TN as a result of MS. As a muscle relaxant, baclofen can help those patients' muscle spasms and cramps as well as their face pain.

How it's taken. Baclofen comes in 10 mg and 20 mg tablets. The usual starting dose is 15 to 30 mg per day, taken over three divided doses. It's typically increased by 10 mg every two or three days until the pain is gone, up to a usual maximum of 80 mg a day. Most people get adequate pain relief on 50 to 60 mg per day, taken in three or four divided doses.

Baclofen needs to be taken three to four times a day because it's a short-lasting drug. Its effects last only 4 to 8 hours because it is absorbed by the body and excreted very quickly.

If taken along with carbamazepine or another anticonvulsant, baclofen is usually maintained at 40 mg per day.

It's best taken with food to limit the possibility of upset stomach.

Key points. The advantage baclofen used to have over older anticonvulsants is that it is a drug with fewer and milder side effects, and it has almost no drug interactions. Now that newer anticonvulsants have been developed with similar side-effect and drug-interaction profiles, it's lost a bit of that advantage.

Because it works differently than anticonvulsants, baclofen remains a good alternative for those who have allergic or troubling reactions to carbamazepine, oxcarbazepine and the others. Dr. Fromm found that 74 percent of his patients who couldn't take carbamazepine or who weren't helped by it improved significantly on baclofen. So it's still a drug that shouldn't be discounted as an "also-ran."

The cost of baclofen also is less than the new anticonvulsants.

It's metabolized by the kidneys. Some doctors order occasional kidney function tests for patients on baclofen for a long time.

Precautions. Baclofen has virtually no serious, life-threatening side effects. Even allergic reactions to it are rare. (Signs of allergic reaction are a skin rash and/or breathing difficulties.)

The main problem to consider is coming off the medication too quickly. Sudden withdrawal of baclofen can lead to seizures, hallucinations, anxiety and rapid heart beat, so it's important to reduce doses gradually before stopping the medicine.

The most common side effects are drowsiness, dizziness, muscle weakness, impaired coordination, twitching, nausea, fatigue and upset stomach. As with most medicines, these side effects often taper off as the patient adjusts to the medication.

Baclofen has only a few known possible adverse interactions with other drugs—primarily tricyclic antidepressants (i.e. amitriptyline, desipramine, imipramine, nortriptyline) and any drug that depresses the central nervous system (i.e. antihistamines, sedatives, tranquilizers and other muscle relaxants). The combinations can lead to troubling sedation.

Baclofen also may raise blood sugar levels (a possible problem for those with diabetes), and the chance of side effects may increase slightly in those with epilepsy, kidney disease, mental problems and stroke or other brain disease.

TIZANIDINE (Zanaflex)

How it's used in face pain. Tizanidine is a muscle relaxant used to control spasms. It's in the same class of medicines as baclofen, but it works in a slightly different way that's not well understood.

Figuring that it may have the same effect on TN as baclofen, doctors began trying it in the mid-1980s. The early feedback was not promising. One study found that only one in six patients who tried tizanidine for face pain was helped. And so it's not used very often these days for TN.

It may be helpful as an add-on to an anticonvulsant if baclofen fails or can't be taken.

Tizanidine also has been used with some success in treating postherpetic neuralgia, migraines and myofascial pain.

How it's taken. Tizanidine comes in 2 mg and 4 mg tablets. It's usually started at 1 or 2 mg a day and increased gradually to a typical dose of 8 mg a day.

At lower doses, it can be taken all in one dose at bedtime. At higher doses, it's normally taken in three doses. The usual maximum is 36 mg a day.

Like baclofen, it's a short-acting medicine that's absorbed and excreted in the space of 3 to 6 hours. So when it's used for pain, spreading it over three doses is usually needed.

It can be taken with or without food.

Key points. The good news is that this is a drug with virtually no serious side effects and only a few drug interactions. The bad news is that it's not a terribly effective drug for TN.

Although tizanidine is certainly not a drug that's high on the use list in TN and related face pain, it at least is an alternative that may help some people some of the time when other drugs have failed or produced allergic or intolerable reactions.

Tizanidine is metabolized by the liver. It's not recommended for those with pre-existing liver or kidney problems, and doctors sometimes order liver function tests early in the course of this medicine.

Precautions. Other than rare cases of liver problems that can lead to acute hepatitis, tizanidine has few side effects. The most common ones are sedation, drowsiness, fatigue, dizziness, dry mouth and nausea. Anxiety and back pain are also occasionally reported. At high doses, fever, lack of appetite and tingling sensations may occur.

It should be used with caution in patients on blood-pressure medications because tizanidine may lead to too much of a drop in blood pressure. It can also be excessively sedating when used with baclofen and other muscle relaxants, tranquilizers and other central nervous system depressants, such as antidepressants and narcotic pain-killers.

Tizanidine also may lessen the effectiveness of oral contraceptives.

• OTHERS •
PIMOZIDE (Orap)

How it's used in face pain. Pimozide is an antipsychotic drug that's most often used in treating the uncontrolled tics of Tourette's syndrome and chronic schizophrenia.

It was tried in TN in the 1980s, and one study in 1989 reported that all 48 of the TN patients who tried it got pain relief.

With that kind of track record, you'd think it would be the most prescribed medication for TN. And maybe it would be if not for this drug's potential side effects and interactions with other drugs.

Pimozide can cause life-threatening heart arrhythmias, a movement disorder that may not go away even when the drug is stopped and, rarely, the potentially fatal neuroleptic malignant syndrome. A host of other drugs can increase the chances of these and other less serious side effects, which also are numerous. At least one death has been linked to use of pimozide.

Because of these potential problems, pimozide is seldom used for TN or any type of face pain. It's also not undergone more widespread testing to determine if its effectiveness is really as high as the single 1989 study found.

How it's taken. Pimozide comes in 2 mg and 10 mg tablets. The usual starting dose is 1 to 2 mg per day, the average dose is 6 mg per day, and the suggested maximum is 10 mg per day.

It should not be taken with grapefruit juice because that can interfere with the breakdown of pimozide and possibly increase the risk of heart rhythm problems.

Key points. The good news is that pimozide is not as sedating and doesn't impair thinking as much as the anticonvulsants. It's also a fairly inexpensive drug – about the same as older tricyclic antidepressants such as amitriptyline.

Beyond that, most doctors feel the side-effect risks are just too great to widely use pimozide in face pain.

"Its adverse reactions make it unacceptable as a routine drug," says Dr. Zakrzewska.

Pimozide is metabolized by the liver.

Precautions. The list of precautions and warnings is long. Potentially serious heart-rhythm problems can occur. The risk of this can be increased by taking pimozide along with a wide variety of drugs that includes antibiotics, anti-fungal medications, phenothiazines (medicines used to treat nervous and emotional disorders) and tricyclic antidepressants.

Rare but possible is neuroleptic malignant syndrome, a potentially fatal condition that features such symptoms as seizures, fast breathing, fast heartbeat, irregular pulse, fever, jumps in blood pressure, sweating, loss of bladder control and severe muscle stiffness.

A third serious possibility is tardive dyskinesia, a movement disorder that can cause fine, "worm-like" movements of the tongue or other uncontrolled movements of the mouth, tongue, cheeks, jaw or limbs. This condition may not go away even if the drug is stopped.

Other side effects include: blurred vision, constipation, dizziness, light-headedness when standing up from a lying or sitting position; dry mouth, difficulty speaking, loss of balance, mood changes, restlessness, a shuffling walk and trembling fingers and hands.

Blood tests should be done periodically, and pimozide is not recommended for those with glaucoma, liver disease, kidney disease, heart disease or heart rhythm problems. An electrocardiogram should be done to rule out heart problems before pimozide is started.

Besides the drug interactions that can increase the chance of heart-rhythm problems, pimozide reacts in other ways with a host of other drugs ranging from other antipsychotics to anti-cholinergics (which treat stomach cramps) to the attention-deficit drug methylphenidate (Ritalin).

Bottom line: check carefully with your doctor and a pharmacist before starting and check again if you start other drugs while on pimozide.

CLONAZEPAM (Klonopin)

How it's used in face pain. Clonazepam is a medication that slows down the nervous system. It's a tranquilizer in the benzodiazepine class of drugs, the same family as the better known sedative diazepam (Valium).

However, clonazepam also has been found to have anticonvulsant properties, which makes it useful for controlling petit mal seizures and also panic or movement disorders such as restless leg syndrome.

It's been reasonably helpful in treating TN and related face pain. Four studies involving 64 people found a success rate of 66 percent.

Because it's not quite so effective as most of the anticonvulsants and because it's also arguably the most sedating of the face-pain drugs, it's typically not a front-line choice.

Clonazepam is often used as an add-on drug as opposed to a stand-alone TN drug, and it's also been used with some success to treat burning mouth syndrome.

How it's taken. Clonazepam comes in 0.5 mg, 1 mg and 2 mg tablets. It's usually started at 1.5 mg per day spread over three doses. It's then increased by 0.5 mg to 1 mg every three days until pain is controlled. Average doses are in the range of 2 to 10 mg a day, usually spread over three doses. The usual maximum is 20 mg a day.

Key points. Clonazepam is used more often for TN in Europe than in the United States. It probably would be used more if it weren't so sedating or if pain relief was greater at low doses.

As with anticonvulsants, doses should be increased and decreased gradually.

It's a fairly inexpensive drug, costing less than most tricyclic anti-depressants.

Clonazepam is metabolized by the kidneys. It's not recommended for those with pre-existing liver disease. Periodic blood counts and liver function tests are often ordered.

Precautions. The most serious side effects (although rare) are a pair of blood disorders (thrombocytopenia and leukopenia) and occasionally breathing difficulties.

The most common side effect is marked drowsiness, sluggishness, fatigue, dizziness, confusion and personality changes or sadness. At high doses, it may cause a slowed heart rate and staggering.

Clonazepam has only a few drug interactions – none particularly worrisome. Carbamazepine and phenytoin can lesson clonazepam's effectiveness, and excessive sedation can occur when clonazepam is taken with other central nervous system depressants such an antidepressants, sleep aids, narcotic pain-killers and some muscle-relaxants.

OPIOIDS
(Morphine, MS Contin, OxyContin, Fentanyl, etc.)

How they're used in face pain. The term "opioids" comes from the poppy flower and its product opium. Morphine and codeine were two of the earliest agents used in pain control, but their main drawback was addiction.

In World War II, researchers began to develop less-addicting synthetic agents such as meperidine and methadone. Many others have come along since, but because all of these medications are interrelated by their "morphine-like" effects, they're as a group called "opioids" or "opiates."

The drugs in this family all interact with three key brain receptors and work by overriding or bypassing the pain signals. That's an entirely different way of coping with the pain than anticonvulsants and the other TN medicines, which work by altering the transmission of the pain signals.

Because of concerns over addiction, overdose, heavy sedation and a few potentially serious interaction with other drugs, opioids are used very sparingly in face pain. Their role is largely as a stop-gap therapy to treat sudden break-through pain for a few days until longer-term medications have a chance to kick in and as a later option when other medicines, surgeries and therapies have failed.

Opioids are sometimes used in severe, chronic face pains such as neuropathies, anesthesia dolorosa and post-herpetic neuralgia when other medications are not helping.

A host of agents fall under this family, including codeine, fentanyl, hydrocodone, methadone, morphine, oxycodone and propoxyphene. Numerous brand names have been developed using derivatives of these or combinations of opioids with more commonly used pain-killers such as aspirin and acetaminophen (i.e. Tylenol). Examples: MS Contin is morphine sulfate, OxyContin is oxycodone hydrochloride, Darvocet is a blend of acetaminophen and propoxyphene napsylate, and Lortabs are acetaminophen and hydrocodone bitartrate.

How they're taken. Opioids can be delivered in every conceivable way: tablets, capsules, liquids, nasal sprays, suppositories, injections, intravenously, by medicated patches worn on the skin and even opioids "lollipops" (i.e. Actiq and Fentanyl Oralets).

Dosing plans should be carefully tailored to each case, and regular checkups should be scheduled throughout the course of opioid treatment. Doses should be followed carefully, and levels should be gradually increased and gradually decreased to avoid severe side effects.

Because opioids are powerful and controlled substances, patient education is important, too. For example, it should be stressed that unused pills should never be given to anyone else. These medications also should be kept in a safe place. Fentanyl "lollipops" look a lot like candy to a child, and the opioid dose in just one can be enough to kill a small child.

Key points. The question of when to use opioids is a hotly debated one in all sorts of pain management. Some doctors are averse to prescribing them at all because of addiction, drug-trafficking and lawsuit issues.

Dr. J. David Haddox, senior medical director for health policy with Connecticut-based drug manufacturer Purdue Pharma LP, is one who says opioids must be used carefully but not totally discounted.

He says studies have shown opioids are usually effective in relieving nerve-related pains, albeit at higher doses than most other types of pain. He says that with proper management and patient education, opioids may be the only effective option for people who have tried other face-pain therapies and found no relief.

Sedation is another issue with opioids. Doses needed to stop pain may rise to a level that's heavily sedating to most people. That may be unacceptable to those who have other options open to them, but people who are in severe pain despite trying everything else may well accept the tradeoff.

Precautions. Lots of points to consider here. Besides potential addiction and the possibility of withdrawal symptoms after long-term use or a sudden stop of the medicine, there are a few serious concerns that are generally dose-related.

At too-high levels, opioids may slow breathing to dangerous levels, leading to a stupor and possibly cardiac arrest. Early signs of that can include cold, clammy skin, confusion, seizures, severe dizziness, low blood pressure, severe nervousness, narrowing of the pupils, severe weakness and slowed breathing.

More common side effects are drowsiness, dizziness, a light-headed feeling when standing up, mental clouding, nausea, constipation and dry mouth.

Opioids interact with a variety of other medications. They should not be taken with MAO-inhibiting antidepressants, and they can be especially sedating when taken with other central nervous system depressants, such as antihistamines, anticonvulsants, sleep aids and muscle-relaxants. Alcohol also should be avoided while on opioids.

Opioids can increase blood levels of carbamazepine, so dose levels may need to be regulated when these two types of medications are taken together to minimize adverse side effects. Increased side effects also may occur when opioids are taken along with tricyclic antidepressants.

Opioids are generally not recommended for those with pre-existing heart, kidney, liver, gall-bladder or lung disease, for those with an underactive thyroid and for those prone to seizures.

A LOOK AT OPIOIDS USED ...

Drug	Available Forms	Typical Dose	Time to Peak Relief
Morphine	T, L, ER, IM, IV	By mouth: 10-30 mg every 4 hours By injection: 5-20 mg every 4 hours	By mouth: 1-2 hours By injection: 30-60 minutes
Codeine	T, L, IM	By mouth or injection: 15-60 mg every 4-6 hours	By mouth: 1-2 hours By injection: 30-60 minutes
Fentanyl	TD, TM, IM, IV	TD: 25-100 mcg/hour TM: 100-1,000 mcg/hour By injection: 50 mcg/ml	TD: 1-3 days TM: 20-30 minute By injection: 20-30 minutes
Meperidine	T, L, IM, IV	By mouth or injection: 50-150 mg every 3-4 hours	By mouth: 60-90 minutes By injection: 30-50 minutes
Oxycodone	T, C, L, ER	By mouth: 5 mg every 6 hours ER: 10 mg every 12 hours	1 hour
Hydrocodone	T, C, L	5-10 mg every 4-6 hours	1 hour

KEY:
• *Available forms.* *T=tablet; C=capsule; L=liquid; ER=extended release; IM=intramuscle injection; IV=intravenous; TD=transdermal (skin patch); TM=transmucosal (lozenge or lollipop) (Note:Route of delivery affects time to peak relief.)*

... FOR CHRONIC FACE PAIN

Duration of Relief	Potentially serious or toxic effects	Other Common Effects
By mouth: 3-6 hours By mouth: 1-2 hours	Slowed heart rate, cardiac arrest, seizures, depressed breathing	Mood change, nausea, constipation, dizziness
By mouth or injection: 3 hours	Slowed heart rate, depressed breathing	Constipation, sweating
TD: varies TM: varies By injection: 1-2 hours	Heart arrhythmia, seizures	Mood changes, confusion, sweating
By mouth or injection: 2-4 hours	Slowed heart rate, cardiac arrest, depressed breathing	Mood changes, dizziness, nausea, sweating
3 hours	Slowed heart rate, depressed breathing	Nausea, dizziness
3 hours	Slowed heart rate, depressed breathing	Nausea, dizzines

KEY:
• *Typical dose.* mg=milligrams; mcg=micrograms; ml=milliliters; TD=transdermally; TM=transmucosally; ER=extended release
• *Side effects.* All of the above also are typically sedating and adversely affect mental clarity.

COMPARING THE MEDICATIONS ...

Drug *(brands)*	Type of Drug	Available Forms
Carbamazepine *(Tegretol, Carbatrol)*	AED	T, L, ER, CH, SC
Oxcarbazepine *(Trileptal)*	AED	T, L
Gabapentin *(Neurontin)*	AED	C
Lamotrigine *(Lamictal)*	AED	T, CH
Topiramate *(Topamax)*	AED	T, C/SC
Phenytoin *(Dilantin)*	AED	T, C, ER, L, I
Levetiracetam *(Keppra)*	AED	T
Tiagabine *(Gabitril)*	AED	T
Valproate *(Depakote, Depakene)*	AED	C/SC, L, ER, I
Zonisamide *(Zonegran)*	AED	C
Amitriptyline *(Elavil)*	AD	T, I
Imipramine *(Norfranil, Tofranil)*	AD	T, I
Nortriptyline *(Pamelor)*	AD	C, L
Venlafaxine *(Effexor)*	AD	T, ER
Baclofen *(Lioresal)*	MR	T
Tizanidine *(Zanaflex)*	MR	T
Pimozide *(Orap)*	AP	T
Clonazepam *(Klonopin)*	T	T

KEY:
* *Type of drug. AED=antiepileptic drug (anticonvulsant); AD=antidepressant; MR=muscle relaxant; AP=antipsychotic; T=tranquilizer.*
* *Available forms. T=tablet; C=capsule; SC=sprinkle capsule; ER=extended release tablet or capsule; L=liquid; CH=chewable tablet; I=injectable or IV.*
* *Dose ranges. Therapeutic dose ranges, listed in milligrams per day.*
* *How metabolized. Tells whether drug is metabolized (broken down) in the liver or kidney.*

...USED FOR TN

Dose ranges	How Metabolized	Suggested Tests?	Cost
300-2400	Liver	CBC at 1 month	$54.31 generic: $15.30
300-2700	Kidney	Electrolytes at 1 month	$179.00
600-4800	Kidney	None	$177.00
25-500	Liver	None	$137.00
50-400	Kidney	None	$177.00
100-800	Liver	CBC, liver function at 1 month	$23.47
250-1500	Kidney	None	$242.22
32-56	Liver	None	$194.00
600-2000	Kidney	Liver function at 1 month	$98.10
100-600	Liver	Liver function at 1 month	$217.00
40-300	Liver	None	$57.99
25-200	Liver	None	$42.75
20-150	Liver	None	$17.22
75-375	Liver	None	$154.10
15-80	Kidney	None	$118.85
1-36	Liver	Liver function at 1 month	$219.78
0.5-8	Liver	EKG before starting, liver function at 1 month	$63.99
1-20	Kidney	CBC, liver function at 1 month	$44.00

KEY:
* **Suggested blood tests.** *Tells what blood tests doctors typically may order at the beginning of or during this therapy. CBC is a complete blood count. Electrolytes refer to levels of blood chemicals, such as potassium, sodium and calcium. EKG is an electrocardiogram test of heart rhythm.*
* **Cost.** *Estimated cost per month at an average dose level, according to Epocrates/Drug Topics Red Book.*

SIDE EFFECTS AND INTERACTIONS ...

Drug (brands)	Sedating Effects	Mental Clarity	Potentially Serious or Toxic Effects
Carbamazepine (Tegretol, Carbatrol)	+++	+++	Allergic reaction (skin rash, fever, mouth sores) depressed bone marrow; drop in white blood count, sodium levels or blood platelets
Oxcarbazepine (Trileptal)	++	++	Allergic reaction (skin rash, fever, mouth sores) drop in blood sodium levels or blood platelets
Gabapentin (Neurontin)	+++	++	Allergic reaction (skin rash, fever, mouth sores) drop in white blood count
Lamotrigine (Lamictal)	++	++	Allergic reaction (skin rash, fever, mouth sores) swollen lymph nodes
Topiramate (Topamax)	++	+++	Allergic reaction (skin rash, fever, mouth sores) kidney stones; glaucoma; tingling
Phenytoin (Dilantin)	+++	+++	Allergic reaction (skin rash, fever, mouth sores) drop in blood platelets or white blood count; liver toxicity
Levetiracetam (Keppra)	+++	++	Drop in white blood count, hostility, suicidal ideas
Tiagibine (Gabitril)	++	+	Weakness at high dose
Valproate (Depakote, Depakene)	+++	++	Liver toxicity (watch for yellow eyes); pancreatitis; depressed bone marrow; drop in blood platelets or white blood count
Zonisamide (Zonegran)	+++	++	Allergic rash; kidney stones; depressed bone marrow; confusion; heat stroke
Amitriptyline (Elavil)	+++	++	Heart arrhythmia, convulsions, tremors, yellowed eyes
Imipramine (Norfranil, Tofranil)	++	++	Heart arrhythmia; drop in blood platelets and white blood count; convulsions; hallucinations

... OF TN MEDICATIONS

Other Common Effects (Besides Sedation and Mental Clarity)	Interactions with Other Drugs
Dizziness, impaired coordination, blurred vision, headache, chest pain (in elderly)	Oral contraceptives, blood-thinners, MAO inhibitors, other anticonvulsants
Dizziness, double vision, impaired coordination	Oral contraceptives, other anticonvulsants
Dizziness, nervousness, clumsiness, rash, tremors, diarrhea, slurred speech	Antacids
Dizziness, double or blurred vision, insomnia, impaired coordination	Valproate, several other anticonvulsants
Dizziness, impaired coordination, eye-twitching, eye-twitching, speech difficulty, tremors, nervousness, double vision	Valproate, several other anticonvulsants, oral contraceptives, acetazolamide
Dizziness, impaired coordination, sore gums, tremors, eye-twitching, double vision, constipation, mood change, nervousness	Antacids, valproate, oral contraceptives, estrogen, some anticonvulsants, bronchodilators and others
Agitation, anxiety, dizziness, headache, impaired coordination, weakness, dry eyes, cough, dry throat	None known
Dizziness, nervousness	Valproate and several other anticonvulsants
Headache, dizziness, double vision, irritability, restlessness, impaired coordination, cramping, nausea, hair loss	Cimetidine, erythromycin, blood-thinners, other anticonvulsants
Dizziness, headache, loss of appetite, irritability, back pain, shakiness	Valproate, carbamazepine, phenytoin
Dizziness, dry mouth, increased appetite, blurred vision, orthostatic hypotension, urine retention, skin sensitivity to sunlight	MAO inhibitors, clonidine, cimetidine
Dizziness, dry mouth, rapid heart beat, orthostatic hypotension, blurred vision, constipation, skin sensitivity to sunlight	MAO inhibitors, clonidine, cimetidine

... Side Effects and Interactions of TN Medications Continued

Drug (brands)	Sedating Effects	Mental Clarity	Potentially Serious or Toxic Effects
Nortriptyline *(Pamelor)*	++	++	Heart arrhythmia; drop in blood platelets and white blood count; convulsions; hallucinations
Venlafaxine *(Effexor)*	+	+	Rise in blood pressure at high doses; increased heart rate
Baclofen *(Lioresal)*	++	+++	Allergic skin rash; hallucinations if drug stopped too quickly; severe muscle weakness; convulsions
Tizanidine *(Zanaflex)*	++	++	Acute hepatitis; tingling; fever
Pimozide *(Orap)*	+	+	Heart arrhythmia; movement disorder (tardive dyskinesia); potentially fatal seizure or heart attack; convulsions
Clonazepam *(Klonopin)*	++	+++	Drop in blood platelets or white blood count; breathing difficulty, slowed heart rate and staggering at high doses; convulsions

KEY:
- *Sedating effects.* Estimate of how tired and drowsy it may make you feel. + is mildly sedating, ++ is moderately sedating, +++ is very sedating.
- *Mental clarity.* Estimate of how much the drug may affect memory, thinking ability and other mental skills. + is a mild effect, ++ is a moderate effect, +++ is a substantial effect.
- *Potentially serious or toxic effects.* These are uncommon, rare or very rare possibilities, but symptoms should be watched for and reported immediately if experienced.
- *Other common effects.* These are less serious but more common side effects that may be experienced other than sedation and mental impairment. Many of these often abate as you adjust to the medicine. (Orthostatic hypotension is a sudden drop in blood pressure when standing up that may make you feel like you're about to black out.)
- *Interactions with other drugs.* These are some of the medications that may cause adverse reactions when used with the listed medication. Check with your doctor or pharmacist before using these together.

Other Common Effects (Besides Sedation and Mental Clarity)	Interactions with Other Drugs
Dizziness, blurred vision, dry mouth, headache, rapid heart beat, constipation, skin sensitivity to sunlight	MAO inhibitors, clonidine, cimetidine
Headache, dizziness, blurred vision, nervousness, insomnia, constipation, dry eyes, loss of appetite, decreased sex drive, agitation, trembling, skin sensitivity to sunlight	MAO inhibitors, levodopa
Dizziness, muscle weakness, impaired coordination, twitching, elevated blood sugar, confusion	Tricyclic antidepressants, other sedating drugs
Dizziness, dry mouth, anxiety, back pain, nausea	Blood-pressure medications, oral contraceptives, other sedating drugs
Blurred vision, constipation, dizziness, orthostatic hypotension, dry mouth, speech difficulty, loss of balance, mood change, tremors	Antipsychotics, anticholinergics, methylphenidate, antibiotics, antifungals, tricyclic antidepressants, heart medications and others
Dizziness, confusion, personality change, depression	Carbamazepine, phenytoin, some antifungals, other sedating drugs

COMPOUNDING:
ANOTHER WAY TO TAKE MEDICINES

Taking a pill or capsule isn't the only way to get medicine into our bodies. We can also get migraine relief from a nose spray, absorb various creams and gels through our skin, even take in pain-killers via medicated lollipops, as we discussed above.

Up until World War II, more than half of our medications were made on site by pharmacists, who used powders, liquids and other raw ingredients to concoct the exact medication we needed. That changed drastically in the 1950s. With the arrival of mass-produced pills in set forms and set doses, the practice of pharmacy quickly went from medicine-making to order-filling.

Most of the time, that's an efficient and effective way to get people what they need. But what happens when one size doesn't fit all? What about the person who's allergic to a dye used to manufacture a drug they need? What if a person needs a dose somewhere between two manufactured doses? What about the person who needs something that just isn't commonly made?

These kinds of special situations have been the domain of specialty pharmacists known as "compounding pharmacists." Compounding is the art and science of preparing customized medications. It's a practice that's making a comeback, in part because of the recent development of "penetrator" agents that help carry medication through the skin that once was stopped by our outer layer of skin.

Compounded medications offer an alternative for people having difficulty taking their face-pain pills and capsules.

Compounding pharmacists say one of the biggest advantages is that most anticonvulsants, steroids, antidepressants and pain-killers can now be formulated into creams that can be rubbed directly on the face. This bypasses having to digest pills, which can eliminate nausea and some of the other side effects that occur when medicines are channeled into the bloodstream for delivery throughout the body.

"A lot of times the creams avoid the side effects that oral medicines produce, especially stomach upsets," says Pennsylvania compounding pharmacist Diane Boomsma.

Because medicated creams are absorbed directly into the tissue or bloodstream at the affected site (called "transdermal delivery"), much less medicine is needed. For example, Alaska compounding pharmacist Bob Niebert said he's found that as little as 4 mg of carbamazepine (Tegretol) cream can sometimes do the job of 1,200 mg of carbamazepine pills. He says these lesser amounts virtually eliminate the possibility of toxic effects and greatly reduce the chance of systemic side effects.

Compounded creams also can be crafted to deliver exact levels that each person needs to get relief – no more, no less. "If we find that a 5 percent formulation didn't work but 10 percent was too strong, we can make a cream that's 7.5 percent," says Boomsma. She says that's easier on patients than having to break small scored tablets to adjust doses.

Another advantage is with patients who have to take more than one medicine. Rather than taking several different pills, compounded mixtures or creams can be made that combine everything into one application.

For TN patients, Boomsma says she's seen success with a cream that blends carbamazepine to quell hyperactive nerves along with the topical anesthetic lidocaine to desensitize trigger points. She's also sometimes added gabapentin (Neurontin), which often helps the more constant, burning pains, and occasionally ketamine (another anesthetic) or clonidine (mainly a blood-pressure drug but one that also depresses the central nervous system).

Niebert told the Alaska Trigeminal Neuralgia Support Group that he's had success with a face cream that combines carbamazepine, the muscle-relaxant baclofen (Lioresal) and the pain-killer ketoprofen.

One disadvantage is that there are few pharmacists who specialize in compounding. The service also is usually more expensive than manufactured pills in a bottle, and not all insurance plans pay for compounded medications. Some will pay only after additional paperwork, such as verification by a doctor that the usual medicine can't be used due to an allergy or that a compounded medicine is needed to avoid a particular side effect.

As with oral medication, compounding may take some trial and error to find a combination and/or dose level that works. Depending on factors such as skin characteristics, degree of pain and the chemical penetration enhancers used, some neuralgians will have better success than others.

Transdermal creams are usually applied three to four times a day. Boomsma says they usually go to work in 1 to 2 hours. Patients using transdermal creams should always wash their hands after application to avoid getting the cream in their eyes.

The International Academy of Compounding Pharmacists is a Texas-based professional organization that can help people locate compounding pharmacists in their area. The group's web site at www.iacprx.org has a page in which users type in their Zip code, and pharmacists within that region are then listed. IACP also can be reached by phone at 281-933-8400 or 1-800-927-4227.

HELP PAYING FOR TN MEDICATIONS

If the cost of paying for TN medications is a burden, help may be available in a variety of ways, including state aid and drug company patient assistance programs.

More than half of America's states have pharmaceutical assistance programs. These plans offer discounted drug prices to seniors on fixed incomes, the disabled, the uninsured and others with limited incomes.

To see if your state has a program, the National Conference of State Legislatures has an excellent web site that lists participating states, their basic guidelines and contact information to apply. The site is www.ncsl.org/programs/health/drugaid.htm. Or call your state legislator for details.

Almost all drug companies also have little known patient assistance programs in which discounted and even free medications are given to needy patients. This aid is generally available only to those who are uninsured, who don't qualify for government assistance and who have limited incomes.

Every company's program is different, and income levels vary. But most companies use a sliding scale that takes into account need, the drug's cost and other medical expenses the patient has. Patient advocates say they've known cases in which people earning up to $50,000 a year have qualified.

In most cases, the paperwork has to be submitted by the patient's doctor, a nurse, social worker or other medical professional. If approved, you may receive a card that can be used to fill the prescription at a local pharmacy, or the company may send the medication directly to the doctor.

Supplies are usually good for five or six months at the most before paperwork must be resubmitted to prove a need still exists. The aid programs are intended more as short-term help, not as long-term solutions. Nevertheless, they can very helpful to someone who's temporarily out of work or someone who has maxed out on insurance coverage for the year.

Patient advocates say these programs are much under-used, mainly because people who could qualify just don't know about them. Others are discouraged by the paperwork. Still, the Washington-based Pharmaceutical Research and Manufacturers of America (PhRMA), a pharmaceutical trade group, says drug companies give away nearly 3 million prescriptions worth more than $500 million each year.

PhRMA has an excellent web site in which patients can type in basic information about their financial situation and drug needs, then find

SEVEN WAYS TO HOLD DOWN MEDICATION COSTS

• Ask your doctor if a lower-cost generic drug or a less expensive alternative might be available.

• Ask if the doctor has samples. If he/she knows your finances are limited, he or she may give you samples each time you come in.

• Start a new medicine with a limited supply. In case you have an allergic reaction or quickly the find the medicine isn't working, you don't want to pay for more pills than you use. Federal law precludes medicines from being returned once they're dispensed.

• Ask your pharmacy if they offer any discount programs or accept discount cards. AdvancePCS, for example, offers a free AdvancePCS RxSavings Plan card that's good for discounts of 13 percent to 25 percent at thousands of participating retail pharmacies. There are no income limits, but applicants must not have insurance coverage. More information is available online at www.advancerx.com or by calling 1-800-ADVANCE. Many pharmacies also accept AARP discounts.

• Once you're sure you need a medicine long-term, ask for 90-day supplies rather than 30-day ones. Most pharmacies offer discounts for larger orders.

• Review your medicines with your doctor periodically to make sure you still need everything that you're taking at the current doses.

• Look into applying for state pharmaceutical assistance or for free drugs or discounts through drug-company patient assistance programs.

— Source: Cost Containment Research Institute

out immediately if they qualify for discounts or free drugs. The site also allows users to access details and contact information for 48 drug companies that offer assistance programs. The site is www.helpingpatients.org, or call PhRMA at 202-835-3400 or write it at 1100 Fifteenth St. N.W., Washington, D.C. 20005.

The Washington-based Cost Containment Research Institute (not a government agency) also offers a 48-page booklet called *"Free and Low-Cost Prescription Drugs."* It lists details on more than 100 assistance programs and includes a variety of tips and techniques for holding down drug costs. The book is available to download online for $4.95 at www.institute-dc.org or can be ordered in printed form by sending a check for $6 to: Institute Fulfillment Center, P.O. Box 210, Dallas, Pa. 18612-0210.

Finally, some organizations offer to help patients apply for low-cost prescriptions, sometimes free, sometimes for a fee. One national program is the New York-based, volunteer-run Free Medicine Program, which supplies information, application forms and help applying for a one-time cost of $5 per medicine. The fee is refundable if the medicine isn't approved. More details are available online at http://freemedicineprogram.com or by calling (646) 205-8000 or writing: Free Medicine Program, 1632 York Ave., New York, N.Y. 10028.

PREGNANCY AND TN

Trigeminal neuralgia can pose a dilemma for women who want to have children. Specifically, how do you keep TN pain under control when most TN medications increase the chance of birth defects?

It's true that studies have found that most anticonvulsants can double or triple the odds of birth defects. Valproate (Depakene, Depakote) in particular should be avoided if pregnancy is planned. Mayo Clinic neurology professor Dr. Keith Campbell suggests that this medication should be avoided altogether in women of child-bearing age unless adequate means of birth control are being used.

Also among the most risky in pregnancies, according to U.S. Food and Drug Administration ratings, are: the anticonvulsant phenytoin (Dilantin), the antidepressant imipramine (Norfranil, Tofranil) and the tranquilizer clonazepam (Klonopin).

Although medication represents an increased risk, it doesn't mean that young TN females have to give up their pain relief to get pregnant. In fact, the vast majority of pregnant females taking anticonvulsants for epilepsy go on to deliver normal, healthy babies.

Because TN is a disorder that occurs primarily in older women beyond their child-bearing years, far fewer face the pregnancy question than do women on anticonvulsants for epilepsy. However, the Trigeminal Neuralgia Association is aware of a handful of women with TN who all had healthy infants despite taking carbamazepine before or during their pregnancies.

Interestingly, each of these women also reported that they did not have TN pain during their labor and delivery. Maybe our nervous systems are capable of dealing with only one type of bad pain at a time!

Options for women who are planning pregnancies and who do not want to take the added risks of birth defects include:

• Consider a surgical procedure to get rid of the pain. This ideally should be done before pregnancy, but otherwise, the best times are within the first four weeks of pregnancy or after the first trimester.
• Consider a non-medication alternative, such as acupuncture, chiropractic, self-hypnosis, hot-pepper cream or other treatments described in Chapters 15-20.
• Switch to other medications that are less likely to cause birth defects. Discuss this with your obstetrician or see the list below.

In any event, pregnant women and those planning on becoming pregnant should discuss all of the options both with their neurologist and obstetrician.

One other issue worth noting is that some anticonvulsants decrease the amount of oral contraceptives in the bloodstream by as much as 40 percent. That means women face an increased risk of unplanned pregnancies while on these medications.

According to a study at Johns Hopkins Hospital in Baltimore, the anticonvulsants most likely to interfere with oral contraceptives are phenytoin (Dilantin), phenobarbital (Luminal), primidone (Mysoline) and carbamazepine (Tegretol).

Anticonvulsants believed not to interfere with oral contraceptives include valproate (Depakote, Depakene), gabapentin (Neurontin), lamotrigine (Lamictal), topiramate (Topamax) and tiagabine (Gabitril).

Those who don't want an increased risk of unplanned pregnancy should consider switching to one of the latter anticonvulsants or using a different or additional form of birth control.

PREGNANCY RISK RATINGS OF TN DRUGS

The U.S. Food and Drug Administration rates medications based on their likelihood of causing birth defects.

A rating of "A" means studies have shown no risk to fetuses.

A rating of "B" means an increased risk has been shown in animal studies but not in humans, or no risk has been shown in animals but testing has not been done in humans.

A rating of "C" means animal studies have shown an increased birth-defect risk but adequate studies have not been done to verify that in humans.

A rating of "D" means there may be an increased risk in humans.

A rating of "X" means studies have shown an increased risk in both animals and humans and the drug should be avoided during pregnancy.

No TN drugs are rated in the least-risk "A" and "B" categories. Neither are any rated "X."

Here's where the 19 TN drugs fall:

- "C" rating: Carbamazepine (Tegretol, Carbatrol); oxcarbazepine (Trileptal); gabapentin (Neurontin); lamotrigine (Lamictal); topiramate (Topamax); levetiracetam (Keppra); tiagabine (Gabitril); zonisamide (Zonegran); amitriptyline (Elavil); venlafaxine (Effexor); pimozide (Orap); baclofen (Lioresal); tizanidine (Zanaflex); most opioids.

- "D" rating: Phenytoin (Dilantin); valproate (Depakote); imipramine (Norfranil, Tofranil); clonazepam (Klonopin).

- Not rated: Nortriptyline (Pamelor).

— Source: U.S. Food and Drug Administration

CHAPTER 8

IF MEDICINES DON'T HELP

"When I tell people I'm about to undergo neurosurgery for a condition that isn't life-threatening, they look at me like I'm mad."
—TN "veteran" Howard Karlitz in The Pittsburgh Press

Medication is the only therapy that roughly half of all trigeminal neuralgians ever use for their pain. Neurologists say they have many patients who go 20 or 30 years or even forever getting satisfactory pain control from one or more TN medications.

Rarely, TN even goes away on its own. "A complete remission can occur, so it's not necessarily a lifelong condition," says Harrisburg, Pa., neurologist Dr. Francis Janton.

But most of the time, TN is a progressive disorder. Attacks tend to occur more frequently as time goes along. The pain may become sharper. Remissions tend to get shorter and shorter. Additional trigger zones may develop, or attacks may start happening without any apparent trigger. Sometimes a more constant, burning, underlying pain seems to begin filling the gaps between the fleeting stabs.

When this happens, patients may find they need to take more medicine – or additional medicines – to maintain adequate pain relief. That may work, at least for awhile, but sometimes the pain breaks through even at high doses of multiple drugs. Other times, the higher doses needed to bring pain relief begin causing intolerable side effects.

At that point, "people get frustrated," says Carol James, lead physician's assistant for Johns Hopkins Hospital neurosurgeon Dr. Benjamin S. Carson Sr. "They don't like feeling like they've had one drink too many. They don't want to feel like they're stumbling down the block and not very sure-footed, or that their speech is slurred or their memory is terrible or that they can't balance a checkbook anymore."

Then there are people who just don't like the thought of taking drugs at all, especially long-term. And there are those who either had allergic reactions to the most effective medications as well as those who just didn't get good pain relief at all from any medication.

These are all cases that prompt looking at other options. And there are many.

Choices, choices and more choices

Beyond medicine, the options break down into two main camps – so-called "complementary and alternative medicine" treatments (CAM therapy) and surgery.

CAM therapies involve a variety of treatments that fall somewhere between pills and surgery. In TN, they include acupuncture, upper-cervical chiropractic treatment, nutrition therapy, herbal remedies, hot-pepper face creams, TENS units, hypnosis and more. (We'll discuss all of these in detail in chapters 15-20.)

With surgery, five different front-line approaches are used to treat TN. All are usually done by neurosurgeons (doctors who specialize in treatments of the brain and spine).

Four of the procedures are typically done on an outpatient basis. Three of these four are done by using a needle inserted into the cheek, aimed at the point in the brain where the three main branches of the trigeminal nerve come together. The idea is to use one of three different methods (heat, glycerol or a tiny balloon) to selectively injure the nerve and stop errant pain signals without causing unwanted effects, primarily numbness.

The fourth procedure is radiosurgery, which uses narrowly focused beams of radiation to injure the trigeminal nerve near its root – the same area where compressing blood vessels are typically found.

The fifth procedure is microvascular decompression (MVD). This is the surgery in which the neurosurgeon goes through the skull and attempts to find and fix the presumed cause of the pain – a blood vessel compressing the trigeminal nerve. It's the only procedure in which the goal is to address the suspected cause without causing any new damage to the nerve. It's also the most invasive option.

None of these are easy choices. Making a decision about surgery is probably the toughest issue most neuralgians wrestle with during their ordeal.

"Am I afraid? Deathly," wrote New York free-lance writer Howard Karlitz in The Pittsburgh Press a week before his MVD surgery. "Aside from the danger associated with any surgery, there's an outside chance that I'll lose hearing on one side. Music is one of my passions. But above all, I'm afraid the procedure won't work." (It did... and without hearing loss.)

Many say that picking up the phone to make that first surgical appointment was the hardest thing they had to do.

Australia TN support group leader Irene Wood says surgeons often do not understand why this seemingly "simple solution" does not appeal to more neuralgians. "Fear of the unknown plays a large part," she says. "People think, 'Rather the devil I know than the devil I do not know.'"

Research by Dr. Joanna Zakrzewska, the London oral-pain specialist, bears out what a wrenching time this can be. She does psychological testing on her face-pain patients and finds "considerable depression and anxiety prior to surgery." When measured after successful surgery, she says, these scores go down markedly.

The decision becomes harder when even the experts disagree. Your neurologist, for example, may suggest surgery only as a last resort, after all possible medications and combinations have been exhausted. One neurosurgeon may tell you you're a perfect candidate for an MVD, and another one may advise you to try one of the through-the-cheek procedures first. A nutritionist may tell you that it might help to try megadoses of Vitamin B-12 before undergoing *any* surgery. A chiropractor may tell you your upper vertebrae are out of line, the acupuncturist may tell you your "Qi" energy is out of balance and so on and so on.

The bottom line is that there are lots of options and lots of opinions, and no one of them is *the* answer for everybody. You don't know which one or ones will work for you until you try it.

It makes sense at this point to learn as much as you can about the various options, sift through the pros and cons, and then choose the one that makes the most sense to *you*. If it works, great. Case solved, and move on with life. If it fails, you've still got Plan B, Plan C, Plan D...

When is enough enough?

So you've tried at least a few medicines, and they either aren't helping or they're causing side effects you don't like. How do you know when it's time to look at other options?

"It really boils down to a personal decision on issues like how much pain you can tolerate, what side effects you can tolerate, and what risks you're willing to take," says Dr. Stephen J. Haines, a neurosurgeon at the University of Minnesota. "You're the only one who knows what level of treatment is acceptable to you."

Those "boiling points" are different for everyone.

Some people are willing and able to tolerate a lot of pain. Others want it to be gone altogether. Some people are willing to tolerate some sedation or mental fogginess in exchange for pain relief. Others may have jobs in which those side effects aren't acceptable. Some dread surgery. Others dread being on long-term medication even more.

If averages help, Dr. Zakrzewska did a study to try and find out how long an average neuralgian takes medicine before turning to surgery. She followed 110 TN patients starting in the late 1980s and found that of that group, the average wait was 12.5 years.

In years past, the nearly universal advice from doctors was that if pain relief and side effects are tolerable using medication, there's no reason to consider anything else. That's still by far the prevailing opinion of most neurologists, non-surgical physicians and even some neurosurgeons.

Veteran neurologists like Dr. James Nelson in San Diego and Dr. Stephen Nadeau in Gainesville, Fla., say they've treated lots of neuralgians with medicine over the years and only a small percentage end up needing another option.

Dr. Nadeau says he's found that if a patient gets good results from a medicine early and tolerates it well, that person usually can expect it to work indefinitely. "In my 20-year career, I have referred only two people for surgery," he said at a 1998 Trigeminal Neuralgia Association conference in Orlando, Fla.

Dr. Nelson points to the greatly expanded TN medication arsenal. He says neuralgians have more medicine choices than ever and are more likely to find an effective alternative if the first drug or two didn't work or produced intolerable effects.

Dr. Nelson suggests trying at least several different medications – giving each at least three or four weeks' trial to build up to therapeutic levels – and then trying a few combinations if one medication isn't doing the job alone.

"There might be a drug you haven't tried that you can add and get three more years of control," he says. "But I'd certainly agree that if you can't stand the pain anymore, it's time to try something else."

University of Florida neurosurgeon Dr. Albert L. Rhoton Jr. says he's had patients get relief on as little as a quarter tablet of carbamazepine a day. "As long as you're pain-free on doses that don't cause side effects, that should be continued," he says. But if medicines aren't controlling the pain or side effects become intolerable, he adds, "then it's time to consider surgery."

Dr. Mark Linskey, a neurosurgeon at the University of California at Irvine, also believes medicine is the front-line treatment…"if it's working. But we don't make patients go through a huge gauntlet of multiple trials of 10 different antiseizure medications, including the newest that comes out every two weeks. If they fail the gold-standard Tegretol (carbamazepine) and at least one other medicine added with that, we move on."

To underscore carbamazepine's effectiveness, Linskey cites a study that followed 143 neuralgians who took carbamazepine over a 16-year period. He says 69 percent got good or excellent relief at first, but 6 percent couldn't take it and 25 percent got inadequate relief. Over the 16 years, the drug became ineffective in another 13 percent.

Researchers at the Harvard Medical School, University of Kentucky Medical Center and University of Michigan Medical School recently took a different approach. They surveyed more than 600 neurologists, pain specialists and primary-care doctors in 27 U.S. cities and asked them how many TN drugs they would suggest their patients try before considering surgery.

The most common answer was three drugs, which was the choice of 37 percent of the doctors. Five drugs and four drugs were the next two most common answers, but 17 percent of the doctors surveyed said they would not consider invasive treatment for TN (i.e. surgery) at all.

Concern over possible complications from surgery is no doubt a big reason for this reluctance. Referring doctors often say they've seen or at least heard about people who have gone through one or more surgeries, only to end up with the same – or worse – pain and maybe numbness or other new pains to boot.

The case for sooner surgery

Neurosurgeons don't deny there are failures and even cases in which surgery creates a worse situation. But they'll also tell you that the odds of that are increasingly rare and that a great majority of patients not only get better but say they wished they would have opted for surgery sooner.

Drs. Zakrzewska (a non-surgeon) and her London colleague, neurosurgery professor Dr. David G.T. Thomas, decided to put this issue before patients by surveying 475 people who had undergone a variety of procedures by a variety of surgeons at three different British hospitals.

Drs. Zakrzewska and Thomas found that most patients were satisfied with their surgical results – no matter which procedure they had undergone – and that nearly three of every four patients would undergo the same surgery again, if necessary.

More recently, Dr. Zakrzewska and three other British researchers surveyed 220 other patients who had recently undergone MVDs. Of those, 89 percent said they were satisfied with their situation, 80 percent said the operation turned out better than they had expected, and 73 percent said they should have had the operation sooner.

"The message from this is very clear," Dr. Zakrzewska says. "You do better from surgery."

Surgeons say that given feedback like that, newer patients should at least be told about the surgical options long before they're in excruciating pain and/or heavily medicated.

"Don't wait until you're 80 and have suffered for 30 years before considering surgery," says Dr. John Alksne, chief of neurosurgery at the University of California's San Diego Medical Center. "I'm very frustrated by how many people have suffered so long."

"Times have changed," says Dr. Ronald Brisman, a neurosurgeon at New York's Columbia Presbyterian Medical Center. "Physicians used to recommend surgery only after the pain of TN became agonizing or the side effects of drugs intolerable. Since the advent of new treatments such as radiosurgery, I believe that if the pain is a bother or the medications are a bother, you should think seriously about neurosurgery... You don't have to wait until you're in agony to see a neurosurgeon."

Waiting to the point of agony also isn't an ideal time to rationally weigh the pros and cons of the various procedures.

"When patients have severe attacks," says Dr. Zakrzewska, "I have found they will accept any form of treatment, whatever the potential complications. These same patients when in remission, however, are much more critical of the different forms of treatment."

Michael Pasternak, president of the Trigeminal Neuralgia Association, knows the feeling well. He says his pain got so bad he would've done anything his family doctor said. "He could've recommended the vet, and I would've gone," Pasternak says.

No one wants to have neurosurgery unless it's necessary. Many people don't even want to think about it until the pain gets so bad that they're forced into it. That's when surgeons end up with severely hurting patients pounding on their doors saying things like, "I don't care what you do, doctor. Whack off my head if you have to. Just get me out of this pain now!"

So even if you have no plans to have surgery now, it never hurts to weigh the options at a time when lightning bolts aren't erupting in your face.

Is there a time window?

Some neurosurgeons also are beginning to believe there's a more pressing reason to consider surgery sooner – the pain may become less "fixable" with time.

Dr. Alksne in San Diego, Drs. Peter Jannetta and Kenneth Casey in Pittsburgh, Dr. Ronald Apfelbaum in Salt Lake City and Dr. Kim Burchiel in Portland are among those convinced there's a window of time in which surgery is most effective.

These surgeons all report that their MVDs are most successful when done in the first seven to eight years of the pain's onset. Success rates start to go down markedly from that point on. Drs. Jannetta and Casey, for example, report that success rates average about 93 percent in the first seven years but drop to between 81 to 85 percent after then.

They theorize this is because blood vessels compressing the nerve continue to cause more and more injury – eventually to the point where the nerve fibers are permanently damaged.

This continual compression also can affect additional nerve fibers as time goes on. So even if a vessel is removed from the nerve later, surgeons say, these fibers may never heal.

Drs. Jannetta, Burchiel and others believe this widening, chronic damage explains why neuralgians' pain often changes character over the years.

"Time is important," says Dr. Jannetta. "As a blood vessel beats on a nerve and stretches it, you start to get burning pain in addition to the sharp, stabbing pain… Another thing you get eventually is numbness. Over time, the numbness and burning can get worse, and you can get into other problems like facial flushing and a runny nose. This can lead to a spectrum of problems."

Another concern surgeons have about putting off MVDs is a pain-processing trait known as "central facilitation." Simply put, it's how the brain can be "trained" to read repeated signals so that even when the input stops, the brain still reads it.

For example, if your finger is poked repeatedly by a paperclip, it won't be much of a problem at first. But after awhile, the pain goes from annoying to hurting as the nervous system ramps up its attention to what is becoming a chronic, albeit minor, threat. At that point, even if the jabbing stops, the finger will hurt for a period afterward.

It's the same reason why someone can feel real pain in their foot even after the foot has been amputated. How? The sensation isn't in their foot… it's been etched into their brain.

The brain may well have the same response to a compressed trigeminal nerve. After years of the nerve being beaten on by a pulsating blood vessel, the brain may continue processing injury signals long after the offending vessel is removed.

A third concern surgeons have is the nervous system's apparent ability to create new pathways for nerve impulses at injured sites. Recent research indicates that nerves often deal with injury by opening new pathways or "channels" for biochemicals such as sodium, potassium and calcium to pass through. (You'll recall from Chapter 3 that the movement of these biochemicals from one nerve to another is what creates an impulse.) These new channels are usually much more sensitive to changes than pre-existing ones, and they may generate pain impulses with little or no provocation.

When injuries heal, some channels close. However, others seem to become permanent, which maintains the nerve's oversensitivity. This might be another explanation why MVDs aren't as effective in later years.

Whatever the explanation, surgeons say their findings suggest that it may be a mistake to try and hold out as long as possible on medication.

Dr. Alksne, for example, has begun telling his patients that if they want the best chance of permanent or long-term relief without lingering problems, they should consider MVD in the first seven years of their pain.

That doesn't mean MVD is not an option after that point. But that seven- to eight-year point is where the outcomes seem to start going downhill.

"Given enough time, I believe a majority of patients will need surgery," says Dr. Burchiel, adding that unfortunately, there is no way to tell at what point the injury is becoming chronic.

"We don't know the natural history of this disorder," Dr. Burchiel says. "If we did, perhaps we could test the condition of the trigeminal nerve every year and could tell that at a certain point it was time for surgery. We know that the more you progress toward constant pain and some degree of numbness, the less likelihood there is that you'll get help from drugs or surgery. But we don't know exactly when to move on to surgery."

He argues that if TN is a progressive pain, it's better to have MVDs done when younger and healthier rather than waiting for the pain to become chronic and less treatable.

"In the surgery world, trigeminal neuralgia is considered a great victory," Dr. Burchiel adds. "It's something that we can readily treat."

Whether patients are ready to accept that treatment – considering its possible risks – is another matter. As some patients have said, it's a lot tougher to make that choice when you're *not* the one holding the scalpel.

CAM options

As we mentioned earlier, the five surgeries aren't the only options if medications aren't working.

Before moving right into surgery, some neuralgians want to make sure they're not overlooking any other less-invasive therapies that might help.

A variety of so-called CAM (complementary and alternative medicine) therapies are options that sometimes give good relief. CAM therapies have become increasingly popular in recent years. The U.S. government's National Institutes of Health has even devoted a division to CAM – the National Center for Complementary and Alternative Medicine.

NCCAM defines CAM therapies as a "group of diverse medical and

WHAT DO PATIENTS WANT?

London oral-pain specialist Dr. Joanna Zakrzewska polled neuralgians attending the 2000 Trigeminal Neuralgia Association conference in Pittsburgh about what they ideally want from TN medications and surgeries. Here's what they said:

From medications:

- At least 75 to 80 percent pain relief.

- Only one and perhaps two side effects, so long as the effects are mild. No severe side effects and none that must be treated by other medications.

- Must be able to work, drive, socialize, sleep and generally carry on a normal life.

- Not a lot of different pills and doses. One long-acting pill taken twice a day is acceptable.

- Not have to worry about things like wind, vibrations, brushing teeth, etc. setting off attacks.

- No memory loss or concentration problems.

From surgeries:

- One procedure and done, or at least a procedure that gets rid of pain for at least 5 to 10 years.

- No profound numbness or other disabling conditions, such as hearing loss, facial paralysis or anesthesia dolorosa (pain and numbness at the same time).

- To be able to avoid taking medication after surgery, or at most, require only a low dose.

- Thorough follow-up by surgeon.

health-care systems, practices and products that are not presently considered to be part of conventional medicine."

NCCAM breaks down CAM therapies into five main categories:

1.) **Alternative medical systems,** which includes homeopathic and naturopathic medicines as well as non-Western medicines such as traditional Chinese medicine and India's Ayurveda system.

2.) **Mind-body interventions,** which includes techniques to enhance the mind's ability to affect body functions, such as hypnosis, prayer, meditation and mental healing.

3.) **Biologically based therapies,** which use substances found in nature, such as herbs, vitamins and food supplements.

4.) **Manipulative and body-based methods,** which involve specialized movements of the body, including chiropractic treatments, osteopathic medicine and massage.

5.) **Energy therapies,** which involve applying energy fields that purportedly influence the body, such as magnets, healing touch and Reiki.

Somewhere between these and conventional medicine are a few other therapies that fall under what's known as "integrative medicine." NCCAM defines these as treatments that combine mainstream medical therapies with CAM therapies and that have some high-quality scientific evidence of safety and effectiveness.

Very few CAM or integrative therapies have had any formal studies done in the use of TN and related face pain. Most of the evidence is "anecdotal" – based on what one or a few patients or doctors report.

Following are some of the more common but "non-mainstream" therapies that have been tried in TN. Some are done by physicians and might be considered more conventional than CAM. Others are done by CAM practitioners or are self-help measures:

- **Hot-pepper cream.** These capsaicin-based creams are rubbed on the painful areas and/or trigger zones three or four times a day in an effort to desensitize the areas.
- **Anesthetic nerve blocks and anesthetic eye drops.** These numbing agents are usually used for quick, temporary pain knock-backs, but they sometimes break pain cycles.
- **Upper-cervical chiropractic therapy.** A specialty within chiropractic, these practitioners attack face pain by adjusting misaligned vertebrae in the neck and upper spine.
- **Acupuncture.** Widely used in Eastern medicine, the idea is to use very thin needles to unblock impeded energy flow through various areas of the body.
- **Botulinum toxin.** One early study has found that the same Botox injections used in cosmetic procedures is sometimes effective in TN pain, at least in the short term.
- **Nutrition-based treatments.** There's some evidence that

Vitamin B-12 injections and supplements may help rebuild damaged nerve myelin. Several other vitamins and minerals also may help quell hyperexcited nerves.

- **Dietary changes.** Some neuralgians say they've been helped by eating healthier diets and specifically by avoiding such foods as fat, salt, sugar, caffeine and the artificial sweetener aspartame.
- **Herbal remedies.** For nerve disorders, recommendations range from oil rubs of St. Johns wort and peppermint to aromatherapy treatments of lavender and basil oils to herbal drinks of St. Johns wort, valerian, scutellaria and/or chamomile.
- **Craniosacral therapy.** Somewhat akin to chiropractic, these therapists use light touch to adjust bones, muscles and other tissue that may be impeding the movement of cerebrospinal fluid.
- **Biofeedback and hypnosis.** Neither are curative but are aimed at harnessing the brain's power to better cope with chronic pain.

Many people find CAM therapies appealing because they're generally not very invasive and carry very low risks. Most of them involve no cutting, little or no pain, no troubling side effects and little chance of making things worse. The main risk is that they just won't work.

Though the risks are generally low, that doesn't mean CAM treatments are completely harmless. As the U.S. Food Administration pointed out when it banned the weight-loss herb ephedra in early 2004, herbs might be natural, but they can sometimes kill.

Too-high doses of some vitamins also can cause harm, and chiropractic neck adjustments have the potential to cause nerve and blood-vessel injuries. So just as in any medical therapy, it makes sense to learn about CAM treatments, ask about potential side effects and seek out experienced practitioners.

For most CAM therapies, there is precious little research that gives patients data on what kind of success they can expect and how long any relief might last.

Roger Levy, chairman of the Trigeminal Neuralgia Association's board of directors, says TNA has heard from numerous people who have been helped to various degrees by all sorts of CAM treatments. However, he adds that the big unknown is how many people fail at the same therapy for every one that is helped. "Failures in the use of CAM tend to go underreported," he says. "The anecdotal evidence suggests that some CAM works for some people but not for others."

Levy says that those with so-called "atypical TN" and "atypical face pain" seem to be particularly interested in trying CAM therapies since standard medical treatments tend to be less effective in these types of cases.

Others, he says, are attracted to CAM because many of these treatments and practitioners deal with mind and spiritual issues in addition to just the physical aspects. "TNA believes that one needs to treat the patient, not just the condition," Levy says. "So we need to take care of the mind and body as well as our specific facial pain condition."

To get a better handle on CAM's value in treating face pain, TNA is assembling a task force to establish guidelines that patients could follow.

In the meantime, TNA offers these bits of CAM advice:

- Keep in mind that little clinical testing has been performed on most CAM therapies that's in accordance with Western scientific standards.
- Always research the safety and effectiveness of a product or treatment before using it.
- Determine the expertise of the provider.
- Establish the cost and the time-frame in which treatment may be expected to work.
- Discuss the proposed treatment with your doctor.
- Ask your local TNA support group or the TNA national office to put you in touch with patients who may have experience with the product or treatment you're considering.

Chapters 15-18 and Chapter 24 also may lead you to sources that can help you decide which treatments seem best suited to your condition.

Some people are more willing to explore the CAM waters than others. Some even prefer CAM therapies as a first-line approach – even *before* trying the standard TN medications or even *if* medications were working well. But for others, their top goal is getting rid of the pain as quickly and completely as possible, even if it means taking greater risks than pills or acupuncture needles.

Making the surgery decision

If you're leaning toward surgery, there are a few questions worth asking at this point.

Dr. Haines, the Minnesota neurosurgeon, offered a list of things he'd be asking if he were facing TN surgery. Here's his list from the Fall 1998 edition of the Trigeminal Neuralgia Association's TNAlert newsletter:

1.) Make sure you've exhausted reasonable non-surgical therapy. Can you take medication and function normally? Is it relieving the pain without intolerable side effects?
2.) Make sure of your diagnosis. Talk with your physician about typical vs. atypical TN (now proposed as TN-1 and TN-2) and other face-pain variations. Surgeries are more likely to be successful in the typical or TN-1 cases.
3.) How much time can you afford to spend recovering from surgery? Recuperation is faster for some procedures.
4.) Are you willing to have a major operation, given your general health and ability to tolerate surgical stress? A microvascular decompression (MVD) is major surgery and requires a small opening in the skull behind the ear to get at the base of the trigeminal nerve. On the other hand, an MVD actually protects the nerve by removing blood vessels that are compressing it. Other procedures are deliberately destructive – radiofrequency lesioning, glycerol injections, balloon compression and radiosurgery all cause some damage to the nerve in order to disrupt pain signals.
5.) Can you tolerate facial numbness? The destructive procedures can cause this, and occasionally, so can MVDs. Most people can tolerate some numbness and say it's far preferable to the pain of TN. However, some patients have found it extremely bothersome.
6.) Does your pain come from the upper division of the trigeminal nerve? If so, there is a slight risk that the destructive procedures will leave the cornea of your eye with no sensation. The MVD has the highest success rate in terms of preserving sensation in the cornea.
7.) Can you tolerate a recurrence of the pain? It is more likely to recur with some procedures than with others. The MVD, which is very slightly riskier because it's major surgery, has the lowest rate of recurrence. Pain is most likely to return following a glycerol injection.
8.) Can you accept the particular risks of the procedure you're considering? Do you know what they are? This is a personal, not a medical, decision. People are different in the way they deal with risks.

9.) Have you considered the distinction between an established procedure with a track record and something that is promising but new? It is especially difficult to assess the risks of new procedures. Make sure your surgeon is very clear with you about the track record of the procedure you're having and the amount of experience he or she has had with it.

Some other questions to ask yourself:
- Are there any other alternatives I feel comfortable trying before trying surgery?
- How many symptoms do I have beyond the classic TN ones? In general, the longer the list of symptoms, the less chance that any treatment is going to be completely helpful.
- Is the pain getting to the point where it's wearing me down or significantly interfering with my life?
- Is the pain becoming more burning and constant or am I still getting some extended remissions?
- Am I starting to get numbness along with the pain?

This is also a point where that pain diary you've been keeping (you *are* keeping one, right?) can help you measure the problem. If, for example, you've been taking gradually more and more medicine yet still having consistently more pain break-throughs, that might be a telling detail.

Ray Land, a neuralgian from Pennsylvania, put his pain ratings in a color-coded graph format, and one look was all that was needed to show how his pain was progressing. That helped convince him it was time to try surgery.

Doctors and psychologists also have various questionnaires that can be given to help quantify the problem. The McGill Pain Questionnaire, for example, is excellent both for measuring the severity of pain as well as helping to sort out whether the pain is more typical or atypical (TN-1 or TN-2).

Pain ratings taken at periodic intervals can determine if the pain is getting consistently worse. This can be done using Visual Analog Scales (in which patients rate their pain on a numerical line) or having patients select which Wong-Baker FACE (sketches of faces depicting various emotions) best matches their situation. And the Beck Depression Inventory is a widely used questionnaire that can show if anxiety and depression are creeping in. (See chapter 23 for more on these.)

One other big help at this point is talking to other people who have been down this road before. The Trigeminal Neuralgia Association has a list of people who have been through the various surgeries and who are willing to talk to others by phone. It also has a network of support groups, which themselves have many members who are willing to share their experiences – good *or* bad.

Information on both of these avenues is available by writing TNA at 925 Northwest 56th Terrace, Suite C, Gainesville, FL 32605, by calling 352-376-9955, by emailing tnanational@tna-support.org or by visiting the TNA web site at www.tna-support.org.

Your doctor also may be able to refer you to other local patients who have or had TN.

Wading through the options

So you're at the point of exploring surgery.

Do you go for one of the through-the-cheek (i.e. *"percutaneous"*) treatments, hoping to get lasting relief without the bothersome numbness that sometimes results? Do you try radiosurgery, even though the jury isn't out yet on how effective it's going to be in the long run? Or do you go for the "big one" – the microvascular decompression surgery that carries greater promise but also greater risk?

"There is no procedure in which 100 percent of the people who get that treatment are cured," says Cincinnati neurosurgeon Dr. John M. Tew. "All of these procedures are relatively safe, but all have side effects."

All of the procedures have different pros and cons, and even surgeons disagree about which surgery is "best." Thus it wouldn't be unusual to go to three different surgeons and get three different opinions. Some surgeons just prefer one type over another, and others have differing criteria on when it makes sense to do which procedure.

"I think it's important to fit the approach to the patient, not fit the patient to the approach," says Dr. Linskey, the California neurosurgeon. "Not all patients are best served by one approach. But if all you have is a hammer, everything looks like a nail. This is *not* how to handle patients."

"There is no overall agreement on the 'correct' operative approach for the treatment of TN," adds Dr. Jeffrey A. Brown, a neurosurgeon at Wayne State University School of Medicine in Detroit. "Clearly, the most appropriate procedure is the one that carries the smallest risk for the patient while providing satisfactory pain relief with minimal side effects. This, of course, may vary from patient to patient and also from surgeon to surgeon because the best treatment for the surgeon may well be the technique the surgeon can perform the best."

Although surgeons don't always agree on the specifics, most will tell you each of these surgeries has a role in the overall armory of weapons used to fight TN. The tough part is deciding which one best suits which case.

And that comes down to such factors as age and health, the type of pain, the location of the pain, the patient's personal feelings about the varying risks and any prior procedures that have been tried.

"You have to select the right weapon for the right patient," says Dr. Jamal Taha, a Cincinnati neurosurgeon. "Every person is different."

NEED MORE HELP DECIDING WHAT TO DO?

Another whole book is devoted entirely to the question of how to determine which treatments to try when facing a medical problem.

It's called, *"Port in the Storm: How to Make a Medical Decision and Live to Tell About It,"* by Dr. Cole Giller (Lifeline Press, 2004).

Dr. Giller is a neurosurgeon who battled cancer. His book offers advice on tracking down the information you'll need to make a good decision, and it guides you through the sometimes anguishing process of deciding what to try and what to skip.

Which kind of surgery?

All of the surgical procedures have a few things in common. As Dr. Tew pointed out above, none are guaranteed to work in all cases. All also carry varying types and degrees of risks.

Not surprisingly, the greatest risks come with the most invasive procedure, the MVD. In this procedure, the surgeon goes inside the skull through a half-dollar or smaller size hole behind the ear and attempts to correct the presumed cause of the pain by putting a small pad between the nerve and a compressing blood vessel.

MVD carries a scary list of potential problems ranging from infections and hearing loss to "worst-case scenarios" such as paralysis and death. But as York, Pa., neurosurgeon Dr. Joel Winer puts it, "The chance of something God-awful going wrong is slim."

The risk of a potentially serious complication or permanent problem from an MVD (such as meningitis, spinal fluid leak and hearing loss) is along the order of 1 to 2 percent. The chance of death is about one-half of 1 percent.

Dr. Carson, the Johns Hopkins Hospital neurosurgeon, tries to put MVDs into perspective for his patients by telling them that "on a 1-to-10 scale of brain surgery (where 1 is the worst), this is a 10." In other words, there are a lot of worse procedures you could have than this one.

The benefit of this risk, however, is the best odds of complete and long-term pain relief without numbness.

MVD risks are highest for those in poor health to start with. For that reason, MVDs are usually not recommended for those with serious heart or lung problems or other conditions that would make this surgery overly risky.

Age used to be a determining factor as well. The general rule was that if you're over age 65, MVD was not an option. However, these days most surgeons are much more interested in health than chronological age. Successful MVDs have even been done on patients as old as the early 90s.

If health is an issue, all three of the through-the-cheek procedures may still be options. All three of these are normally outpatient procedures that involve only short periods of anesthesia, if any.

The radiofrequency lesioning procedure involves inserting an electrode through a catheter in the cheek and heating the nerve where its three main branches come together.

Glycerol injections involve injecting a small amount of an oily, alcohol-like substance into a tiny cavity in that same area. Glycerol is mildly destructive to nerve fibers.

Balloon compression uses a tiny balloon to compress the nerve against an adjoining bone, also in this same area.

If even a short course of general anesthesia is too risky, the radiosurgery procedure requires no anesthesia at all. Patients are administered the painless doses of radiation while wide-awake, with optional sedating medications to relax them.

While these procedures are less risky than the open-skull MVD, they are not risk-free. Partial numbness is somewhat common in the needle procedures, and there even have been a few reports of death in cases where the surgeon's needle punctured an artery or a sudden rise in blood pressure caused cerebral bleeding. Numbness also can occur in radiosurgery treatments, and there's also concern about delayed consequences since this procedure is still fairly young.

Dr. Alksne, the San Diego neurosurgeon, said he uses life expectancy to give his patients some general guidelines on which procedure to choose.

For those with a life expectancy of less than 10 years, he suggests sticking with medications, unless the pain or side effects are intolerable. If surgery is needed, he usually recommends radiosurgery or possibly one of the three through-the-cheek procedures.

For those with a life expectancy of between 10 and 20 years, Dr. Alksne suggests considering any of the above four procedures, even for those not having severe medication side effects.

For those with a life expectancy of more than 20 years, Dr. Alksne suggests considering an MVD.

AVERAGE LIFE EXPECTANCIES	
Current Age	Expected Additional Years
50	33
55	28
60	24
65	20
70	16
75	12
80	9
85	5
90	5
Source: Internal Revenue Service Publication 590	

The nature and location of pain

The type of pain you're having also can make a difference in the choice of treatment.

Dr. Brisman, the New York neurosurgeon, first of all makes sure his patients really do have TN and not some other face pain. "There are lots of other face pains that do not respond well to neurosurgery," he says.

He also says that he looks for at least some sharp, stabbing pains as a good clue that the pain will be helped by any of the TN procedures. The more the case tends to stray from sharp stabs to the more constant burning pains, he says, the less likely surgery is to be helpful.

Dr. Anthony Kaufman reported the same thing in a 2002 study he conducted at the University of Manitoba in Canada. Dr. Kaufman looked at the results of 129 consecutive patients who had MVDs for classic TN (TN-1) and 27 other consecutive patients who had MVDs for "atypical" TN (TN-2). He found that 82 percent of the classic-TN group had excellent or good results while only 74 percent of the "atypical" group had that level of relief.

Drs. Jannetta and Casey in Pittsburgh have been finding similar results. While more than 85 percent of classic TN cases bring excellent or good results, the "atypical" MVD success rate is more in the 65 to 75 percent range. They also looked at balloon compression success rates in "atypical" cases and found only a 60 percent good-or-excellent rate.

University of Pittsburgh researchers found that people with "atypical" cases also are more likely to get pain back following surgery. They looked at the five-year, long-term results of 1,188 patients who had had MVDs and found that while 80 percent of the "classic" TN patients were still having good or excellent results at that point, only 51 percent of the "atypical" cases had that level of relief.

The bottom line is that the odds are better than 50-50 in all of these cases, but there's more of an argument for surgery in the classic cases.

For cases related to multiple sclerosis, radiosurgery and the through-the-cheek procedures make more sense than MVD because the underlying cause is a self-sustained nerve injury – not a compressing blood vessel. This assumes that an MS patient doesn't also happen to have a compressing vessel.

Face pains related to nerve injuries, such as trauma or surgery, are generally not helped by any of the above surgeries. Most doctors try to treat these with medication or other non-surgical options. (We'll take a closer look at treatment in MS and nerve-injury cases later in this chapter.)

As for location of pain, it makes no difference in the case of MVD, radiosurgery and glycerol. All three of these are good options for pain in any of the branches.

However, the radiofrequency procedure can be targeted very well for pain in the jaw or cheek, but for pain in the eye area, it's more likely to cause numbness of the cornea (the surface of the eyeball). The balloon compression, on the other hand, is very unlikely to cause that problem, so it's a better option for eye-area TN pain.

Complications and recurrence

The overall degree of a surgery's risk sometimes isn't the only risk factor worth considering. Sometimes it's the particular type of complication that can make a difference.

For instance, some degree in hearing loss in the operation-side ear can occur in less than 1 percent of MVD surgeries. When the auditory nerve is monitored during surgery, there's an even more minute chance. That may be an acceptable risk for a majority of MVD candidates, but a musician may want a procedure with *no* risk of hearing loss.

Numbness might be a bigger worry for others. In that case, MVD offers the least risk, followed in order by radiosurgery, glycerol injection, balloon compression and then radiofrequency lesioning.

For still others, the success rate for complete relief might be the main goal. In that case, MVD and radiofrequency lesioning are highest on most lists, closely followed by glycerol injection and balloon compression and then radiosurgery.

Then there's the issue of how long pain relief can be expected to last. Pain can come back following any of these procedures, but it's most likely to come back with glycerol injection, followed by balloon compression, radiofrequency lesioning and then MVD. The recurrence rate of radiosurgery is a bit less certain because of its relative newness, but the early numbers show it comparable to balloon compression.

As you might have noticed, no procedure topped every list. So all surgical decisions come down to tradeoffs.

Are you willing to accept bigger risks in exchange for the best odds at long-term relief? Then MVD is the way to go.

Are you in poor health or would you rather go with the least-invasive approach even if it means slightly lower odds of success? Then radiosurgery is a good choice.

Are you willing to trade a greater likelihood of numbness for an improved chance of success? Then consider radiofrequency lesioning.

Would you rather avoid open-skull surgery and limit the chance of dense numbness even if it means greater odds of the pain coming back? Then a glycerol injection might be the way to go.

Or do you have eye-area pain and don't want to risk major surgery to get rid of it? Then the balloon compression might be your best answer.

We'll discuss the pros and cons of each of these procedures in more detail in the next five chapters. Also see the charts that follow Chapter 13 for a quick comparison of success rates, complication rates and recurrence rates.

Prior procedures?

One last factor in the choice of surgeries is whether any prior procedures have been done.

Most neurosurgeons say the best results from MVD come when that procedure is the first one tried. They say it's best to work on anatomy that's "pristine," or in other words, nerves that haven't already been damaged by heat, glycerol, balloons or radiation. Some also argue that it's best to get a compressing blood vessel off of the trigeminal nerve as soon as possible rather than stringing out an ongoing compression injury by covering over its effects with either medication or one of the destructive procedures.

A few surgeons say they've had nearly as good MVD success when operating after a failed other procedure. In fact, some prefer to try one of the less-invasive procedures first and see if that gives long-term or permanent relief before moving onto something more risky.

Radiosurgery and the three through-the-cheek procedures are all options following a failed MVD, assuming the MVD didn't create a new problem that these four can't address.

And all five of the surgeries are, in most cases, repeatable if the pain comes back after one try. (See Chapter 14 for more details on what to consider if an initial procedure fails.)

Whatever procedure is ultimately chosen, patients want to have a role in selecting it, says Dr. Linskey. "Our patients are equally satisfied as long as they are properly prepared and counseled pre-op," he says, adding that in his practice, nearly 100 percent of post-operation patients say they were satisfied with their choice no matter which procedure was done.

Which came first... the surgery or the surgeon?

Most people start their surgical journey by picking a surgeon first and then listening to the recommendation that doctor makes. For reasons of time, cost, insurance, doctor availability and more, very often patients only get one opinion from one surgeon. Ideally, that game plan will work out if it's not possible to get other opinions.

But because TN surgeries are such specialized procedures that aren't commonly done even by most neurosurgeons, a better option may be to figure out which surgery suits you best and then find the best surgeon you can who specializes in that procedure.

As Dr. Gerhard Fromm, the late Pittsburgh neurologist, once wrote, "The choice of a neurosurgeon who is skilled in a given procedure is at least as important as the choice of procedure itself."

Very few surgeons and practices offer all five of the procedures. Most surgeons tend to favor one or two of the techniques over the others. And so they may give you only that one or those two options. They may not even tell you about other options.

You'll find a healthy dose of information about all of the TN surgeries in this book. There's also a surprising wealth of data in the medical literature and on the Internet on success rates, complications, complication rates, pain-recurrence rates and just about anything else you'd want to know.

The problem is that it can be hard for a layperson to track down and then understand all this information that has been written primarily by doctors for doctors. It can also get pretty confusing because many of the studies seem to show conflicting results. (See Chapter 23 for tips on tracking down reliable medical information.)

Dr. Zakrzewska recently took a close look at 219 TN surgical articles and was not only struck by the conflicting results but by how lacking many of these studies were.

Using standards set by 13 experts, she found that only 70 percent of the studies met the standards. And even in those, there were numerous drawbacks and inconsistencies, such as:

- Most were written by the surgeons themselves without independent observers.
- Some studies sorted out the different variations of TN and others did not.
- Definitions of success varied from study to study. For example, one study might classify "success" as no pain and no medications while another might classify "success" as pain that's improved enough that medicine controls it again.
- Complications were reported differently from study to study. Some papers divided numbness, for instance, into different degrees while others lumped all degrees of numbness into one number.
- Definitions of what constituted a pain recurrence varied.
- The length of time and manner in which patients were surveyed following surgery varied. Many studies had only limited patient follow-ups, raising the possibility of complications and recurrences going underreported.

"There is no internationally agreed format for the reporting of these results and yet the need for such a format has been highlighted," says Dr. Zakrzewska, who developed a model format that she's urging surgeons to begin following.

There's also some evidence that the numbers that show up in the medical journals are a little on the "rosy" side to start with. When Boston neurosurgeon Dr. William Sweet directly *polled* 140 neurosurgery groups on their experiences with TN surgeries, he found more deaths, a higher rate of complications and generally less optimistic results than those being reported in the medical journals.

Dr. Zakrzewska and Dr. Thomas came up with similar findings in their survey of 475 patients who had had surgery at three different institutions by a variety of doctors. They suggest several explanations for this possibly overly optimistic reporting, including:

- Poor patient follow-up.
- A reluctance of surgeons to publish sub-par results.

• And a possible tendency for patients to more willingly admit negative results to independent reviewers rather than their own doctors (perhaps out of fear of what treatment they might be offered next).

Picking a skilled surgeon

Once you've decided on the surgery, how do you find a surgeon who is skilled in that procedure? It's an important question because outcomes vary based on the surgeon's skill and experience.

Dr. Sweet found in his survey of 140 neurosurgery groups that the more experienced the surgeon, the fewer the complications.

Four researchers from Massachusetts General Hospital and Harvard Medical School verified that in a 2003 study. The researchers studied the MVD results in 1,326 cases done by 277 different surgeons at 305 U.S. hospitals between 1996 and 2000.

They found that outcomes were better and complications fewer at the high-volume hospitals and with the high-volume surgeons. They also found that of the four deaths that occurred in this MVDs, three occurred in surgeries performed by surgeons who performed only that one MVD that year.

"It's important to see someone who treats TN frequently, not rarely," says Dr. Alksne, the San Diego neurosurgeon.

That makes sense. As with any skill, the better training you get and the more experience you have, the better you become at it.

"The best results are done when the surgeon you are using has been trained by a master in the technique," says Dr. Linskey. "There is a learning curve for each (of these procedures), and so you need to be finding surgeons when they're over that learning curve. And surgeons need to be doing a regular minimum case volume in order to maintain their technical proficiency."

Some suggest that a good minimum to go by is at least 20 to 30 of a particular procedure per year to be proficient.

So two good question to ask a surgeon are: "How many of these procedures have you done?" and "How many do you do in an average year?" But even more important is, "How many *successes* do you have?"

Surgeons should be able to tell you where they trained, how many of these procedures they do, what their track record has been, what kind of complications they've been seeing and what kind of recurrence rates their patients have had.

You might also get good advice by seeking referrals from your family doctor and other specialists you've seen. Nurses sometimes have useful "inside" information to share on surgeons' abilities. And some states have government agencies or private health-consumer organizations that keep tabs on performance of doctors and institutions.

But often the best referral source turns out to be other patients. If you know enough people and do enough asking around, you're bound to turn up at least a few informed opinions on just about any doctor in your community.

If your area is fortunate enough to have a TN support group (the Trigeminal Neuralgia Association can provide you with a current list), that may be your best source of all for surgeon information. Support groups almost always have "veterans" who have experience with practically every surgeon in their area.

TNA also can provide names of doctors on its Medical Advisory Board as well as the names of others who are some of the best at each of the TN procedures in the country. That may mean travel and extra costs that insurance won't cover, so patients have to weigh whether the extra trouble and expense is justified.

Seeing the cause

One thing that would help surgeons immensely – not to mention patients – is knowing before surgery exactly what is causing the TN pain.

If the problem is a blood vessel compressing the trigeminal nerve, it would be nice to know that for sure before deciding to open a person's skull to have a look.

"In a way it's disconcerting for the surgeon because you're going in there blind," says Dr. Winer, the York, Pa., neurosurgeon. "An MVD is not like many surgeries where you can see from the X-ray what's causing the problem. Then all you do is go in and cut at the spot marked X. This isn't like that. Sometimes you go in and find an absolute array of Andy Warhol-looking vessels. Other times you go in and everything looks fine."

That may change. Researchers are working on improved magnetic resonance imaging (MRI) techniques that are giving doctors a better look than ever at the brain's array of vessels and nerves.

An MRI is a device that creates computerized images of the head. But instead of using radiation as in X-rays, MRIs involve collecting a rapid series of data while the subject is inside a magnetized chamber. The computer gathers the data and compiles it in "slices" to give a finished picture.

MRIs give a fairly clear look at the trigeminal nerve, which is the biggest of the 12 cranial nerves. Sometimes some of the vessels that surround it also can be seen. The drawback is that standard MRIs aren't refined enough to reliably show if vessels are compressing the nerve. They also don't pick up small blood vessels that could be compressing the nerve.

A newer approach called a "thin-cut MRI" is a refined MRI that uses less than 1 mm slices of data instead of the standard 3 mm slices. When gadolinium dye is injected into the bloodstream before the test and other enhancements are done to make the finished view three-dimensional (a technique known as "3-D volume acquisition"), the view of even small vessels is much better.

To see how accurately thin-cut MRIs could pick up artery and vein compressions of the trigeminal nerve, Dr. Burchiel and his team in Oregon looked at thin-cut MRIs of patients who then went on to have MVDs. The thin-cut MRIs picked up 100 percent of the artery compressions found during the ensuing surgery, 100 percent of the combined artery-and-vein compressions and 82 percent of the vein-only compressions.

Dr. Alksne says that while the new technique may not be 100 percent across the board, it's good enough to serve as a valuable bit of pre-surgery information.

"I use it in decision-making," he says. "If you can't see a vessel, there's less case to go with an MVD, and you may opt for another surgery."

He adds that this test also may be very helpful in determining whether a person with "atypical" TN or TN-2 has a blood vessel compressing his or her nerve.

"This is not a screening exam to help find a tumor or multiple sclerosis," Dr. Alksne stresses. "It's not a way to diagnose TN. TN is a diagnosis made by clinical observation and symptoms... But I think this will help the patient make a decision. It takes the guesswork out of whether you have a vessel on the nerve or not."

Dr. Apfelbaum, the Utah neurosurgeon, cautions that just because a thin-cut MRI does *not* show a compressing blood vessel doesn't mean there isn't one.

"Certainly, if a vessel is seen, it adds assurance," he says, "but if not, it would, in my opinion, be a mistake not to explore the nerve in cases with distinct classical TN."

Most standard MRI scanning devices can be used to do a thin-cut MRI, but it takes different software, different protocol, more time and, of course, a technician who knows how to do this enhanced procedure.

Decisions in "atypical" or TN-2 cases

Since not everyone agrees on what's causing these kinds of pains, the decision-making gets a bit cloudier here.

Some surgeons say the cause is usually the same thing as classic TN or TN-1 – a compressing blood vessel – and, therefore, the same surgery options are available. Others argue that these cases are better handled by medications or CAM therapies.

Both camps agree that the surgical results are not as good with "atypical" and TN-2 cases as with the classic, TN-1 cases.

Pro-surgery doctors argue that the results are still in the 50 to 75 percent range, which is good enough to solve a lot of problems. But the anti-surgery doctors point to cases in which surgery not only didn't help but made patients' pain worse or added numbness to the pain.

Medication-wise, doctors seem to get the best response from a combination of medicines: anticonvulsants for the sharp pains (i.e. carbamazepine, oxcarbazepine, gabapentin) and tricyclic antidepressants for the more constant pain (i.e. amitriptyline, nortriptyline, desipramine, imipramine).

Other options include hot-pepper cream and the whole range of CAM therapies discussed in chapters 15-18. For troubling cases that aren't responding to any of these, some surgeons have begun offering procedures such as motor cortex stimulation, which is directed at disrupting the pain-reading signals in the brain instead of focusing on the trigeminal nerve itself. This and several other procedures for hard-to-solve cases are discussed in Chapter 14.

Decisions in multiple sclerosis cases

Because the cause of pain in multiple sclerosis patients usually stems from lesions on the trigeminal nerve rather than a compressing blood vessel, the decision-making strategy is a bit different for these patients.

The same medications that are used to treat other types of TN also can be used to treat MS-related TN. "The most effective medicine for TN is carbamazepine (Tegretol, Carbatrol), which usually relieves TN in patients with or without MS," says Dr. Brisman, the New York neurosurgeon.

One other medication that some doctors have used for MS/TN patients is misoprostol (Cytotec), an anti-ulcer medication that doesn't have the sedating effects of most anticonvulsants.

Researchers around the world are looking for a therapy that will either stop MS damage to healthy myelin or help the body regenerate damaged myelin. The research includes medicines, nutrition regimens and gene therapy. If a breakthrough occurs there, it could also play a role in TN pain.

If myelin can be encouraged to "stay ahead" of the damage being caused by a compressing blood vessel, pain might be prevented without having to undo the compression. (For more on this research, see Chapter 22.)

MVD is not the surgery of choice in MS cases since the aim of that is to find and move an errant blood vessel. One of the through-the-cheek methods – which aim to short-circuit the pain signals – is the preferred type of surgery for MS patients who aren't getting relief from medications.

Most surgeons recommend glycerol injections as the best choice for MS surgery, and some also recommend balloon compression. Radiofrequency lesioning and radiosurgery results have not been as high in MS cases as in non-MS cases, although both are options.

MS-related pain is more likely to recur than classic TN because new lesions can occur anywhere along the nerve as the disease progresses. MS patients also have a higher percentage of constant "atypical" pain (which is more difficult to control in general than the classic cases of spearing, stabbing pain). And MS patients are more likely to have pain on both sides of their face and more likely to have pain that migrates into a second or third branch of the nerve.

Besides medicine and surgery, MS cases also may respond to some of the CAM therapies discussed in chapters 15-18.

The thin-cut MRI may help rule out a blood vessel compression. Keep in mind, there are cases in which MS patients also have compressing blood vessels that are correctable by MVD surgery.

Decisions in post-herpetic neuralgia cases

During an outbreak of herpes zoster or "shingles," the usual treatment is a one- to two-week course of an anti-viral medication such as acyclovir (Zovirax), valacyclovir (Valtrex) or famciclovir (Famvir). Doctors also may suggest non-steroidal pain-killers such as ibuprofen or naproxen for the pain and drying agents such as calamine lotion or corn starch for the rash. For severe pain, prescription pain-killers – including narcotics – are sometimes prescribed.

Recent research has found that steroids, which were sometimes used in the past, are of little help and may even worsen the outbreak.

If post-herpetic neuralgia persists after the rash, that pain seems to respond better to antidepressants such as amitriptyline (Elavil), desipramine (Norpramin), nortriptyline (Pamelor) or imipramine (Norfranil, Tofranil).

In cases that have a sharper pain quality, some of the same medicines that work for TN also may help. These include the anticonvulsants gabapentin (Neurontin), carbamazepine (Tegretol, Carbatrol) and oxcarbazepine (Trileptal).

Dr. Steven Graff-Radford, a face-pain specialist at Cedars-Sinai Medical Center in Los Angeles, says if one medicine isn't working, sometimes adding a second one will do the trick. He says topiramate (Topamax), lamotrigine (Lamictal) and tizanidine (Zanaflex) are three he finds helpful as post-herpetic neuralgia "add-ons."

Anesthetic nerve blocks and using patches or creams of the topical anesthetic lidocaine also may help. Some doctors prescribe Lidoderm patches for their post-herpetic neuralgia patients. These lidocaine-containing patches can be worn for up to 12 hours at a time.

Some patients also are helped by hot-pepper cream, TENS units (electrical devices that "distract" pain signals) and some of the other CAM techniques described later.

Decisions for trigeminal neuropathic or deafferentation pain

These are the types of pain caused by injury to the trigeminal nerve.

In most cases, nerve injuries are treated with medicine. Sometimes the same medicines used to treat classic TN help neuropathic pain, especially gabapentin (Neurontin), oxcarbazepine (Trileptal) and carbamazepine (Tegretol, Carbatrol). These tend to work best for sharper, stabbing pains.

Lamotrigine (Lamictal) may help in neuropathies caused by diabetes. And Dr. Graff-Radford says he's had good success with such antidepressants as amitriptyline (Elavil), nortriptyline (Pamelor) and venlafaxine (Effexor).

Some patients also have been helped by using hot-pepper cream (Zostrix, Capsazin-P and others) five times a day for five days, then three times a day for three weeks.

Depending on the nature and location of the injury, surgeons sometimes are able to relieve pain by cutting out injured nerves (a procedure called a "peripheral neurectomy" that's described in Chapter 14). The idea is to remove malfunctioning sections of nerves and to give the rest of the nerve a new chance to heal itself correctly.

In really troubling cases, doctors may try therapies such as TENS units that send competing signals that overload the brain, thereby distracting it from the face pain. And motor cortex stimulation and other procedures discussed in Chapter 14 are also new options.

No two cases alike

The bottom line is that TN affects different people in many different ways. No two cases are exactly alike.

California neurosurgeon Dr. Robert Wayner put it this way in a talk to a TN support group: "Some people have a very mild case, some people have a very severe case. Some people respond easily, some people don't respond at all. Some people have hardly anything done for it, and some people have had everything done for it, including having most of their teeth pulled out and drilled, all to no avail."

Dr. Burchiel says the prevailing opinion, at least among neurosurgeons, is that MVD is the "gold standard" for getting rid of TN in patients who are willing and able to have that procedure done. He considers the three through-the-cheek procedures to be "important adjuncts" for people who can't or won't undergo MVDs or who fail MVD. Others would add radiosurgery to that list. And if they all fail, there are partial nerve cuts, brain stimulation and a host of other medical procedures as described in Chapter 14. And the entire field of CAM therapies.

The promising news is that the vast majority of trigeminal neuralgians do ultimately find relief for their pain, whether it's medication, surgery or something in between.

Says Dr. Zakrzewska: "Trigeminal neuralgia is one of the few neuropathic pains in which 100 percent pain relief can be obtained."

WHAT TO DO ABOUT SURPRISE ATTACKS

The fact that TN pain runs in cycles is both a blessing and a curse. Those pain-free periods are a welcome relief and often allow patients to reduce or cut out medication.

The problem is that the pain doesn't always return gradually and with advance notice. Sometimes it comes back sharply and swiftly.

Because it takes several days for the standard TN medications to build up to helpful levels, patients sometimes find themselves on no medication and in sudden agony.

The same can happen to patients who haven't yet been accurately diagnosed and who haven't yet been started on TN medications.

When overwhelming pain strikes, don't try to grit and bear it until the next appointment. Call your doctor immediately and let him or her know the severity of the attacks. There are immediate measures that can be taken to knock back the pain until longer-term controls can be put into place.

Dr. Jeffrey Cohen, a neurologist at New York's Beth Israel Medical Center, said the best advice is to do what you can to head off emergencies in the first place. That includes complying with prescribed doses, closely following your doctor's recommendations on increasing and decreasing medications and avoiding known factors that aggravate attacks.

"You may not be able to avoid washing your face, shaving or eating, but certainly avoid what you can," Dr. Cohen says.

If pain starts breaking through, call your doctor before it gets to unbearable proportions. If that's not possible or if your doctor can't be reached, Dr. Cohen says the following are times when a trip to the hospital emergency room may be warranted:

- The pain is so severe you can't eat or sleep.
- Your medicine has suddenly stopped working.
- You've developed apparent side effects, especially soon after starting a new medicine. Pay particular attention to a bad skin rash.
- You've been off medication and the pain suddenly came back full-force.

When going to the emergency room, it helps to have a prepared one-page rundown of your condition, your doctor's phone number, what medications you're taking and what has worked or not worked in the past. Also consider having your regular doctor write a note of what treatment should be given in case of a sudden flare-up when he or she can't be reached. Dr. Nelson, the San Diego neurologist, suggests getting the instructions written on your doctor's prescription pad.

Keep in mind that ER personnel may not be terribly well versed in TN, so having instructions from a specialist – especially one who is familiar with your particular case – can be extremely helpful. A short, written report also may save time and unnecessary testing.

Without a clear read on the problem, emergency-room doctors may do blood tests, imaging and consultation before deciding on a course of action. "This can lead to a big delay in treatment before you actually get something that's helpful to you," says Dr. Cohen.

A prepared report can be especially important if a severe attack has made it difficult or impossible for you to talk.

"This is probably the most important thing you can do for yourself," registered nurse Jim Herbert told a TN support group in northern Florida. "If you're in a situation where you're not able to communicate ... they may do something to try to help you that may be doing you harm."

It also helps immensely if one or more people who are close to you fully understand TN. In case an emergency attack happens, these people can "go to bat" for you and make the phone calls, drive you to the doctor or ER and help you to make care decisions.

In emergency situations, doctors can take several steps to get a quick pain knock-down.

One option is an injection of a local anesthetic, which at least buys time to get a longer-acting therapy in place.

Another option is an injection or intravenous infusion of an opioid, such as morphine sulfate. Dr. Cohen says this usually relieves pain in 10 to 30 minutes, and individual doses can last for 3 to 4 hours.

A third option is an IV "loading dose" of an anticonvulsant. Most anticonvulsants come only in pill or capsule form and must be built up in dose over a few weeks, but fosphenytoin (Cerebyx) and valproate (Depacon) are two that can be given in quick, immediately therapeutic IV doses. These also may start to bring relief in as little as 15 minutes, Dr. Cohen says.

"You can't do this everyday," he adds. "This isn't for maintenance, but it can break a cycle and get you out of pain."

IV treatment may require an overnight stay in the hospital.

Before leaving the ER, make sure you have instructions on what to do in the short-term until you can talk to your regular doctor about your options. "Just because you got rid of the pain at that moment, don't ignore what happens 6 hours from now or tomorrow," Dr. Cohen says.

Keep in mind that it is in these emergency situations that patients are most vulnerable to despair and irrational actions. That's why when unbearable or sudden attacks come on, it's best to get help and not suffer in desperation at home.

HEALTH INSURANCE AND DISABILITY ISSUES

In a perfect world, neuralgians could pick whatever doctor or treatment they want and not have to worry about affording them. Unfortunately, our health-insurance system seldom covers all expenses and often limits choices.

Under managed-care plans, for example, the insurer may only pay for "in-network" doctors or may deny coverage for particular procedures, especially if done out of state or out of network. This doesn't mean you're not free to go where you'd like and do what you want. But it does mean that if you do, you'll be paying more of and possibly the entire bill out of pocket.

Considering that TN surgeries typically range between $10,000 and $30,000, that's an option many people can't afford. Even just the co-pays and deductibles on covered expenses can be daunting.

With most Health Maintenance Organization (HMO) plans, patients must first get a referral from their primary care physician to see a specialist. Non-emergency surgeries also usually need to be pre-approved by the insurer. The same is also sometimes true for tests such as MRIs and CT scans.

Those who have coverage for prescription drugs may find that their insurer has a "closed formulary" in which only listed drugs are covered. Others have a "preferred formulary" in which the insurer will pay only part of drugs not on their list, meaning patients may have to pay more out of pocket for some TN drugs than others.

These kinds of details can be found in your insurance policy or by checking with your employer's benefits person. Some of the factors that go into reimbursement decisions include: what kind of coverage you or your employer has; whether the insurer considers the treatment medically necessary; whether the treatment has been demonstrated to be safe, effective and better than other possible therapies, and whether you've first tried other more conservative (and presumably less expensive) treatments.

If you feel you've been turned down unfairly, your doctor may be willing to explain the situation to the insurer and have the decision reversed. If you can provide convincing evidence that the out-of-network or uncovered treatment offers a level of care or a viable option that the covered option doesn't, you may get approval. All insurers have a review process that allows patients to appeal claims decisions that may have an adverse effect on them.

Insurers normally will want one or more medical opinions to support your request. It's not good enough that you believe out-of-network Doctor A will do a better job than in-network Doctor B, for example.

Some tips that insurance attorneys offer: be persistent; put your requests and arguments in writing; get names, dates and other details of correspondence, and if your appeal is turned down, ask for the clinical reason and find out if that decision included input from a medical expert in the relevant field. For instance, if you're being denied a particular type of surgery, was a neurosurgeon involved in the decision?

If you still are getting nowhere, you can appeal the insurer's decision to your state's insurance department. State legislators also may be able to help, especially if you have a compelling case.

These days, all five TN surgeries are commonly accepted enough that they shouldn't be denied outright. Several years ago radiosurgery was sometimes denied as being "experimental" because it was still a fairly new procedure. Now that it's been done for thousands of TN cases, it's almost universally accepted as a viable option. However, that doesn't mean an insurer still won't insist on a less-expensive procedure first.

If you're without insurance or not covered by any government plan, most hospitals have social workers who may be able to arrange discounted or even free surgeries. Most hospitals do a percentage of these every year.

Sometimes the pain or side effects from medication or surgery become such a problem that people are unable to work. That raises the issue of another type of insurance – Social Security disability.

This isn't an easy safety net for face-pain patients to qualify for, but there have been people deemed incapacitated enough to get it.

Whether you qualify isn't a question of how bad it hurts. It boils down to two main points: 1.) Does the effect of this pain prevent you from doing any job you've done in the past 15 years? and 2.) Are there any jobs you *can* do, given your age, education and work experience?

Your state Social Security office will judge based on a detailed form you fill out and an interview with Social Security Administration personnel. The form asks details about your condition as well as work history, education, training, medical history, medications and tests you've had.

Some medical conditions are obviously disabling and are included in SSA's Listing of Impairments. TN is not on that list. So to gain disability approval, applicants have to show that their daily activities, social interactions, concentration levels and the like are similar to disabilities that *are* on the list.

Roughly 60 percent of all claims are turned down at the initial application. Those who believe they were unfairly denied have 60 days to appeal. An attorney is usually a good idea at this point.

If your request for a reconsideration is turned down, you can then seek a hearing before an administrative law judge. And if that fails, you can appeal to SSA's Office of Hearings and Appeals. Beyond that, only legal issues can be appealed to federal courts – not the merits of how disabled you may or may not be.

For help finding a lawyer who specializes in disability issues, the National Organization of Social Security Claimants' Representatives is a professional group that can give referrals of members throughout the country. It can be reached at toll-free 1-800-431-2804. More information on the group is available online at www.nosscr.org.

Now let's take a closer look at each of the five types of TN surgery.

PROCEDURE	COMPARING THE FIVE ...
	PROS
RADIOFREQUENCY LESIONING	• Very high initial success rate (about 96%) • Level of nerve injury is controllable • Can target location well, especially in lower two divisions • When it works, pain relief is usually immediate • Recurrence rate lower than all but MVD
GLYCEROL INJECTION	• High initial success rate (about 91%) • Severe numbness and serious complications unlikely • Mild type of injury to nerve fibers • Available to those in poor health; general anesthesia not needed • Readily repeatable four times before success rate falls
BALLOON COMPRESSION	• High initial success rate (about 92%) • When it works, pain relief usually immediate or within days • Effective in eye area; hardly any chance of corneal numbness • Normally done with patient asleep; no feedback needed • Almost no chance of anesthesia dolorosa
RADIOSURGERY	• Can be done on practically all, regardless of poor health • Easiest on patient: no needles, anesthesia or incisions • No recuperation needed; resume normal activities right away • Severe complications extremely rare • Most have no numbness; usually only mild when happens
MICROVASCULAR DECOMPRESSION	• High initial success rate (about 93%) • Best chance of long-term relief without pain recurring • Most have no numbness; mild and temporary when occurs • Only procedure that attempts to undo presumed cause of pain • May help "atypical" cases 50-65% of time

... MAIN TN SURGERIES

CONS

- At least some numbness is highly likely
- Severe numbness and anesthesia dolorosa possible (2%)
- Corneal numbness possible, especially when treating eye-area pain
- Temporary jaw-muscle weakness possible
- Can be discomforting procedure if kept awake to give feedback

- Pain most likely to return with this option
- Corneal numbness, anesthesia dolorosa possible
- Not as controllable and targetable as radiofrequency
- Can be temporarily painful for some shortly after glycerol injected
- May take several days for pain relief to occur

- Pain more likely to return than with MVD and radiofrequency
- Repeatable, but results not as good as in first-time procedures
- Temporary jaw-muscle weakness somewhat likely
- Almost all get at least some numbness, usually mild and temporary
- Experienced surgeon needed for correct balloon placement

- Rates of complete relief less than other procedures
- Pain relief is delayed, usually a few weeks to 3 months
- Long-range effects of radiation uncertain
- More expensive than all but MVD
- Units not widely available; may need to travel to metro area

- Most invasive procedure
- Patients must be in relatively good health to undergo major surgery
- Serious complications, including death & hearing loss, rare but possible
- Recuperation time of several weeks, maybe more
- Most expensive of the procedures

CHAPTER 9

RADIOFREQUENCY LESIONING
Fighting face pain with heat

"All patients develop numbness in the face after a succcessful procedure,
which, in the majority of patients, is tolerable...
Pain is immediately relieved in 99 percent of patients."
—Cincinnati neurosurgeons Dr. Jamal M. Taha and Dr. John M. Tew Jr.
in "Techniques in Neurosurgery"

The concept that heat can alter the function of a nerve is a long-standing principle in neuroscience. The anatomy of nerves makes some nerve fibers more susceptible to heat than others, since the insulation around them differs.

More than half of the 125,000 fibers in each trigeminal nerve are without an insulating layer (myelin). The fibers also differ in size. Smaller and unmyelinated fibers react to temperature changes more quickly than larger and myelinated fibers. That means it's possible to damage one type of fiber but not another depending on how much heat is applied.

When heat is applied long enough to a nerve, damage occurs that leads to a reduction in the number and intensity of pain signals being delivered to the brain.

This concept is useful in TN because the heat-induced damage can be enough to prevent the triggering of pain attacks.

Surgeons used heat from electric current to treat TN pain as early as 1931. At that time, however, surgeons were using cautery needles, which didn't have very precise control over the degree of heat generated by the current. Nor did pre-World-War-II surgeons have the technology to accurately guide the current-generating electrode into the Gasserian ganglion – the spot where the trigeminal nerve's three main branches come together. As a result, early radiofrequency procedures led to much dense numbness and some troubling complications, including infections and loss of eyesight.

That changed in 1965 when Boston neurosurgeon Dr. William H. Sweet took advantage of new technology to improve the procedure. He used a fluorescent X-ray device called a "fluoroscope" to help guide the electrode safely and accurately into the ganglion, and he began using a radiofrequency device that delivered much more controlled heat to the targeted area.

Dr. Sweet also used a short-acting anesthetic so the patient could be awakened during part of the procedure to give the surgeon feedback on pain location, pain relief and degree of numbness being generated by the radiofrequency current. His technique showed that patients could get good and lasting pain relief without dense numbness.

Dr. Sweet called the technique "radiofrequency rhizotomy." (A rhizotomy is a surgery to cut or damage a nerve so as to interfere with the transmission of the pain signals to the brain or spinal cord.)

This procedure – also called "radiofrequency gangliolysis," "radiofrequency lesioning" and "radiofrequency thermo-coagulation" – quickly became the most widely used surgery to treat TN.

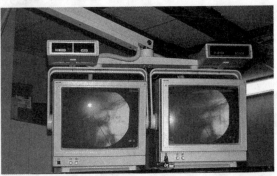

These fluoroscope monitors help surgeons guide needles to the right spot during radiofrequency and other through-the-cheek procedures. (Photo by George Weigel)

How it's done

Radiofrequency lesioning, as we'll call it, is typically a less-than-1-hour procedure done either in a hospital operating room or radiology suite.

Two techniques are currently in use. One involves heating the nerve for a predetermined time at a predetermined temperature with the patient asleep. The other involves keeping the patient lightly sedated so he/she can wake up after each application of the current. That allows the surgeon to assess the patient's blink reflex and facial sensation to determine when enough heat has been given.

With the patient asleep under a short-lasting general anesthetic and lying on his or her back, a hollow needle is inserted through the cheek, past the jawbone and into the ganglion with the aid of the fluoroscope.

Once the needle is in place, the electrode is inserted into it. The patient then is awakened, and the surgeon triggers light radiowaves through the electrode so the patient can tell the surgeon exactly which area of the face the stimulated section of nerve serves. This stimulation feels like a tingling sensation.

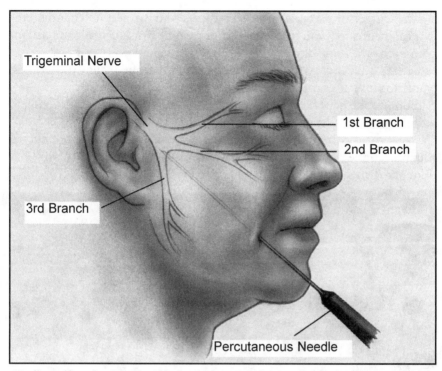

Needles used in the three through-the-cheek or "percutaneous" procedures are inserted into the cheek, just beside the mouth. The target is the point where the trigeminal nerve splits off into its three main divisions. (Sketch by David Peace, University of Florida)

The area of the face that triggers TN pain seems to be the best main target of the procedure. Once the surgeon has located that precise spot on the nerve, the patient is put back to sleep so the nerve can be heated to the point where a lesion (an area of damage) is created. This is where some deliver the heat all at once with the patient remaining asleep and others deliver it in several 15- to 20-second steps with patient feedback in between.

The lesion is made by allowing the current to flow between the tip of the needle electrode and a ground point on the patient's shoulder. A thermocouple on the radiofrequency device keeps the temperature below the point where uncontrolled damage can occur. Generally, the temperature used is between 60 and 90 degrees centigrade.

The goal is to make the trigger zone less sensitive to sharp pin stimulation. In an ideal procedure, patients afterward should be able to feel a safety pin in the affected area of the face – just not as sharply as before.

After surgery, the cheek may be a bit sore from the needle. That discomfort can be treated with ice packs and/or pain-killers. Normally the patient goes home the same day and can resume normal activities right away.

There's a bit of a balancing act involved in radiofrequency procedures. Make too much of a lesion and you damage the sensory nerve fibers in addition to the pain fibers, creating dense numbness. Don't heat it enough and the pain persists or possibly returns sooner.

"I try for a compromise that will relieve pain without producing too much numbness," says Cincinnati neurosurgeon Dr. John Tew, who has done more than 3,000 radiofrequency lesioning procedures.

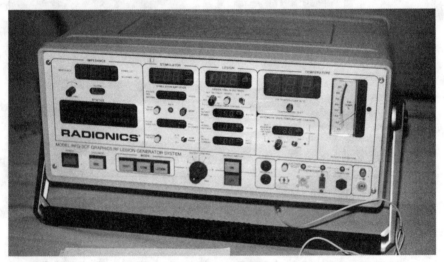

A radiofrequency unit that's used to generate heat during a radiofrequency lesioning procedure.   (Photo by George Weigel)

Radiofrequency's role in TN

The aim of radiofrequency lesioning is to injure the nerve in the right place at just the right amount so the pain is no longer triggered – but without causing troubling numbness.

It's usually reserved for people who have failed medication, either because of poor pain relief or unacceptable side effects.

While this procedure has been used in several variations of face pain, including multiple-sclerosis and nerve-injury cases, radiofrequency lesioning is most effective against classic TN (TN-1). It's not as effective when there's already a loss of sensation or when the person has persistent pain and/or multiple trigger zones in different branches of the nerve. There's also the risk that it may make pain worse when used in cases in which the nerve has been injured (neuropathic and deafferentation pains).

Radiofrequency's strong suit is that this is a controllable, targetable type of injury. The surgeon can locate precise spots on the nerve and decide how much or how little injury to create. That makes it possible to target just the lower branch or just the middle branch, thereby limiting possible complications to those areas. And it allows surgeons to "go light" in cases in which the patient is willing to trade better pain relief for less numbness.

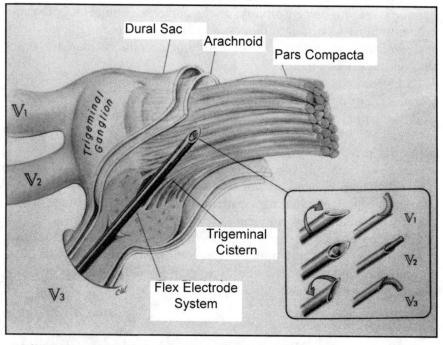

An electrode is used to heat the nerve in a radiofrequency lesioning procedure. Note how the trigeminal nerve is actually a bundle of smaller nerve fibers.

(Sketch reprinted with permission of W.B. Saunders Co., from *Operative Neurosurgical Techniques* by Drs. H.H. Schmidek and William H. Sweet, 1988)

Radiofrequency is usually not the top choice for pain in the upper nerve branch – the area that serves the eye – because the heat injury may cause corneal numbness. If the cornea (the surface of the eyeball) is numb, people may not know if there's an object in the eye that could cause serious damage.

Doctors who prefer radiofrequency procedures over other surgeries like it because it has a very high initial success rate, a lower recurrence rate than the other through-the-cheek procedures and it gives quick pain relief.

It's also repeatable if the pain comes back, and it doesn't carry the risks of open-skull surgery. It also can be done following a failed MVD or other through-the-cheek procedure.

Proponents also like it because the degree of numbness can be controlled thanks to patient feedback and the accuracy of heat delivery.

On the other hand, some doctors don't prefer radiofrequency lesioning because it is a "high-energy injury" to the nerve that's more likely to cause severe numbness, corneal numbness and anesthesia dolorosa (a troubling and hard-to-treat combination of pain and numbness) than the other through-the-cheek procedures.

Radiofrequency detractors also say this procedure can be discomforting for the patient because he or she is awake during parts of the procedure. And they point out that this isn't a curative procedure. It's using one injury to overcome another, which although is usually successful, it isn't as preferable as fixing the underlying cause.

There's also more expertise required by the surgeon for this procedure. It takes experience, good judgment and sometimes the ability to acquire accurate feedback from a groggy patient to do just enough damage to stop the pain without causing problems.

University of Florida neurosurgeon Dr. Albert L. Rhoton Jr. says that radiofrequency is a good option for someone who can't undergo or doesn't want the major surgery of MVD and who is willing to accept the likelihood of at least some numbness.

Success rates and recurrence

How effective is radiofrequency lesioning? Worldwide data suggest initial success rates of at least 85 to 90 percent. That's the low end. Most clinics report 95 to 98 percent success rates, and a few have reported 99 to 100 percent success rates.

These rates put the initial success on a par with microvascular decompression and a notch above the other three nerve-injuring procedures.

If the surgery is successful, the TN pain is often gone right away or within a few days. The former trigger zones can be touched without setting off attacks.

However, only about 75 percent of radiofrequency patients are pain-free after an average of six years, according to Dr. Tew's review of 5,705 cases from nine medical centers.

Dr. Tew says an average of about 3 percent of the patients per year get their pain back during the first five years following surgery. He says that drops to about 1.4 percent each year in years six through 10 following surgery and then to less than 1 percent per year after that. Other reports have placed recurrence rates as high as 9 percent per year, primarily in the first few years after surgery.

The possible drawbacks

Radiofrequency procedures, although very safe in a large majority of cases, aren't without complications.

The most common unwanted effect is facial numbness. Almost everyone has at least mild numbness, but it often becomes less bothersome after the first two or three weeks and then fades to a level that most people find barely noticeable.

"An overwhelming majority feel the numbness is far more preferable than the intense tic pain," points out Dr. Rhoton.

He says that in cases prior to surgery where people aren't sure how they'd feel about numbness, he sometimes gives a series of temporary, local-anesthetic injections. "That enables the patient to live with a numb face for awhile and find out what it's like," he says.

In Dr. Tew's review, about 6.6 percent of patients reported numbness or facial sensations that remained troubling. Some studies have reported the rate at about 10 percent. These feelings can range from annoying or dense numbness to tightness, burning, crawling or itching feelings. Sometimes these troubling sensations also subside in time, but more often than not they're permanent. Antidepressants and/or anticonvulsant medications may help treat them.

In another 2 percent or fewer cases, anesthesia dolorosa occurs. This is a very uncomfortable and sometimes intolerable feeling that patients describe as a combination of numbness and constant and severe pain. It's also very difficult – if not impossible – to treat. (More on dealing with this condition in Chapter 14.)

Another concern is numbness of the cornea – the membrane covering the eye. This happens in about 6 percent of the radiofrequency cases, according to Dr. Tew. It's most likely to happen in cases where the surgeon is trying to treat pain in the eye/forehead area, but it has happened even when the TN pain was in the lower jaw.

In itself, corneal numbness is not a problem. But without feeling in the eye, a foreign body or infection can invade the eye and cause damage without being detected. Patients with this complication must regularly inspect their eyes for redness and other signs of possible eye trouble, such as blurring. Eye drops are sometimes needed when the surgery also causes a decrease in tearing.

In about one in five cases, radiofrequency patients find they have weakness in their jaw muscles or a "looseness" in their jaw joint. That complication usually goes away by itself in three to eight months. However, the problem can be permanent for about 1 percent of patients.

Occasionally, patients get an outbreak of cold sores or facial blisters a week or so after their surgery. This happens in about 5 to 14 percent of the cases. These sores go away on their own and can be treated with topical medications.

Occasional double vision, buzzing sensations or "fullness" in the ear also almost always go away on their own in a matter of weeks.

And occasionally, infections can occur a few days after surgery. Patients should report fever, stiff neck, headache, inflamed eye, confusion or lethargy to their doctor. If an infection is occurring, it almost always can be controlled quickly and easily with antibiotics.

Although it's extremely rare these days, there have been deaths related to radiofrequency lesioning. In his informal poll of 8,000 surgeons, Dr. Sweet turned up more than a dozen deaths as of 1986.

Most of the deaths were due to cerebral bleeding caused by a sharp rise in blood pressure during the point in the surgery where the surgeon heated the nerve. That risk is largely avoided today by giving a drug intravenously that controls these sudden blood-pressure rises during surgery.

Other deaths resulted from bleeding caused by the electrode puncturing a vessel, from meningitis and from heart attack during surgery.

Dr. Tew says he's found the likelihood of many of the complications can be cut in half through the use of newer curved-tip electrodes that allow smaller and more precise lesioning.

In more than 500 patients he's treated with that approach, severe troubling sensations occurred in only 2 percent of the cases and minor troubling sensations occurred in only 9 percent, accompanied by a 98 percent success rate in relieving pain.

Also being tested is a new type of radiofrequency electrode system that measures electrical activity in the nerve. This can help the surgeon correctly position the electrode without needing feedback from the patient. For patients, it would mean not having to be awakened during parts of the radiofrequency procedure.

CHAPTER 10

GLYCEROL INJECTIONS
Fighting face pain with a liquid

"Glycerol (injection) is an easily performed, well tolerated procedure that provides excellent relief for most patients with trigeminal neuralgia. It usually produces only modest trigeminal sensory loss."
—Salt Lake City neurosurgeon Dr. Ronald Apfelbaum

Surgeons have been injecting various chemicals into the trigeminal nerve since the 1800s in an effort to stop TN pain. The substance of choice in recent years is a viscous alcohol called "glycerol" that's similar to the consistency of honey.

Glycerol, which is a component of fats, is toxic in direct contact with nerve fibers. It's the most effective injected substance found yet in stemming pain without completely disabling the nerve.

Glycerol's use in TN came about accidentally in 1975 when Swedish surgeons Dr. Sten Hakanson and Dr. Lars Leksell were exploring the use of cobalt radiation in treating TN (see Chapter 12 on radiosurgery for more on this approach).

Dr. Hakanson was looking for a way to mark the site on the trigeminal nerve for radiosurgery. One of the attempts was to use tantalum dust (a metallic substance) that would later be easily seen on an X-ray. To carry the dust in solution and make it easy to place into the Gasserian ganglion, he used several fluids, one of which was glycerol.

At that time, several weeks would pass between the time of marking the patient for the procedure and the radiation treatment. What Dr. Hakanson found was that the patients who received the glycerol were often free of pain when they came back for their radiosurgery treatment. He reported this observation in 1981.

Research eventually determined that glycerol causes the cells in the protective coating (myelin) of nerve fibers to swell and "slough off." The damage also can affect the nerve fibers themselves. The result is that these injuries interfere with the transmission of signals through the nerve.

Boston neurosurgeon Dr. William Sweet and University of Pittsburgh neurosurgeon Dr. L. Dade Lunsford were among the first to try glycerol injections in the United States. It's been a widely used technique in treating TN since the early 1980s.

Prior to that, surgeons had been injecting alcohol into the Gasserian ganglion. That was the substance of choice dating back to 1909, when Dr. Wilfred "Soreface" Harris – so nicknamed because of his lifelong interest in treating facial pain – first injected it.

Although alcohol helped, it was making just about everyone numb – including complete numbness in one out of three cases. Alcohol also was causing eye inflammations in about a third of the cases, a few of which were bad enough to lead to blindness.

Pain relief from alcohol wasn't very lasting either. In most cases, pain was returning within 12 to 18 months. And alcohol was found to cause significant scarring of the nerve, which limited how often it could be successfully repeated.

Glycerol is a major step forward in each of those areas. Although it's still the procedure in which pain is most likely to come back, troubling side effects are uncommon, most patients tolerate the procedure well, and it's repeatable.

How it's done

Glycerol injections (also called "glycerol rhizotomy," "glycerol rhizolysis" and "glycerol chemoneurolysis,") are done by inserting a needle through the patient's cheek and through one of the three openings in which the trigeminal nerve branches enter the skull. (The opening is called the "foramen ovale," and it's the same opening that's targeted in radiofrequency lesioning.)

Just inside this opening there is a depression in the bone with some ligaments around it. These form a little cave (called the cave of Meckel) which houses the Gasserian ganglion, where the three branches of the nerve come together.

After the patient is heavily sedated and the cheek numbed with a local anesthetic, the surgeon inserts the needle with the patient lying down. With X-ray help, the needle is advanced into the cave. "When spinal fluid leaks out of it, I know it's in the right place," says Portland neurosurgeon Dr. Kim Burchiel.

At that point, the patient is moved into a sitting position so the surgeon can measure how much glycerol will be used. Spinal fluid is drained from this little pea-sized cistern and then filled with Omnipaque (a liquid solution that can be seen on X-ray). The Omnipaque solution helps determine the size and shape of the cistern.

The Omnipaque is then allowed to drain out of the cistern, and the glycerol is injected. The volumes are typically 0.3 to 0.9 ml of glycerol.

In cases of eye-area pain, some of the Omnipaque may be left in the cistern. That's because this is a heavier liquid, and the glycerol will float on it, allowing the glycerol to come into contact only with the upper-division nerve fibers. This gives the surgeon a way to target glycerol's effects to the upper fibers without harming the fibers serving the uninvolved lower part of the face.

Only pure, anhydrous glycerol should be used, not diluted forms or types used in some ophthalmic agents.

Once the glycerol is in place, the patient must remain sitting up for two hours so the glycerol doesn't drain out of the cistern before it has a chance to work.

Some people experience a mild burning sensation and a few have more intense pain for about 5 or 10 minutes, Dr. Burchiel says.

Patients can either be heavily sedated or put asleep with a general anesthesia during the 25- to 40-minute procedure. Dr. Hakanson originally had used a general anesthetic to put everyone to sleep, reasoning that the patient's feedback isn't needed as in radiofrequency lesioning.

Surgeons who use sedation say this approach is somewhat less risky and has fewer lingering effects afterward.

Glycerol injections are usually done on an outpatient basis, but some doctors keep their patients overnight for observation. Pain relief is occasionally immediate, but most often it's several days before the results are apparent.

In up to about 5 percent of the cases, a glycerol procedure can't be completed because the surgeon isn't able to extract fluid or be sure of the proper needle placement.

Glycerol's role in TN

As with radiofrequency lesioning, glycerol injections seek to stop face pain by injuring the nerve just enough to interfere with the nerve signaling while not causing troubling complications. It doesn't address the presumed underlying cause of a blood vessel compressing the nerve.

This is a mild type of injury that has the advantage of holding down the odds of serious, unwanted effects, such as severe numbness and anesthesia dolorosa. It's also very effective up front, working well initially in about 90 percent of the cases. However, the main tradeoff seems to be that the pain is more likely to come back than with the other procedures.

Glycerol injections work best in classic, TN-1 cases, but they also can be used to treat multiple-sclerosis (symptomatic TN) cases. Glycerol is less successful in treating "atypical" or TN-2 cases and, like any destructive procedure, has the potential to make neuropathic or deafferentation pains worse.

Doctors who prefer glycerol injections say they like the procedure because of its limited risk of troubling numbness and other serious complications. It's also a relatively quick and easy procedure, and it's readily repeatable. Some people have had six or more injections in cases where the pain kept returning after a few years. However, a few reports suggest that the procedure can become up to 20 percent less effective in repeated cases.

Glycerol also can usually be done after a failed MVD or other through-the-cheek procedure.

Because glycerol injection does not require general anesthesia, it can be a good option for someone with heart or lung problems and others who don't tolerate general anesthetics well.

And because of the low chance of jaw-muscle weakness, glycerol also might make good sense for someone already having jaw problems on the other side, such as from a previous TN surgery on that side or a temporomandibular joint problem.

On the other hand, many surgeons aren't keen on glycerol because of the slightly lesser initial success rate, the fact that pain relief isn't immediate in half of the cases and especially because of the greater chance that the pain will return within a few years. Some also are concerned about the possibility of corneal numbness.

The other "rap" against glycerol is that it's not as controllable a way to damage the nerve. It can damage nerve fibers in any of the nerve's three divisions if it comes into contact with them.

Besides targeting upper-division nerve fibers by using the Omnipaque solution, it's also possible to somewhat regulate glycerol's effect depending on how the patient's head is tilted. But when it comes down to it, the surgeon injects what appears to be the right amount in the right place and then hopes for the best.

Salt Lake City neurosurgeon Dr. Ronald Apfelbaum says glycerol is a good choice for those who can't undergo or don't want an MVD and who also don't like the prospect of a permanently numb face. If they're willing to accept the tradeoff of lower long-term success rates for those two factors, then glycerol is a good option.

"I've never had anybody say, 'I'd rather have the numbness gone and the pain back,' but it's nice not to have either," says Dr. Apfelbaum.

Success rates and recurrence

Initial pain-relief results for glycerol have varied widely, from as low as 74 percent to as high as 98 percent. The average comes out to about 90 to 91 percent – a bit less than radiofrequency lesioning and microvascular decompression and almost on a par with balloon compression.

Pain relief also is not immediate in many cases. About half of the patients come out of the glycerol procedure with at least some relief, but for the others, relief is normally a matter of days. Some have gone three weeks and even as long as six weeks until the pain let up.

Follow-up studies on glycerol patients have found that their pain is more likely to return than in those who have had one of the other four commonly used TN procedures. Some people do get life-long control from one injection, but in the majority of cases, the results start to go downhill at two years and beyond.

On average, a little more than 12 percent of glycerol patients get their pain back each year.

Reviews of surgical reports by Cincinnati neurosurgeon Dr. John Tew and Detroit neurosurgeon Dr. Jeffrey Brown found that only about 55 percent of glycerol patients are pain-free after three years and only 46 percent are pain-free after five years.

A review of 1,363 patients' outcomes by London oral-pain specialist Dr. Joanna Zakrzewska found an even lower long-term success rate. Her study found that only 45 percent of glycerol patients were pain-free two years after their surgery.

The possible drawbacks

Numbness is the most common unwanted effect of glycerol injections, but it's usually less of a complaint than with radiofrequency and balloon procedures. About two-thirds of glycerol patients report either no numbness or only light numbness that's not enough to be annoying.

"Most people have very mild numbness, just a little bit around the corner of the mouth," says Dr. Apfelbaum.

Only 4 percent of the 1,751 patients in Dr. Tew's review reported severe or troubling numbness. In most cases of numbness, it tends to become less over time as the nerve attempts to heal itself (the same reason that pain can return).

Glycerol also can cause some other altered sensations – sometimes a blend of numbness along with tingling, crawling and/or burning sensations. About 10 percent of glycerol report this unwanted effect.

Anesthesia dolorosa, that hard-to-treat combination of numbness and pain, also can occur, although rarely. Reports place that risk at anywhere from less than 1 percent to about 2 percent.

Corneal numbness also can occur. It doesn't happen quite as much with glycerol as radiofrequency lesioning, but reports still place the risk at between 3 and 7 percent. That's significantly higher than the three other procedures (balloon compression, radiosurgery and MVD). Sometimes corneal feeling comes back, but in the meantime, patients need to take special care to avoid eye injuries, eye irritations and eye infections that they won't be able to detect because of the lack of a pain warning.

Patients also are likely to experience bruising or swelling and occasional minor bleeding at the needle insertion point. Within a few days that discomfort is gone.

Another possible reaction that happens 1 to 4 percent of the time is an outbreak of cold sores on the lips, which go away on their own or are treatable with topical medications. (These sores are thought to occur because the procedure activates the dormant herpes zoster virus that resides in the trigeminal ganglion of many people.)

The jaw-muscle weakness that sometimes occurs after radiofrequency lesioning and balloon compressions happens only rarely with glycerol injections. Dr. Tew's review found it happens less than 1 percent of the time – and even then, the weakness almost always resolves itself in a matter of months.

There have been a few reports of death related to glycerol injections, mostly involving accidental puncture of an artery and in at least one case, a recovery-room heart attack.

Other occasional and temporary post-surgery effects include a headache, double vision, ringing of the ears, nasal congestion, a runny nose and "fullness" in the ears.

CHAPTER 11

BALLOON COMPRESSION
Fighting face pain by squeezing the nerve

"Balloon compression relieves pain by turning off the 'switch'
that triggers the pain."
—Detroit neurosurgeon Dr. Jeffrey Brown

A third through-the-cheek procedure is the balloon compression, also called "balloon gangliolysis" or "percutaneous microcompression."

The roots of this procedure date back to the 1950s when Danish surgeons were investigating the belief that at least some TN pains were being caused by too-small openings at the point where the trigeminal nerve exits the skull and enters the face.

Their solution was to cut a hole in the skull to get at the opening, then drill away some of the bony tissue to widen the opening. The procedure seemed to work.

But what surgeons soon discovered was that it wasn't the wider opening that was giving pain relief. It was the inadvertent "squeezing" of the nerve during the procedure that was doing the trick.

Although the procedure was somewhat successful, it never became very popular because: 1.) It involved major, open-skull surgery and the potentially serious complications that go along with it, and 2.) The pain relief wasn't very lasting.

It wasn't until the late 1970s that Chicago neurosurgeons Dr. Terry Lichtor and Dr. Sean Mullan resurrected the basic idea – this time using a much-less-invasive through-the-cheek approach.

Drs. Lichtor and Mullan used a tiny balloon inflated at the end of a hollow tube (stylet) to do the nerve-squeezing. They introduced the stylet through a hollow needle inserted in the cheek, much like in the radiofrequency and glycerol procedures.

That approach eliminated the need for open-skull surgery and made the nerve-compression approach much less risky.

How it's done

A larger needle is used for balloon compression than either radiofrequency lesioning or glycerol injections because the balloon-carrying stylet must be inserted through it to reach the ganglion.

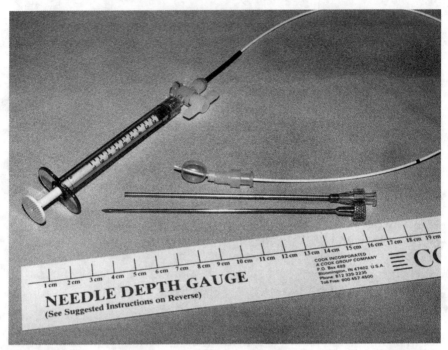

This photo shows the instruments and the tiny balloon (center) that are used in a balloon compression procedure.   (Photo by George Weigel)

The patient is typically asleep throughout this procedure for two reasons. One is that patient feedback is not needed. The other is that the bigger needle would be a bit more painful to an awake patient. However, a few surgeons offer the procedure without general anesthesia to patients who either can't tolerate or don't want that type of anesthesia.

With the patient lying down, the surgeon inserts the needle and guides it toward the Gasserian ganglion – the same target as in the radiofrequency and glycerol procedures. However, in this case, the needle is stopped just short of the opening leading to the ganglion (the foramen ovale).

A stylet with a tiny balloon in the end is then threaded into the hollow needle, along the side of the nerve and ganglion and finally into Meckel's cave, that tiny bony cavity that houses the ganglion.

Instead of damaging the nerve fibers with heat or glycerol, the surgeon inflates the tiny balloon with a small amount of liquid that can be seen on the fluoroscope. When situated in the right spot, the balloon inflates into a pear shape.

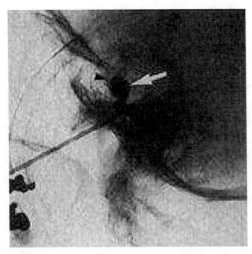

This image from a balloon-compression procedure shows how the tiny balloon inflates into a pear shape when it's in the right area.

(Image courtesy of Dr. Jeffrey A. Brown, neurosurgeon, Wayne State University School of Medicine, Detroit)

The idea is to squeeze the nerve against bony tissue and damage it enough to disrupt the misguided pain signals without causing bothersome numbness.

Surgeons have been experimenting with the balloon pressure and inflation times to find an ideal balance. Most use a balloon pressure of between 1 and 1.5 atmospheres (760-1,100 mm/HG) and keep the balloon inflated for between 1 and 7 minutes. Some prefer the lower time because of a concern that longer inflation times will increase the chance that the patient will have abnormal facial sensations. But not all have found that the longer times lead to more unwanted effects.

After the balloon is deflated, the stylet and needle are removed, and the patient is allowed to wake up. The whole procedure takes about 20 minutes.

Research has found that the squeezing injury selectively damages the larger, myelin-coated nerve fibers as opposed to the smaller nerve fibers without myelin. These larger fibers are the ones that trigger pain attacks, not ones that carry pain signals themselves. That's different from the heat-caused damage in radiofrequency lesioning, which directly damages the pain-carrying fibers.

Why is that important? Because by avoiding damage to certain types of nerve fibers, it becomes possible to avoid complications that relate to those fibers. For example, corneal numbness and anesthesia dolorosa are two complications that are hardly ever seen with balloon compression because this procedure usually does not injure the nerve fibers involved in those problems.

After balloon-compression surgery, the patient gets ice to hold down any swelling and discomfort at the injection site and then usually goes home the same day. Some go home the next day.

Most surgeons attach an external heart pacemaker during this procedure or give atropine prior to surgery (especially for those with heart rhythm problems) because patients' heart beats often slow during needle placement and balloon inflation. That's seldom a problem, but these precautions can virtually eliminate heart problems during surgery.

In rare instances, balloon compression can't be completed because the patient's foramen ovale is too small to accommodate the stylet. That happens about 1 percent of the time.

Balloon compression's role in TN

As with radiofrequency lesioning and glycerol injections, balloon compressions use a controlled injury to interfere with the nerve's ability to transmit signals. And as with those other two procedures, balloon compressions are most effective in classic, TN-1 cases. They also can be used to treat face pain related to multiple sclerosis.

Balloon compressions are not as helpful in "atypical" or TN-2 cases or in treating post-herpetic neuralgia. They also are generally not recommended for neuropathic or deafferentation pains, which could be worsened by the squeezing injury of the balloon.

This procedure is one of the options offered to patients who haven't found adequate relief from medication. Balloon procedures also can usually be done after a failed microvascular decompression surgery or other through-the-cheek procedures.

It's a procedure that also can be repeated if pain comes back after a failed balloon compression. However, Detroit neurosurgeon Dr. Jeffrey Brown, one of the pioneers in this procedure, says he's found that repeat balloon compressions don't have quite as high a success rate as first-time compressions and also are more likely to cause more bothersome numbness.

Doctors who favor balloon compression like it because it's low-risk, technically quick and easy to perform, and effective initially for nine out of 10 patients.

When the procedure works, pain relief is usually immediate, which can be a big plus to a patient in extreme pain. The procedure itself also is painless for the patient since he or she is usually asleep.

Although there is a greater chance of mild numbness and jaw-muscle weakness than other procedures, corneal numbness and anesthesia dolorosa are very unlikely with balloon compression.

Perhaps the biggest advantage is that balloon compression can be used in eye/forehead cases without the threat of corneal numbness and eye infections. Those are particular concerns when using radiofrequency lesions and glycerol injections to treat eye/forehead pains.

Doctors who don't favor balloon compression point to the high rate of mild numbness and to its slightly higher rate of pain recurrence than radiofrequency lesioning or microvascular decompression.

Although jaw-muscle weaknesses usually go away in a few months, it's permanent for 4 to 5 percent of patients – higher than other procedures. That can be a particular problem for someone who already has chewing difficulties on the other side, such as temporomandibular joint problems or damage from a previous TN treatment on that side.

Balloon-compression damage also isn't as controllable as radiofrequency lesioning. Although the balloon selectively damages the right kind of nerve fibers, it's not as selective by location. By slightly changing the positioning of the balloon, some targeting of particular nerve branches can be done but not as precisely as with radiofrequency lesioning.

Finally, the use of general anesthesia for this procedure can be a drawback for patients not in good health or for those who have reactions to anesthesia.

Success rates and recurrence

Although different surgeons have reported initial success rates ranging from 64 to 100 percent, Dr. Brown's review of hundreds of reported cases found an average initial success rate of 92 percent.

How long pain relief lasts also has varied widely from study to study. The average works out to about 25 percent of the people getting their pain back within the first three years.

Like the other procedures, pain recurrences are likely to continue as time passes, although the rate seems to slow after the first three years. After about 10 years, an estimated 30 percent of patients are likely to have their pain back, says Dr. Brown.

If pain comes back, balloon procedures can be repeated one or more times. However, Dr. Brown's study found that the success rate of repeat procedures is down around 68 percent compared to the 92 percent average success rate of first-timers.

The possible drawbacks

Surgeons have been able to reduce complications by refining the balloon inflation pressures and times over the years.

Still, numbness is by far the most common unwanted effect. Dr. Brown reports that just about everybody can expect some degree of numbness afterward. He says about 80 percent of patients classify it as mild numbness, 14 percent say they have moderate numbness and about 6 percent say they have severe numbness.

About 13 to 14 percent of patients report minor troubling sensations such as tingling or crawling, while 5 to 6 percent say they are left with troubling sensations that are severe.

Jaw-muscle weakness is something else that's seen more often with balloon compression than with other procedures. As many as two-thirds of patients may have at least a little chewing difficulty, which usually goes away within a few months. However, this jaw-muscle weakness can be permanent for about 4 to 5 percent of patients, according to Dr. Brown's review of cases.

Corneal numbness and anesthesia dolorosa have occurred, but both are very rare in balloon procedures. Eye infections and other infections also are very rare.

Some patients occasionally come out of surgery with double vision or in about 1 percent of the cases, develop cold sores. Both of these almost always go away on their own shortly.

Very few serious or life-threatening problems have occurred with balloon compression. The main threat is if the surgeon inserts the large needle too far and accidentally punctures the carotid artery.

Overinflation of the balloon also can destroy the nerve and leave permanent numbness.

There has been only one reported death with this procedure. That involved a 62-year-old man who died seven months after surgery as a result of complications from unexplained cranial bleeding.

CHAPTER 12

RADIOSURGERY
A no-incision surgery using radiation

"You don't feel anything. There's no pain. The only discomfort I had was a headache from where they attached the 'halo.'"
—Joe Anderson, founder, International
Radiosurgery Support Association

It was shortly after World War II that Swedish neurosurgeon Dr. Lars Leksell developed a patient head-frame to help surgeons guide needles and electrodes into precise spots of the brain.

A few years later, in 1951, Dr. Leksell and Swedish biophysicist Dr. Borje Larsson got the idea to pair this frame with a device that delivered radiation to targeted spots of the brain. These precisely controlled beams of radiation, they found, could stop tumors or create therapeutic injuries without the use of needles, scalpels and electrodes.

And so was born the "bloodless brain surgery," or what Dr. Leksell termed "stereotactic radiosurgery."

"Radiosurgery" refers to medical treatment that involves the use of beams of ionizing radiation. "Stereotactic" means the treatment is guided by some sort of imaging, whether by X-ray, by computed tomography (CT scans) or, as in this case, by magnetic resonance imaging (MRI).

The combination of these technologies has made it possible for doctors to treat tumors and brain blood-vessel disorders without making a cut. Radiosurgery also has given new hope to patients with previously inoperable tumors and those with problems in parts of the brain that would cause serious deficits if removed by scalpel.

Because radiosurgery does not involve any incisions or general anesthesia, it's an option open to practically all patients, including those with heart, lung and other serious health problems.

In the world of face pain, radiosurgery has been found to be effective in treating TN – especially the classic or TN-1 types. In fact, the first two patients that Dr. Leksell treated with his radiosurgery device both had TN, and both got rid of their pain.

The general goal of radiosurgery is the same as in the three through-the-cheek surgeries – injure the nerve just enough to disable those errant pain signals without causing troubling complications. Only in this case, highly focused beams of radiation are used to do the controlled damage instead of heat, glycerol or the squeezing action of a balloon.

Since radiation travels through skin and bone, there's no need to insert a needle or otherwise make any openings. That alone is appealing to patients.

Radiosurgery involves one other key difference – the area targeted for injury. In radiofrequency lesioning, glycerol injections and balloon compression, the target area is the Gasserian ganglion – that point just beyond the jawbone where the trigeminal nerve's three main branches come together.

That was the original target zone of radiosurgery as well, but surgeons soon found that they could get much better results by aiming the radiation near where the trigeminal nerve enters the brainstem. This is the same area where blood vessels are usually found compressing the nerve. It's an area near the center of the skull that's not readily accessible to needles but *is* easily targeted by radiation.

Two types of radiosurgery devices are used to treat TN – Elektra Inc.'s "Gamma Knife" and the linear accelerator, or "linac," which includes a variety of versions manufactured by several different companies.

The Gamma Knife

Nearly two decades after Dr. Leksell's first experimentation with radiosurgery, the world's first Gamma Knife went into full-time operation in 1968 in Stockholm, Sweden.

Despite its name, the Gamma Knife actually isn't a knife at all. Doctors using it don't even make an incision.

The Gamma Knife is a large globe device – picture a Volkswagen-sized football helmet – with a sliding couch attached to it. It looks somewhat like an MRI unit, only just the patient's head goes into the globe. Inside the globe is radioactive cobalt, which is the source doctors use to deliver a series of narrowly focused beams of cobalt-60 radiation to a target within the brain.

Patients wear a helmet with 201 adjustable holes in it during the procedure. These are what allow the radiation to be precisely targeted and controlled. By themselves, none of the 201 fine beams of radiation that come through these holes is enough to significantly damage tissue. But where the beams converge, the dose becomes potent enough to disrupt blood vessels in the targeted area. That injury cuts off the nerve tissue's blood supply and causes sections of the tissue to scar and die.

In the case of brain cancer, the beams are aimed around the periphery of the tumor. In the case of TN, the beams are focused on the trigeminal nerve a few millimeters out from where it connects to the brainstem.

It became possible to target this nerve "root" when imaging improved to the point where the trigeminal nerve could be clearly seen on MRI pictures.

Thanks to MRI and the aid of a computer, it's possible to aim the Gamma Knife with extreme precision – down to one-tenth of a millimeter.

Partly because of their relative newness and partly because of their expense, Gamma Knife units are not readily available in all parts of the country. As of 2001, 66 Gamma Knife units were in use in the United States and 153 were in use worldwide, according to its manufacturer, Elekta Inc. Most of these locations are university or research hospitals in large metropolitan areas, but Elekta officials say units are now starting to become available in some mid-size metropolitan areas.

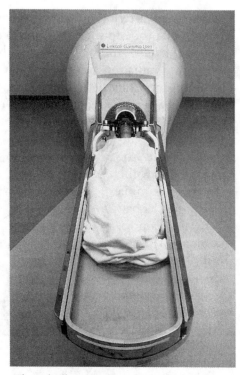

The Leksell Gamma Knife unit looks a bit like an MRI unit with a sliding couch attached to it. The couch slides into the globe, where the radiation is delivered.

(Photo courtesy of Northwest Hospital Gamma Knife Center, Seattle, Wash.)

More than 120,000 people have been treated worldwide with the Gamma Knife, and of that number, about 8,700 have been TN cases, according to Elekta's figures.

Linear accelerators

The linear accelerator or "linac" is another radiation device that became popular in the 1980s. It was developed primarily as a tumor-fighting tool.

Unlike the Gamma Knife, which was built exclusively for treatment of the head, the linac originally was built to treat cancers elsewhere in the body. In 1986, an add-on piece of equipment was developed to treat brain tumors, arteriovenous malformations (abnormal brain blood vessels that are prone to sudden rupture) and other brain disorders.

The linac looks and works differently than the Gamma Knife. Instead of shooting radiation beams through a helmet, the linac is a moving overhead gantry that delivers radiation in a series of arcs. Where the arcs intersect is where the most damaging radiation occurs.

The radiation sources also are different. While the Gamma Knife delivers gamma rays from a cobalt 60 nuclear source, the linac is more similar to X-ray radiation – only at a higher energy level. Linac radiation is created when electrons are accelerated and then sent crashing into a metal target.

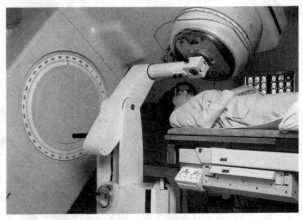

A modified Linac Scalpel can be used to treat TN or tumors of the head. This radiation unit travels in an arc above the patient's head.

(Photo courtesy of Sofamor Danek Surgical Navigation Technologies)

Linacs are made by several different companies. Various institutions may have them under such names as the Clinac 600, the XKnife, the CyberKnife, the Peacock, the Precise, the SRS 200XK and the Novalis Shaped Beam Surgery unit.

Linacs are still used primarily for treating cancers, and not all centers that have linacs use them for TN. Although there have been a few published reports on linac's use in TN, the numbers are far fewer than with Gamma Knife.

How Gamma Knife is done

A team approach is used for radiosurgery, usually consisting of a neurosurgeon, radiation therapist, medical physicist, radiation oncologist and/or a nurse.

The first step is to attach a halo-like metal frame to the patient's head. This is the only potentially painful part of the procedure since the surgeon must use a few small pins to securely fasten the frame to the skull.

Patients are usually offered a mild sedative before this step and are given a local anesthetic at spots on the head where the frame will be attached. The frame is needed to position the head inside the Gamma Knife unit and ensure that the radiation beams will be aimed precisely.

Patients typically say this attached frame doesn't hurt so much as gives a feeling of pressure, much like a "tight band" tied around the head.

Once the frame is in place, the patient undergoes an MRI or other imaging procedure so that doctors can precisely locate the nerve's root. If the patient can't undergo an MRI because of having a pacemaker, a metal implant or other reason, other imaging tests can be done instead to locate the nerve root (such as a computed tomography scan and/or CT cisternography).

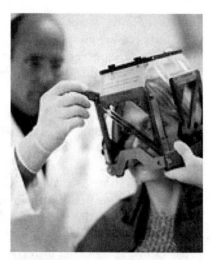

A metal frame is attached to the patient's head in preparation for a Gamma Knife treatment.

(Photo by Dr. Kenneth Casey, neurosurgeon, Allegheny General Hospital, Pittsburgh, Pa.)

The location information goes into a computer, which doctors use to plot the radiation dose and exact radiation targets of the 201 gamma rays. This plotting phase usually takes the team of doctors one to two hours.

When the treatment plan is ready, the patient lies on the Gamma Knife couch, and the head frame is secured inside a large helmet with 201 holes in it. The helmeted patient is then slid into the globe where the cobalt-60 radiation is directed precisely to the target through the 201 holes.

The actual treatment is painless, bloodless and over in 20-50 minutes, depending on the age of the unit's cobalt. (Cobalt becomes less radioactive over time and so longer dose times are needed as the material ages.) The entire process – from the time of the frame placement to the end of the radiation treatment – normally takes about four hours.

Most patients have no immediate side effects (other than an occasional upset stomach or headache), and most go home the same day. Some centers prefer to keep their patients overnight for observation before discharging them the next day.

Normal activities can be resumed right away.

Sometimes the spots where the pins were attached are sore for a day or two. And occasionally, patients report that their pain gets worse immediately soon after the surgery before getting better a few weeks down the road. That's most likely due to temporary nerve swelling from the treatment.

How a linac treatment is done

This procedure also starts by attaching a head frame. Once the frame is in place, the patient undergoes an MRI (or CT scan), and the medical team computes the target and doses – just as in Gamma Knife.

The main difference is the way in which the radiation is delivered. Instead of being fitted with a helmet with holes and lying still in a non-moving chamber, the patient lies on a treatment couch with his or her head frame fastened to it. Then the linac unit moves over and around the patient's head in a programmed series of arcs.

The treatment couch also rotates to complete the process. The actual treatment typically takes 40 to 60 minutes, and the whole process takes about the same four hours as Gamma Knife.

Most patients go home the same day, and the after-effects are similar to Gamma Knife – temporary soreness at the pin sites, a possible headache, maybe some tiredness, and occasionally, some increased pain due to temporary nerve swelling.

In both types of radiosurgery, patients must lie flat on their back and be still during the radiation phase. Some people are relaxed enough that they fall asleep during the procedure, which is fine since no patient feedback or cooperation is needed. For more anxious people or those who have trouble lying still, mild sedatives can be given to help them relax.

Linac treatments are done more out in the open, which is less discomforting for people with claustrophobia who get anxious even in a semi-enclosed unit such as the Gamma Knife.

Radiosurgery's role in TN

Radiosurgery is the newest of the five TN surgeries. It also takes a different approach than the other four procedures. As is often the case with anything new and different, radiosurgery has been met with a variety of views on its usefulness and effectiveness – as well as some controversy.

Some surgeons like the success rates and non-invasiveness enough that they think radiosurgery should be the front-line surgery choice for most people – and maybe even an option instead of medicine. "The results are so good and the side effects so little that (Gamma Knife) can be an alternative to treatment with medicines," said San Diego neurosurgeon Dr. Kenneth Ott at a 2002 Trigeminal Neuralgia Association conference.

Others have nagging concerns about issues such as how long the pain relief will last, what the long-term effects of radiation might be and the possibility that delayed side effects will turn up.

Most doctors' views seem to fall somewhere between those two – that the early results are reasonably good, that radiosurgery has at least a limited role to play in TN, and that the jury is still out on the procedure's long-term performance.

Just about everyone agrees on a few things.

First, as in each of the other procedures, radiosurgery seems to work best in classic or TN-1 cases, when most of the pain is sharp and stabbing. Dr. Ronald Brisman, a neurosurgeon at New York's Columbia Presbyterian Medical Center, says his best Gamma Knife results are in classic, TN-1 patients whose MRIs show obvious blood-vessel compression of their trigeminal nerve.

Most surgeons have reported excellent or good pain relief in better than 90 percent of their TN-1 Gamma Knife patients, but the rates drop to 50-60 percent in multiple-sclerosis cases and under 50 percent in "atypical" or TN-2 cases. Dr. Brisman says Gamma Knife often relieves the sharp, stabbing pains of people with mixed cases, but it's much less effective against the more constant, burning types of pain.

Radiosurgery is not normally used in post-herpetic neuralgia and in cases of neuropathic and deafferentation pains in which the nerve already has been significantly injured.

Almost all surgeons also agree that radiosurgery results are best when it's the first surgical procedure tried. Some also have reported that it works best early in the course of pain as opposed to many years down the road.

However, radiosurgery is almost always an option despite any other procedures that have been tried before. Although success rates aren't quite as high as when radiosurgery is the first procedure, the drop-off rate isn't so much as with the other surgeries, which can be up to 30 percent less successful when they follow a failed other procedure. Radiosurgery seems to be only slightly less effective when it follows one of the through-the-cheek procedures and about as effective as the first time when it follows an MVD.

One possible explanation for this lesser drop-off is because radiosurgery involves targeting a different spot on the nerve for selective injury. In repeat radiofrequency, glycerol and balloon procedures, the same area of the nerve is targeted – the ganglion. So whether you heat it, inject it or squeeze it, the nerve is being subjected to injury in the same area over and over again. When radiosurgery is used following a failed other procedure, the radiation is directed at an entirely different site that hasn't yet been injured – the nerve's root.

If the pain comes back following an initial radiosurgery, a second radiosurgery can be done. Most surgeons advise waiting at least four to six months after the first one, both to avoid giving too much radiation in too short a time and to give adequate time to see if the first radiosurgery is going to work. Results in these repeat cases are slightly less than in first-time radiosurgeries.

Just about everyone agrees that radiosurgery is a good surgical option for those who are too sick, too old or unwilling to undergo a microvascular decompression surgery. It's the easiest and least invasive procedure on patients.

Differences of radiosurgery

One of the biggest differences between radiosurgery and the other TN surgeries is that pain relief is almost always delayed. It usually takes several weeks and often as long as two to three months for the pain to get better. A few people have waited as long as six months after surgery before improvement occurred.

This delayed reaction occurs because radiosurgery's radiation doesn't "zap" living tissue – it interferes with the nerve's blood supply and the growth of new cells. Some researchers theorize that abnormal and already-injured nerve fibers are more sensitive to radiation, which might explain how radiosurgery can work without causing widespread numbness.

"People often ask, 'Is this like a laser?'" says Dr. Ronald Young, a Seattle neurosurgeon and director of the Northwest Hospital Gamma Knife Center. "And I say, 'No, it isn't. Laser produces immediate vaporization of tissue. The Gamma Knife does not do that. It has an effect on growing cells. And so it normally takes some time before the effects are noticed."

That can be a big drawback for people in excruciating pain, especially considering that the other four surgeries offer either the prospect of immediate relief or relief within days.

Dr. Ott says what he sometimes does in this case is offer a glycerol injection to get patients out of immediate pain and then follow that with a Gamma Knife treatment.

The main unknown for now about radiosurgery treatment for TN is whether it will stand the test of time.

"We do not know the long-term results," says Dr. John M. Tew, the Cincinnati neurosurgeon. "Moreover, the long-term side effects of radiation are still not known."

Among the questions that only more time and more patients can answer:

- How likely is it that pain will return years down the road? So far, most published radiosurgery studies have followed up patients for only 5 to 6 years.
- Will any unexpected side effects crop up later? Numbness occasionally appears more than a year after treatment, but Dr. Brisman says that no life-threatening complications have occurred in more than 30 years of Gamma Knife procedures.
- Are doctors using the best target zone and the best radiation doses to do the job? Most Gamma Knife surgeons recently have decided on the best dose range (between 75 and 85 "gray," a measure of radiation) and the best target area (the nerve root). The ideals are less certain with some of the newer models of linac machines. As Dr. Brisman points out, there are enough differences that ideal dosing on one linac machine doesn't necessarily equate to an ideal dose on another machine. In other words, a new machine may ultimately claim the advantage of more pinpoint targeting, but it also may take surgeons some trial time to zero in on the best dosing strategy.

In the short term, radiosurgery has offered the advantage of relatively few unwanted effects. Numbness and sometimes abnormal sensations like tingling and crawling occur but at a somewhat lower rate than the through-the-cheek procedures. Some studies say that more than four out of five Gamma Knife patients report no numbness or other unwanted effects at all. Others say it's more like two out of three.

The ones who do report numbness and other abnormal sensations generally find that it's mild and improves with time. On the other hand, some patients started out with no numbness at all and gradually developed it months down the road.

Serious complications are extremely rare. Other than an approximate 6 percent risk of some permanent numbness (usually mild), a few patients have experienced corneal numbness and annoying abnormal sensations (about 3 percent of the cases). Beyond that, there has been no anesthesia dolorosa, no hearing loss and no deaths.

Because there is no incision, radiosurgery eliminates threats such as infection, hemorrhage, spinal fluid leak and meningitis. That makes radiosurgery a good option for people with bleeding problems and those taking blood thinners such as warfarin (Coumadin).

Since patients are awake throughout the procedure, there are none of the reactions and risks that go with general anesthesia either.

At the end of the procedure, patients normally go about their usual activities without any recuperation time needed.

There's been disagreement over exactly how effective radiosurgery is in comparison to the other four surgeries – both initially and long-term.

One camp says the early numbers are showing that radiosurgery is not as effective at completely knocking out people's pain up front. They point to success rates in the range of 60 to 70 percent when "success" is defined as being pain-free and off medicines. That's significantly less than the initial pain-free rates of 90 percent or so that's typically reported in the four other procedures.

This has led some surgeons to tell people that if they're willing to accept a slightly lower chance of complete relief in exchange for avoiding the rigors of open-skull surgery or limiting the risk troubling numbness that sometimes occurs in the through-the-cheek procedures, then radiosurgery is a good choice. Otherwise, they recommend MVD to those who are younger, healthy and willing, and one of the through-the-cheek procedures for those who want to maximize the odds of complete relief but without open-skull surgery.

Dr. Brisman points out that some of Gamma Knife's apparently lower success rates can be traced to early cases that used a dose of less than 70 gray – the minimum level now thought to be effective. He says that if therapeutic doses are used, radiosurgery success rates are comparable to the other four procedures.

The pro-radiosurgery camp adds that even if the success rates turn out to be a bit less, it's still a procedure that offers a very good chance of getting out of pain or greatly improving it. And that, they say, is a fair trade-off for the non-invasiveness and the fairly low risk of unwanted effects.

"This is a relatively simplistic treatment with few side effects, and it does a lot of good," Dr. Young says of Gamma Knife. "These people feel well, they've been treated, and they can go back to work... After medical therapy, I prefer this option. If it doesn't work, you can always go onto the other procedures."

One other possible down side of radiosurgery is that units are not available everywhere. Many patients, especially those in rural areas, may find they have to travel a distance to get to the nearest radiosurgery for evaluation and treatment.

For help finding the nearest radiosurgery unit, a good source is the Harrisburg, Pa.-based International Radiosurgery Support Association. Its web site at www.irsa.org lists both Gamma Knife and linac units operating throughout the United States along with contact information for the centers using them. Its phone number is 717-260-9808, and its mailing address is IRSA, 3005 Hoffman St., Harrisburg, Pa. 17110.

Almost all insurers now routinely pay for radiosurgery, assuming the insurer is convinced it's needed in your case. That's changed drastically from the 1990s when some insurers refused to pay for it, arguing that the technique was still experimental.

Radiosurgery is significantly more expensive than the through-the-cheek procedures but not as expensive as an MVD surgery.

Success rates and recurrence

How effective is radiosurgery? It depends how you look at the numbers.

As we mentioned above, different studies measure success in different terms. One study may define success as at least 90 percent relief with no medications and everything else as a failure. Another may break success down into grades, such as "excellent," "good," "fair" and "failure."

In general, "excellent" results are usually defined as no pain and no medications. "Good" results are usually defined as at least a 50 percent reduction in pain, even if a low dose of medication is needed to achieve that.

When you lump the "excellents" with the "goods," radiosurgery success rates usually come out around 90 percent success – and sometimes slightly higher. That's comparable to the other four procedures.

However, when you separate the "excellents" from the "goods," only about two-thirds of radiosurgery patients get complete relief. Another 20 or 25 percent get at least a 50 percent reduction in their pain, but they often need some medication to maintain that. About one in 10 patients get no relief at all.

Dr. Young's reported results on 743 Gamma Knife patients are fairly representative. Measuring success rates six months after surgery, he found 67 percent of his patients reporting "excellent" results, 24 percent with "good" results and 9 percent with little or no relief.

Dr. Mark Linskey, a neurosurgeon at the University of California at Irvine, looked at Gamma Knife results in a slightly different way. He says that when you ask people if they're completely pain-free after radiosurgery, the results are in the 50 to 60 percent range. But when you ask them if they're getting at least 90 percent relief – either without medication or on a low dose – the success ranges from 75 to 95 percent.

To illustrate, Dr. Linskey and two colleagues compared the results of 28 MVD patients and 36 Gamma Knife patients who underwent surgery at the University of Arkansas between 1999 and 2002. Nearly 91 percent of the MVD patients were completely pain-free and off medicines 14 months after surgery compared to only 50 percent of the Gamma Knife patients.

However, when evaluating the same group of patients based on being at least 90 percent improved with or without medication, the results were still 91 percent for the MVD patients but 82 percent for Gamma Knife.

Dr. Young compared first-time Gamma Knife patients to those having repeated procedures and found the repeat success rates to be a bit less. He found "excellent" results in only 53 percent of the repeat cases (compared to 67 percent of the first-timers), 28 percent "good" (compared to 24 percent) and 19 percent failures (compared to 9 percent).

There's also been some disagreement about whether Gamma Knife and linac are equally effective.

Dr. Brisman, for example, argues that the linac is much better suited for use on tumors and other larger structures than on small targets such as nerves.

While the Gamma Knife can be targeted to within one-tenth of a millimeter, many linacs can be targeted only down to about three-tenths of a millimeter. Newer units have been modified to focus as finely as two-tenths of a millimeter, and at least one study found that linacs are equally precise as the Gamma Knife.

When five researchers at the University of California at Los Angeles (UCLA) recently compared the two types of radiosurgery instruments, they concluded that "equally excellent clinical results are obtained for small lesions with Gamma Knife and linac. There are only minor differences... for small, spherical-shaped targets."

Dr. Tew says the initial success rates he's seen from several linac studies have been about 80 percent..

A pair of 2003 studies from UCLA show linac rates comparable to Gamma Knife. One study of 25 classic-TN patients treated by linac at UCLA between 1999 and 2001 found that 76 percent were pain-free after an average of two months and the remaining 24 percent got pain relief of at least 50 percent.

The other UCLA study looked at linac on 41 patients with classic TN, 12 with multiple sclerosis and seven with "atypical" TN. After nearly two years, 56 percent of the classic cases had "excellent" results, 32 percent had "good" results and the remaining 12 percent had no little or no improvement.

The 12 multiple-sclerosis patients fared worse – only 58 percent had "significant" relief nearly two years out – and the "atypical" cases were helped in less than half of the procedures.

In most studies – Gamma Knife and linac both – the median time it takes for relief to occur is about six to eight weeks after surgery. "If a patient doesn't get results in six months," says Dr. Young, "in all likelihood they're not going to."

As with each of the other surgeries, pain can return following radiosurgery. Reported rates have varied.

In Dr. Young's 743 Gamma Knife patients, 67 percent started out with "excellent" results and 24 percent started out with "good" results. After five years, 56 percent were still reporting "excellent" results, 18 percent were reporting "good" results, and 17 percent got their pain back. (The remaining 9 percent failed up front.)

That rate is similar to what Dr. Brisman is finding. He reports that about 15 percent of his patients get their pain back over the first four years.

A few other studies haven't been as optimistic, reporting average recurrence rates of about 10 percent a year.

Looking at a variety of reported studies, London oral-medicine specialist Dr. Joanna Zakrzewska concluded that 75 percent of Gamma Knife patients can expect to be pain-free at two years but only about 58 percent at five years.

With linac, Dr. Tew says the initial 80 percent success rates drops off to between 50 and 70 percent in the studies he's reviewed.

In the 25-patient linac study at UCLA, surgeons reported that 32 percent of the initial successes had their pain back within 13 months – a bit higher rate than in the Gamma Knife reports.

The possible drawbacks

Because there is no cutting and no general anesthesia involved in Gamma Knife therapy, this treatment virtually eliminates the most serious risks of other surgeries. And at least in the short term, there have been very few troubling, unwanted effects. Numbness is the main concern, and even that isn't common.

In Dr. Young's 743 Gamma Knife patients, 17 percent experienced temporary numbness and 6 percent reported permanent numbness (usually mild to moderate). Like the pain relief, this numbness typically does not occur until a few weeks or even months down the road. "The facial numbness is very mild and nothing like that seen with the radiofrequency or glycerol methods," Dr. Young says.

Dr. Linskey reports similar numbness rates – about 15 percent of patients – and he says none of those have involved severe numbness.

"The larger dose you give, the more risk of numbness," says Dr. Young, who has found that numbness also goes up when more of the brainstem is irradiated.

For this reason, precise targeting of the 3 millimeter trigeminal nerve is critical – not only to avoid numbness and other potentially serious consequences if radiation hits the wrong target but also to ensure that the procedure works. "Errors of a few millimeters could mean inaccurate targets," says Dr. Zakrzewska.

The odds of numbness also are slightly greater in repeat radiosurgeries.

More troubling complications are rare. Dr. Young reported corneal numbness in 1.6 percent of his 743 Gamma Knife patients and troubling tingling, crawling or other abnormal sensations in 1.8 percent of his patients.

He, Dr. Linskey and Dr. Brisman report no anesthesia dolorosa from Gamma Knife.

The only other reported problem has been a few isolated cases in which patients experienced altered taste after radiosurgery.

Complications have been a bit more common in the few linac studies.

In the 60-patient UCLA linac study, 25 percent of patients reported numbness (none severe), 33 percent reported problems with dry eyes and 6.7 percent reported eye irritations. In the 25-patient UCLA linac study, 32 percent reported numbness (none severe).

In the 30-plus years radiosurgery has been used, there have been no reported deaths and no evidence that the radiation caused new tumor formation or other life-threatening problems.

Says Linskey: "It's not a free lunch, but it is a safe procedure."

"There are failures," Dr. Brisman says of Gamma Knife, "but 90 percent of our patients are doing extremely well. It works. And there are practically no complications."

CHAPTER 13

MICROVASCULAR DECOMPRESSION
Attacking the root of the problem

"It's incredible that such a small nerve and a small vessel
can have so much effect on a person's life."
—Pittsburgh neurosurgeon Dr. Peter Jannetta

When Dr. Peter Jannetta began to propose attacking TN by going inside the skull to "insulate" the trigeminal nerve with a mini-cushion, the idea wasn't wholly embraced by the medical world.

More than a few fellow neurosurgeons openly questioned the wisdom of risking serious complications and even death when: 1.) TN is not a fatal condition, and 2.) There are other less risky and reasonably effective treatments.

A lot of patients weren't crazy about having their head opened either.

Four decades later, Dr. Jannetta's microvascular decompression procedure has become widely accepted, and many surgeons consider it the patient's best chance at long-term pain relief without numbness.

"If you're young and healthy and willing, this procedure is a more definitive cure than anything else," says Dr. Joel Winer, a York, Pa., neurosurgeon.

Microvascular decompression (or MVD as it's commonly called), is a fundamentally different procedure from the other four surgeries we've discussed.

"MVD is the only treatment that addresses the purported cause of most TN," says California neurosurgeon Dr. Mark Linskey.

In an MVD, the aim is to find and fix an offending blood vessel as opposed to altering the pain-transmission ability of the nerve with a new, surgically induced injury.

The idea actually is to be as *non-destructive* as possible. The only problem with that is that MVD requires an opening in the skull before the surgeon can try to undo the damage the body is causing itself. If all goes well, though, the surgeon will get in and out with no lasting problems.

The aim of MVD is to hunt down one or more blood vessels compressing the trigeminal nerve and move the two apart. A small pad is inserted to keep the vessels and nerve apart.

That move essentially takes the offending mechanical force – a pulsating blood vessel – out of play. That alone is often enough to stop the pain in its tracks. With the vessel no longer beating on the nerve, the patient wakes up and finds the pain is gone completely.

Other times, moving the vessel out of the way gives some improvement at first, but the nerve needs to gradually heal over days or weeks before the pain fully subsides. The longer a person has had TN pain before having an MVD, the less likely it is that pain relief will be immediate, some surgeons believe.

Numbness sometimes occurs with MVD, but it's not a necessary or intentional effect. In the through-the-cheek procedures, more numbness usually means better and longer-lasting pain relief. But that's also more annoying to the patient. And so surgeons try to strike that perfect balance of injury – enough to help but not so much as to harm.

In an MVD, there is no such balancing act. Having numbness doesn't mean better pain relief. In fact, one study found that the majority of patients with "excellent" relief (no pain, no medicines) had no postoperative numbness at all.

In the early years of MVD, some surgeons speculated that it wasn't really the padding action of this procedure that was stopping the pain.

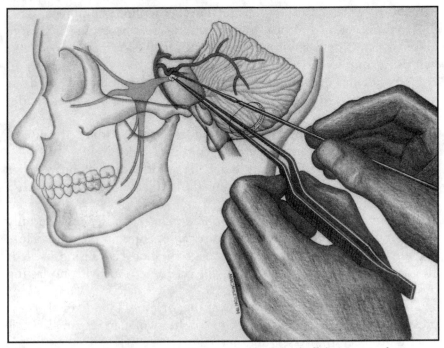

This sketch shows where surgeons work to move a blood vessel off the trigeminal nerve during a microvascular decompression procedure.

(Reprinted with permission of the Mayfield Clinic, University of Cincinnati)

They theorized that the mere action of moving the vessel off of the nerve was causing mild injury to the nerve and stopping pain much like a balloon compression, only at a different spot on the nerve.

Long-term studies have discounted that theory. In fact, it's now thought that irritating the nerve during surgery might be behind the numbness that sometimes occurs. Sometimes vessels can be "decompressed" easily, but other times the surgeon has to do some tugging and manipulating to separate a vessel that has adhered to the nerve or that has wedged itself tightly behind the nerve.

When numbness occurs after MVD, it's usually mild and clears up within a few weeks.

How MVDs are done

MVDs are done under general anesthesia. Prior to surgery, patients must be tested and screened to make sure their overall health is good enough to tolerate the stress of major surgery and the two to three hours of anesthesia that an MVD may require.

Once the patient is asleep, a 1-inch by 3-inch area of hair is shaved, behind the ear on the side of the pain. Positioning is important at this point. The head is secured in a surgical clamping device to prevent any movement during the procedure. After surgery, this may give patients a feeling of having a band around their head.

With the head in place, the surgeon cuts a half-dollar-sized hole (sometimes smaller) in the skull just behind the ear on the painful side. The waterproof covering of the brain (the dura) is then opened to expose the brain.

Using an operating microscope, the surgeon works next to the brain to locate the cranial nerves. Technically, this is cranial surgery, not brain surgery since nothing is being done to the brain itself. "It's *almost* brain surgery," is how Minnesota neurosurgeon Dr. Stephen J. Haines put it.

What the surgeon is looking for is the root zone of the trigeminal nerve – the point where it connects to the pons or brainstem. That's the spot where arteries and veins are normally found to be compressing the nerve. (An artery is a vessel that carries blood from the heart to various parts of the body; a vein is a vessel that carries blood back to the heart.)

During this part of the procedure, another doctor monitors a device that tests the nearby auditory nerve. This nerve lies in the path between the skull opening and the trigeminal nerve. The surgeon has to work around the auditory nerve, and if it's irritated too much, hearing damage can result.

Monitoring keeps track of whether the auditory nerve is being overly stressed so the surgeon can take corrective action before damage occurs. This step has greatly reduced the threat of hearing problems. Many surgeons require a hearing test as part of the pre-operation screening so a baseline reading is available to determine if the MVD affected hearing.

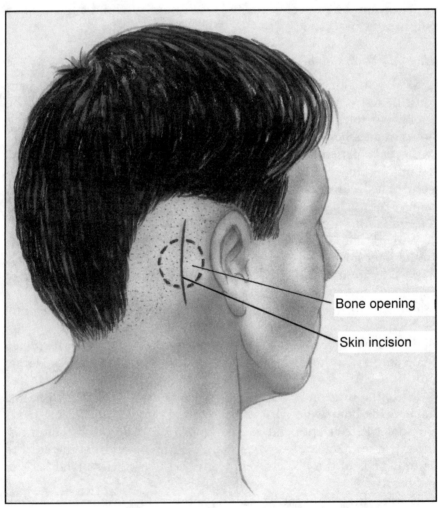

Bone opening

Skin incision

In a microvascular decompression procedure, surgeons enter the skull behind the ear through an opening that's slightly larger than a quarter.

(Sketch by David Peace, University of Florida)

While exploring the trigeminal nerve root through the operating microscope, the surgeon hopes to find one or more offending blood vessels. A pre-surgery MRI sometimes gives surgeons an idea ahead of time where they're likely to find compressing vessels.

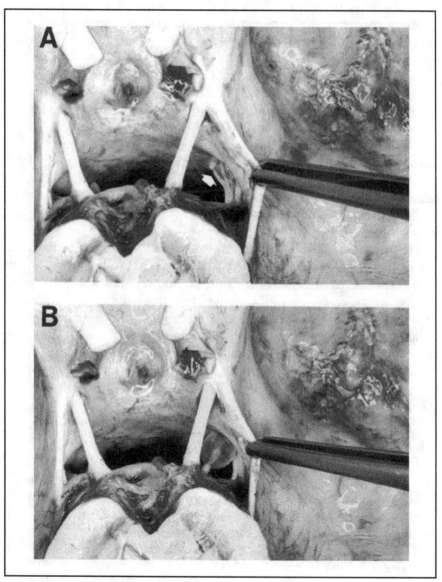

These two photos are actual views of what a neurosurgeon sees through the operating microscope during an MVD procedure.

(Photos courtesy of Dr. Jeffrey A. Brown and Dr. Kenneth Casey, neurosurgeons from Detroit and Pittsburgh, respectively.)

"Ninety percent of the time, it's blatantly obvious," says Dr. Jannetta. "Five percent of the time it's subtle, and 5 percent of the time it's *very* subtle... I've had three patients with veins growing right in the middle of the nerve."

In about 55 percent of the cases, there is more than one vessel compressing the nerve. Dr. Jannetta says it's critical that surgeons look for and find *all* of the offending vessels and not just assume it's one obvious vessel causing the trouble.

In as many as 10 to 15 percent of the cases, surgeons fail to find or recognize compressing vessels. When that happens, most surgeons cut some of the sensory nerve fibers in an effort to bring relief without troubling numbness. (More on this below.)

Failure to find a compressing vessel means one of two things: either something else is causing the patient's pain or the surgeon simply hasn't been able to locate the troublesome vessel. Dr. Jannetta believes it's almost always the latter.

"The problem is not whether a vessel is there or not, but am I good enough to find all of the vessels that *are* there," he says.

He argues that the better a surgeon's training and experience, the fewer "nothing-found" cases there are. In recent studies, some of the most experienced surgeons now report finding vessel compressions in 99 percent of the cases – significantly higher than even a decade earlier.

In recent years, some surgeons have begun using a camera device called an "endoscope" to give a magnified look inside the skull. Some use it in conjunction with the operating microscope and a few use it exclusively. (See Chapter 22 for more details on this new device.)

Dealing with the vessels

Most surgeons use small pieces of Teflon sponge or shredded Teflon felt as a pad between the vessels and nerve.

Other materials such as Dacron felt and Ivalon (a hard sponge) have been used in the past, but these had a tendency to irritate the nerve. Slivers of transplanted muscle, dura and periosteum (a fibrous connective tissue) also have been tried, but most surgeons do not use them because the body has a tendency to break them down.

Teflon also occasionally has caused some scarring and adhesions on the trigeminal nerve, and there have been a few reports recently about this padding causing abnormal growths called *"granulomas"* that can cause gradual hearing problems. But at present, Teflon has been found to be the best, least irritating material.

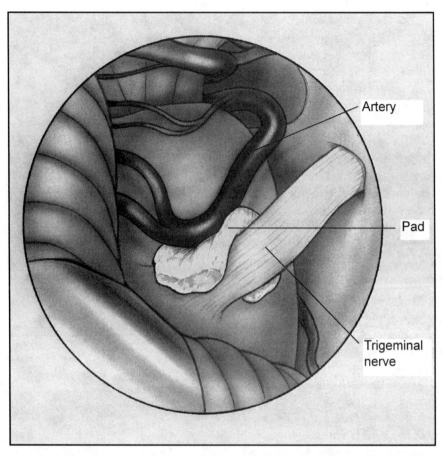

Close-up of how a sponge or pad is inserted between a blood vessel and the trigeminal nerve during a microvascular decompression procedure.

(Sketch by David Peace, University of Florida)

When a blood vessel is found to be compressing the nerve, it's an artery in two-thirds to three-quarters of the cases. It's important to make a distinction because arteries cannot be cut or removed and must be padded off of the nerve.

Veins, however, can be divided by sealing them off and cutting them out rather than padding them. Blood that had been traveling through the removed veins will find its way back to the heart through other veins.

The problem with compressing veins is that in about a third of the cases, new branches can form, causing a new compression. Women between the ages of 35 and 52 seem to have a higher prevalence of veins causing their pain than other groups. Dr. Jannetta and his colleagues found that veins are involved in 37 percent of women in that age group as compared to only 21-27 percent of men.

In an effort to avoid some of the higher pain recurrence in vein cases, some surgeons have begun padding veins even though they could more easily just eliminate them. The early feedback is that this seems to reduce recurrence rates.

Patients sometimes ask why surgeons don't just remove all veins found anywhere near the trigeminal nerve. That can't be done because these veins return blood to the heart from the brain, and removing too many of them (or too big of one) could lead to a stroke.

Once the padding is in place or the vein has been eliminated, the surgeon closes.

The dura is sutured together, and the skull opening is

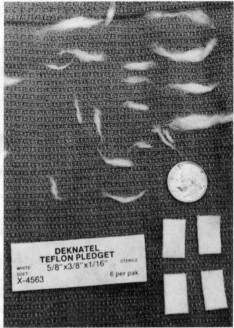

Teflon implants. Teflon pads are pulled apart to make cotton-like "fluffs" of insulating material that are inserted between a compressing artery and the trigeminal nerve. This is the most common cushioning material.

(Photo by George Weigel)

covered with a small titanium mesh plate. Some surgeons replace the skull fragments, which in a few weeks scar together. And a few use nothing, preferring to allow scar tissue to cover the opening.

Steroids are usually given post-operatively to guard against brain swelling, and mild narcotics or other pain-relievers are given as needed for surgical pain. The patient usually spends the first night in intensive care. Coordination and other neurological tests are done at regular intervals for the first 24 hours. If all goes well, the patient goes home on the third day of hospitalization.

The entire MVD procedure typically takes two to four hours, although the actual repair takes more like 90 minutes.

Many patients are able to return to work within two weeks (longer for physically demanding jobs), and most say they are completely recovered in about two months.

MVD's role in TN

Although MVD is no longer as controversial as it was in its early years, there's still plenty of disagreement over exactly who should have it and when.

Neurosurgeons often tell their patients that MVD is a procedure that sounds worse than it really is. Improvements in technique, anesthesia and technology over the past 40 years have greatly reduced the serious risks.

Still, complications such as hearing loss, meningitis, spinal fluid leaks and even death do occur. As Duke University Medical Center neurosurgeon Dr. Robert Wilkins cautions, MVD is not a benign procedure that should be taken lightly.

On the other hand, this is the only procedure that attempts to fix the underlying problem. And it offers a high probability of complete pain relief (sometimes as much as 98 percent) with the best chance that the pain won't come back.

What it boils down to is weighing the potential risks vs. the potential benefits and carefully selecting patients who are best able to tolerate the surgery.

As in each of the other procedures, MVD works best in classic TN – cases that have sharp, stabbing pain and definite trigger zones. The more the pain gravitates away from that, the lower the success rates.

"Atypical" or mixed cases are often helped, but the success rates for these are more in the 50 to 65 percent range as opposed to 90 percent and up. What often happens is that the MVD helps the sharp, stabbing component of a person's pain but not the more constant, burning, underlying pain.

MVD is generally not recommended for neuropathic and deafferentation pains (these are caused by injured or disabled nerves, not blood-vessel compressions), and it's usually not helpful for face pain related to multiple sclerosis. The exception is if a person with MS-related pain also happens to have a blood vessel compressing their trigeminal nerve. This sometimes can be picked up on an MRI.

Most surgeons used to limit MVDs to patients aged 65 and under, but that's loosened in recent years. "Health is more important than chronological age," says Dr. Jannetta.

That new approach has been buoyed by a Canadian study showing that MVD patients over the age of 70 did just as well as those under 70. Some surgeons have even performed successful MVDs on patients in their 90s.

The bottom line: a healthy 70-year-old is probably a better MVD candidate than a 60-year-old with heart problems.

Besides those with heart problems, people who have breathing or lung problems and those with bleeding disorders are poorer risks.

Since the whole idea of an MVD is to find and correct a compressing blood vessel, it's important to make sure of the diagnosis before operating. Face pains that really aren't TN and therefore not being caused by a compressing blood vessel are *not* going to be helped by MVD.

Most surgeons also do not advise MVD unless medication has been given a fair trial and failed or is causing the patient unacceptable side effects.

In years past, MVD was often suggested as an option of last resort – something that one should consider only if in agony or if having debilitating side effects on a handful of medicines.

That's also been changing, at least in the world of neurosurgery. As we discussed in Chapter 8, several recent studies have found that MVD success rates seem to start dropping off after people have had their pain for more than seven or eight years.

Some surgeons are beginning to argue that that suggests a prime "window of opportunity" before irreparable damage is done to the nerve. They say that younger patients in particular should think about earlier MVDs, even if they're not in severe pain or having troubling side effects to their medicine.

Not all agree with this more aggressive approach. More conservative surgeons say the success rates are still good enough in the long term that it isn't worth the extra risk of subjecting people to MVD any sooner than necessary.

Others say that radiosurgery and the through-the-cheek procedures are successful enough and repeatable enough that their lower risk outweighs MVD – at least in older, less healthy patients. They argue that if the less risky procedures fail, then MVD should be considered – even if the success rates are a bit lower at that point.

Even at a 1 or 2 percent risk of death or serious complication in MVD, that's too much for a non-fatal pain condition, contends Chicago neurosurgeon Dr. Sean Mullan. "This is not a trivial figure for a disease with no spontaneous mortality or fixed disability when there is a successful alternative," he says.

On the other hand, pro-MVD surgeons argue that the other surgeries have their risks as well – problems such as anesthesia dolorosa, corneal numbness and severe numbness that are all but eliminated in MVD.

And they point to several recent studies showing that MVD success rates are about 30 percent lower when MVD follows one of the nerve-injuring surgeries.

MVD surgery is routinely covered by insurance, but for those without insurance, this is easily the most expensive of the five TN surgeries.

Success rates

Almost all of the medical literature reports initial MVD success rates of at least 85 to 95 percent – sometimes in the 95 to 98 percent range. Detroit neurosurgeon Dr. Jeffrey Brown's review of 2,318 cases from 20 different surgery practices found the average initial success rate to be 92.7 percent.

In most cases, pain relief is immediate. Once the pressure of the blood vessel is removed from the nerve, the fibers are no longer compacted together and signals from the light-touch nerve fibers stop jumping onto the pain-signaling fibers.

In some cases – especially in those who have had pain for a long time – the pain may take a few days or even weeks to resolve.

What isn't always spelled out in the studies is whether "successes" mean no pain or whether it also includes people who are significantly improved but still in some pain.

One of the few to try and sort out the "pain-frees" from the "much-improveds" is a prospective, long-term 1996 study of 1,185 patients who underwent MVD surgery at the University of Pittsburgh by Dr. Jannetta and colleagues.

That study found that 82 percent of patients had no pain and 16 percent had at least a 75 percent reduction of pain. The remaining 2 percent either had no relief or only minor improvement.

In a study of MVD patients by patients themselves, the Australia TN support group surveyed 71 Australians, Americans and Canadians who had undergone MVDs and found that 80 percent of them were pain-free immediately after surgery.

Pain recurrence

As with the percutaneous procedures, TN pain can return after an MVD.

When the pain comes back, it tends to come back fairly soon after the surgery. Several studies have found that more than half of the people who ultimately get their pain back after an MVD get it back within the first two years.

Long-term studies have found the MVD "drop-out" rate goes down as time passes. On average, about 6 percent of MVD patients get their pain back in the first year, 3 percent a year get it back in years two through four, less than 2 percent get pain back in years five through nine, and then less than 1 percent per year get pain back from the 10th year on.

Counting the initial failures along with those who recur, London oral-pain specialist Dr. Joanna Zakrzewska came up with the following prospects for MVD patients: 81 percent are pain-free at two years, 76 percent are pain-free at five years and 71 percent are pain-free at 10 years.

"If you follow these patients, you're going to get recurrences," says Dr. Jannetta.

He says initial failures may happen for several reasons, such as the surgeon was unable to find the offending vessel (or vessels), the nerve wasn't sufficiently cushioned, or the patient didn't really have TN in the first place.

When pain recurs, he says, it's not because the effects of the MVD "wear off." Rather, he says the most likely reason is that a divided vein sent out new branches and set up a compression problem all over again.

Or it could be that a different vessel elongated with age and caused an altogether new compression point. Sometimes these vessels don't cause a new compression but push an implanted cushion out from between the nerve and the offending vessel.

Or it could be that adhesions have formed to cause new damage to the trigeminal nerve. Adhesions are fibrous growths that sometimes occur along with scar tissue around the surgical site and implanted pad.

Or it could be that the implant failed. Muscle implants, for example, can be absorbed by the body.

Dr. Jannetta's 20-year study found that those with vein compressions were more likely to find their pain returns. Female patients and those who didn't get immediate pain relief also were slightly more likely to have their pain return.

Although MVDs can be done following failed other procedures, the success rates are about 30 percent lower. The best MVD results seem to be when MVD is the first procedure done.

Repeat MVDs also can be done following a failed MVD. Those success rates also are a bit less than the first time – down around 80 percent compared to the 85 to 95 percent range for first-timers.

The possible drawbacks

MVD patients can expect to be stiff, have a headache and some pain around the incision for the first couple of weeks. Those after-effects are common.

Occasionally, patients experience one or more of the following – blurred or double vision, muffled hearing, an outbreak of cold sores, nausea, dizziness, incoordination, fluid in the middle ear or ringing in the ears. These almost always go away on their own in a matter of days or weeks.

A few other possible complications may require medical treatment. These may include meningitis (an infection of the membranes covering the brain), cerebrospinal fluid leaks, lung difficulties and wound infections. A review of 2,540 MVD cases by Cincinnati neurosurgeons Dr. John Tew and Dr. Jamal M. Taha found that one or more of the above problems happen about 16 percent of the time. These also are almost always short-term problems.

Serious and lasting complications are less common, but a lot of things *can* go wrong. Among the more serious risks are hearing loss on the surgery side, brain swelling, intracranial bleeding, stroke, blood clot, facial paralysis and even death.

Hearing loss is the most likely of the serious complications. Some reports have placed the number up around 10 percent, but with more widespread monitoring of the auditory nerve during surgery, the number has dropped to about 2 percent. The most recent reports estimate hearing loss at 1 percent or less.

Dr. Tew and Dr. Taha estimate the chance of non-fatal stroke or cranial bleeding at about 1 percent.

As for the chance of dying, that rate also has been dropping. In recent years the rate has been ranging between 0.4 and 0.7 percent. That averages out to roughly one in every 200 patients. Deaths have occurred due to brain seizures, cranial bleeding, heart attack, stroke and pulmonary embolism.

Facial numbness occurs, on average, between 10 and 30 percent of the time. But this is almost always mild and almost always greatly improves or clears up within a few weeks. Permanent facial numbness in any part of the face occurs less than 2 percent of the time.

About 5 percent of MVD patients report sensations of tingling or crawling in the face.

As we discussed in Chapter 8, success rates can be maximized and complications minimized by picking a well trained, experienced TN surgeon.

In his 1986 poll of 45 neurosurgical services doing MVDs, Boston neurosurgeon Dr. William Sweet found that the incidence of serious complications was "far higher among most less-experienced surgeons."

Dr. Jannetta, who has done more than 4,000 MVDs over more than three decades, also points out that those who are most experienced at MVDs not only have fewer complications but become more adept at finding vessel compressions. "As careful as I like to be," he says, "I still miss subtle vessels."

Partially cutting the nerve

There's one more surgical procedure that's sometimes used short of completely disconnecting the trigeminal nerve at its roots. It's called a *"partial root section"* or *"partial sensory trigeminal rhizotomy."*

The idea of this procedure is to cut enough trigeminal nerve fibers near where the nerve first exits the brainstem to stop or lessen the pain while preserving at least some feeling in the face. This was a common surgical treatment for TN from the early 1900s until the 1960s.

Partial root sections are primarily employed today as a backup strategy in case an MVD surgeon finds no offending blood vessel to decompress. Rather than do nothing, one option (hopefully discussed with the patient beforehand) is to cut some of the nerve fibers near their roots.

A partial root section also may be done if a vessel or vessels are found that can't be safely moved off of the nerve. That may be the case, for example, when a vessel has managed to grow within the nerve fibers.

Another time a partial root section may be done is when pain comes back after a prior surgery and the surgeon goes back in, only to find no new compression or a situation that's unlikely to be helped by a second MVD.

Occasionally it's used when all other procedures have failed and the patient is willing to trade the almost-certain numbness for pain relief.

In a 1993 report by Dr. J.N. Young and Dr. Robert H. Wilkins, 70 percent of 83 patients who underwent this partial cutting of the trigeminal nerve root had no pain or well controlled pain for an average of six years after surgery. About half of these patients reported mild numbness, 18 percent had severe numbness, but the remaining one-third had little or no loss of feeling.

Dr. Zakrzewska and three colleagues did a comparative study of 220 MVD patients and 53 partial-root-section patients in 2003. She found that 89 percent of MVD patients were satisfied with their situation five years later compared to only 72 percent of the partial-root-section patients.

More than one in five of the partial-root-section patients said they were worse off than five years earlier. Dr. Zakrzewska attributed that largely to dissatisfaction with complications, primarily numbness.

As with the through-the-cheek procedures, partial root sections involve a bit of a balancing act. The more nerve fibers that are cut, the greater the chance of lasting pain relief but also the greater the chance of dense and permanent numbness. Lighter cuts may limit numbness but increase the chance that pain will come back.

A few surgeons routinely do partial root sections along with an MVD because they believe it reduces the chance that the pain will come back. Dr. Jack Carey, a now-retired Maryland neurosurgeon who used that approach, said he found that up to 30 percent of the nerve can be selectively cut with little or no loss of feeling to the patient.

Others, like Salt Lake City neurosurgeon Dr. Ronald Apfelbaum, say that's a "belt-and-suspenders approach" that needlessly increases the chance of numbness. "If you cut a little too much, you may produce numbness," he says. "And there's no way to tell how much is too much."

Since this is an open-skull procedure much like an MVD, a partial root section is an option open only to those healthy enough to undergo major surgery.

A COMPARATIVE LOOK ...

Procedure	Initial Pain Relief	Pain-Free at 3 years
RADIOFREQUENCY LESIONING (RHIZOTOMY)	96% (usual range: 85-99%)	68-94%
GLYCEROL INJECTION	91% (usual range: 74-98%)	45-55%
BALLOON COMPRESSION	92% (usual range: 64-99%)	68-75%
RADIOSURGERY (GAMMA KNIFE)	67% pain-free, 24% at least 50% improved	62% pain-free, 21% at least 50% improved
MICROVASCULAR DECOMPRESSION	93% (usual range: 80-98%)	80-81%

Source: Figures are based on a compilation of reported results from published studies around the world as well as comparative analyses by Drs. Jamal M. Taha and John M. Tew Jr. at the University of Cincinnati, Dr. Joanna M. Zakrzewska at the University of London and Dr. Mark Linskey at the University of Arkansas.

Initial pain relief: The single numbers are medians from all studies analyzed. The ranges are the highs and lows reported from most of these studies.

Pain-free numbers: These refer to the generally expected percentages of people who are out of pain at the listed time intervals. Numbers often vary greatly from study to study for a variety of reasons, including differences in reporting, differences in surgical skill and experience and particularly in the case of radiofrequency lesioning, the level of heat injury used. (More heat injury means better results but also more chance of numbness.)

... AT SURGICAL SUCCESS RATES

Pain-Free at 5 years	Pain-Free at 10 years
48-85%	40-75%
36-46%	NA
64-69%	62-63%
56-58% pain-free, 18% at least 50% improved	NA
75-76%	68-70%

	Radiofrequency Lesioning	Glycerol Injection
A LOOK AT POTENTIAL ...		
Numbness (mild or temporary)	++++++	++++++
Numbness (severe or permanent)	+++	++*
Outbreak of cold sores	+++	++
Abnormal facial sensations	+++	+++
Jaw-muscle weakness	Temporary: ++++ Permanent: +++	++ (Temporary only)
Corneal numbness	++	+++
Anesthesia dolorosa	++	++
Hearing loss	0	0
Meningitis	+	+
Other cranial problems	0	0
Death	<0.1%	<0.1%

What the ratings mean:
+ is a very rare complication, occurring less than 1% of the time
++ is a rare complication, occurring approximately 1-5% of the time
+++ is an occasional complication, occurring approximately 5-10% of the time
++++ is a somewhat likely complication, occurring approximately 10-25% of the time
+++++ is a complication that occurs fairly often, approximately 25-50% of the time
++++++ is a common complication, typically occurring in 50% or more of the cases
* Primarily related to repeat procedures, not first time
Details on the complications: Facial numbness is broken down into two classes by how troubling patients find it to be. Cold sores may occur around the lips and usually go away quickly and without permanent consequence. Abnormal facial sensations include new sensations other than pain and numbness, such as "itching," "crawling" or "tingling." Jaw-muscle weakness may affect chewing to different degrees; it usually resolves in weeks or months but sometimes can be permanent. Corneal numbness refers to loss of feeling to the surface of the eyeball and can range from mild to complete numbness.

... UNWANTED EFFECTS OF SURGERY

Balloon Compression	Radiosurgery (Gamma Knife)	Microvascular Decompression
++++++	++++	+++
++	++	+
++	NA	+++
++++	++	++
Temporary: ++++++ Permanent: ++	0	0
+	+	0
+	0	0
0	0	++
++	0	++
0	NA	++
<0.1%	0	0.4%

Details on the complications: Anesthesia dolorosa is a hard-to-treat combination of dense numbness and constant, burning pain that results from nerve injury. Hearing loss can range from slight to complete on the operative side only. Meningitis is an infection of the membrane that covers the brain and spinal cord and can usually be treated with antibiotics. Other cranial problems include such problems as cerebrospinal fluid leak, movement deficits, facial palsy, stroke and cranial bleeding. Death is extremely unlikely but has occurred due to brain seizures, artery punctures, heart attack, stroke and pulmonary embolism.
NA= data not available

CHAPTER 14

IT STILL HURTS... NOW WHAT?

"All five neurosurgical procedures relieve pain in most patients,
but recurrence may occur with any of them."
—New York neurosurgeon Dr. Ronald Brisman

OK. So about half of those with trigeminal neuralgia find their answer with medication. And the majority of those who go on to surgery get relief from that. But what about the rest?

You might have noted in the last five chapters that none of the five main TN surgeries works 100 percent of the time. Or sometimes surgery knocks out the original TN pain but leaves troubling consequences in its wake, such as severe numbness or a new, burning pain – or both. Or as Dr. Brisman points out above, surgery may help initially, but the pain might return later following any of the procedures.

That's what we'll look at in this chapter... why these things happen and what can be done next when both Plan A and Plan B didn't work out the way you hoped.

Why did surgery fail?

A good place to start is to figure out why the surgery you chose didn't work. That reason might be an important clue regarding what to do next.

Sometimes it's a technical problem that prevented the surgeon from completing the procedure. For instance, some people have unusually small openings in the bone around the trigeminal nerve (the foramen ovale), which precludes the surgeon from being able to properly inflate the balloon in a balloon compression procedure. Or in glycerol injections, sometimes surgeons are unable to extract spinal fluid from the trigeminal cistern, where the glycerol is to be injected.

Technical failures might rule out that one particular procedure, but it doesn't mean you can't try one of the others. Just because a small foramen ovale prevented you from having balloon compression, for example, doesn't prevent you from having a completely successful radiosurgery. Or just because a surgeon didn't find spinal fluid in your trigeminal cistern doesn't mean you won't get relief from radiofrequency lesioning.

In the case of microvascular decompression (MVD) surgery, the main "technical failure" is that the surgeon located the trigeminal nerve but didn't find any vessels compressing it. When that happens, some surgeons pad the nerve anyway, supposing that perhaps a nearby vessel might have temporarily moved away. Others will rub the nerve root in an effort to create a mild injury that might have the same pain-disrupting effect as one of the through-the-check procedures. But many will do what we mentioned at the end of the last chapter – cut some of the nerve fibers.

MVDs also may fail because the surgeon did not find a hidden compressing vessel in a hard-to-find spot. Or the surgeon may find and pad off one vessel but miss additional, less obvious compressing vessels. As Pittsburgh neurosurgeon Dr. Peter Jannetta points out, all it takes is even a very small vein to create some rather big pain. In as many as half of the cases, more than one vessel may be compressing the nerve.

A third reason that an MVD may fail is that the padding material was insufficient or wasn't implanted in a way that solved the entire compression.

The four other surgeries also may fail even when the procedure can be carried out according to plan.

In radiofrequency lesioning, going "too light" on the heat in an effort to limit numbness might fail to fully zap the pain. Or the surgeon might not have selected the prime target to create the electrode's injury.

In glycerol injections, it's possible for the glycerol to drain out of the trigeminal cistern before it's had a chance to sufficiently injure the nerve fibers, which is why patients must sit still and upright for two hours after the procedure. Or perhaps the glycerol stayed in the right place but just didn't create enough of an injury to fully relieve the pain.

In balloon compressions, inflating the balloon a few millimeters away from prime placement might make the difference between complete relief and no help. Inflating it at too little pressure or for too little time also can cause failure.

In radiosurgery, even slightly inaccurate targeting can miss the nerve partly or maybe even miss it altogether. Delivering too low of a radiation intensity or not radiating for a long-enough time also can lead to failure.

This is why we can't emphasize enough how important it is to pick a surgeon who's been well trained and has plenty of experience in whatever technique you choose. All of the above reasons for failures tend to occur least in the most experienced hands.

That said, even the best surgeons have their failures… everything seems to go technically well during the operation, but the patient wakes up and still has pain anyway.

If that happens, first keep in mind that pain relief is not always immediate. Sometimes it takes a few days for the glycerol or balloon to do its damage or a few weeks for the nerve to heal after an offending blood vessel has been moved off the nerve after an MVD. And it's the norm for pain relief to occur weeks and even months following radiosurgery. So don't hit the panic button right away.

But if all seemed to go well and enough time passes without relief, sometimes you may never know exactly why the procedure didn't work for you.

What if it worked but the pain comes back?

Sometimes surgery knocks out the pain initially but over a period of weeks, months or years, it comes back.

Step one is to make sure you're really having a recurrence of the original pain and not some new, unrelated problem.

Cincinnati neurosurgeon Dr. John M. Tew Jr. tells of one of his surgical patients who came back to the office fearing that his TN had returned. After examining the man, Dr. Tew found that the pain really was coming from a bad tooth.

So just as getting an accurate diagnosis is critical the first time around, it's equally as important with any new pain after surgery.

Tests such as the McGill Pain Questionnaire that measure exact qualities and levels of pain can help determine if it's the same pain again – especially if the results closely match tests taken prior to surgery.

Very often, surgeons find that recurrent TN pain is not as severe as it was before the surgery. In many cases, this pain responds well to fairly low doses of carbamazepine or other TN medications.

"The first step is usually to go back on medicine," says Salt Lake City neurosurgeon Dr. Ronald Apfelbaum. "Patients might say they've tried that and it didn't work. But if the pain comes back, you often only need just a little bit of medicine to finish off the pain."

Even if medication doesn't solve the problem, at least it might provide some relief until it's determined whether or which other steps are needed.

Be aware that recurrent pain also might not have the exact quality as the original pain. Or the trigger zones may be different. Or what seems like some nerve "rumblings" behind an apparent return of the pain might turn out to be a false alarm or just some temporary, innocuous fluttering.

After all, anyone who has been through TN is quick to notice *any* new facial sensations. Before being too quick to automatically go back for more surgery, make sure the new pain really is a true recurrence and that action is warranted.

"Every recurrence doesn't mean you're going to go down the full-blown path again," Dr. Apfelbaum says.

Why pain might come back

Pain can come back after a successful surgery for a variety of reasons.

In MVDs, the most common reason is that a surgically dissected vein grew new branches, putting pressure once again on the trigeminal nerve. This is often the problem when pain comes back within the first year.

This is also why anatomy-savvy TN patients hope that if they have a compressing vessel, it's an artery, not a vein. Arteries are padded, not cut, and they don't send out new branches.

Occasionally, a blood vessel or other sharp head movement dislodges the padding between a compressing blood vessel and the nerve.

Sometimes the pad itself can cause scarring, compression or irritation, especially if the surgeon used solid Teflon felt pads instead of shredding and "fluffing" the felt into a softer form.

When pain returns later, it's often a new compression caused by a different vessel. With aging, blood vessels continue to elongate and the brain continues to sag, opening the way for new vessel/nerve contacts to occur. In other words, nothing happened to the original problem... a new one cropped up.

Later pain recurrences also can happen when the body breaks down natural implants, such as muscle or periosteum. That's why most U.S. surgeons have switched to persistent materials such as Teflon felt.

In the four other procedures, the main reason pain returns is that the nerve fibers heal themselves enough to allow nerve signals to be transmitted again.

Not surprisingly, the procedure that creates the mildest injury to the nerve fibers – glycerol injections – is also the procedure that accounts for the highest rate of pain return. That's no doubt because the nerve recovers quicker and better from this type of injury.

In each of the three through-the-cheek surgeries, patients with more numbness also tend to have better and longer-lasting pain relief. Again, that's evidence that lesser injuries mean greater healing (but greater chance pain will return) and greater injuries mean less healing (and less chance pain will return).

Healing normally is a good thing. But it's not in this case when pain relief depends on nerve signals remaining disrupted.

It's less clear whether numbness correlates with longer-lasting pain relief in the case of radiosurgery.

In MVDs, numbness does not go hand-in-hand with better and longer-lasting relief. As we mentioned earlier, one study even found that the best MVD results were in those who had no post-surgical numbness at all.

In all of the procedures, pain is more likely to come back in "atypical" or TN-2 cases than in classic, TN-1 cases. And pain is more likely to come back in patients who already failed a previous surgery.

Surgery repeats

If the new pain turns out not to be a false alarm and isn't helped by a new round of medication, another surgery is an option. None of the TN procedures are once-and-done propositions. They all can usually be repeated.

Some glycerol patients, for example, have had six or more injections, each done every few years apart after their pain came back. The injections sometimes become a bit harder to carry out technically over time, and there have been some reports of glycerol's efficacy going downhill after the fourth time. But otherwise, if the procedure can be done and it's helping, there is no limit.

Radiofrequency lesioning is easily repeated, and ensuing results are usually comparable to the first. But the main limiting factor is that the more you do, the odds keep accumulating that you'll at some point end up with dense numbness and possibly anesthesia dolorosa (that troubling and hard-to-treat combination of pain and numbness).

Balloon compressions also can be done repeatedly, but denser numbness and jaw-muscle weakness become more and more likely. Most surgeons prefer to limit these to no more than three or four procedures over a 7- to 10-year period.

As long as patients are willing and healthy, there's no limit to how many MVDs can be done. But as a practical matter, most people figure one or two of these are plenty.

San Diego neurosurgeon Dr. John Alksne says he tries to assess the likelihood of finding a readily fixable problem before doing a second MVD. For example, if a thin-cut MRI clearly shows failed padding or a blood vessel still compressing the nerve, he believes that's a good argument to go back in.

"But if I'm convinced the person who did the operation did it the proper way, found a blood vessel and moved it, and used Teflon," he says, "the chances that I'm going to find something by going back in are very slim."

Surgeons say repeat MVDs sometimes are a bit more technically difficult because of the scarring and adhesions of the first surgery, but patients often tolerate it better, perhaps because they're more familiar with the procedure.

The success rate for repeat MVDs is slightly less than that of first-time MVDs. Most report that about 80 percent of patients are pain-free after a repeat MVD – slightly under the 85-95 percent averages the first time around.

A few complications also are slightly more likely, including mild hearing loss, spinal fluid leaks and possibly more chance of numbness, especially if the surgeon partially cuts some of the nerve fibers in an effort to maximize pain relief.

In radiosurgery, a repeat procedure is generally not done until at least four to six months have passed. That's primarily to give adequate time to see if the first procedure worked.

Even then, most surgeons use about half the radiation dose on the second try and stop there to avoid giving too much radiation.

One alternative if the pain persists is to move the radiation target from the nerve root to the Gasserian ganglion. The ganglion is farther away from the brainstem and is the area surgeons first targeted before finding that radiating the nerve root gave better results. If the root already has been radiated twice, a repeat radiosurgery can be aimed at the unradiated ganglion to avoid overdosing the root. The tradeoff is that this area may not give as good or long-lasting results.

The down side to repeat radiosurgeries is that the second-time results generally are not quite as good as the first-time ones. The odds of pain coming back also are higher, and the odds of numbness and other troubling sensations also tend to go up in repeat radiosurgeries.

For example, Dr. Brisman, the New York neurosurgeon, did repeat Gamma Knife procedures on 31 of his patients, using half the first-time radiation dose, and found that only 65 percent got a 50 percent improvement in their pain. Less than one in four of these patients reported at least 90 percent pain relief without any medication. One in three went on to have other types of surgery, and nearly one in 10 experienced troubling numbness, tingling, crawling or other abnormal sensations.

Which one next?

If a first procedure fails, most patients have the option of either repeating the same procedure or trying one of the others.

Part of that decision will hinge on how well things went the first time around. If pain relief was good and lasted for at least a few years, and if the procedure was well tolerated, most patients are inclined to have the same thing done again.

On the other hand, if the procedure was uncomfortable or didn't work very well, most prefer to try a different approach.

Another variable seems to be the order in which procedures are done. In recent years, surgeons have been analyzing the results of repeat procedures, and they're finding that the success rates are affected by which procedure follows which.

MVDs, in particular, seem to be significantly less successful when they're done after one of the four nerve-injuring procedures.

Dr. Alksne looked at MVD success following failed glycerol injections and found that the success rate was about 30 percent less.

Dr. Peter Jannetta and Dr. Kenneth Casey in Pittsburgh looked at MVD success following failed Gamma Knife procedures and found a similar 30 percent drop in success rates.

And Dr. Jamal Taha in Cincinnati found the same 30 percent decline in MVD success when MVDs followed radiofrequency lesioning.

No papers have been published on MVD results following failed balloon compressions.

Surgeons suspect there may be two reasons for these drop-offs.

One is that the injuries from the four destructive procedures are counter-productive to the nerve's healing following an MVD. The premise of MVD is to move a compressing blood vessel off of the trigeminal nerve root and allow the nerve to recover from this squeezing injury. The thinking is that the nerve has a better chance to return to normal when the blood-vessel problem is corrected *before* the nerve has been damaged elsewhere.

The other possibility is the delay in having an MVD done. Several studies have shown that MVD success rates go down the longer a person has had pain – most likely because compressing blood vessels continue to cause more and more damage that at some point will never heal completely. None of the four other surgeries prevent this continuing damage from occurring at the nerve's root. So even though damaging the fibers might stop the pain signals from getting through to the brain, the presumed compressing blood vessels are still injuring the root. If years pass while a person tries and ultimately fails several other procedures, the root injury might then no longer be as correctable by MVD.

The opposite, however, seems *not* be true when destructive procedures follow MVDs.

Success rates for glycerol injections, balloon compressions, radiofrequency lesioning and radiosurgery all are similar to the rates when these are the first procedures tried – at least in classic TN cases (TN-1).

The apparent message from this seems to be that if you're ever going to go with an MVD, it's best to have it done as the first procedure rather than after the nerve has been damaged by glycerol, balloon, heat or radiation.

Not all surgeons agree with that, of course. Some say they've seen little or no difference in repeat rates among all of the procedures and would much prefer to try a more conservative approach first. They contend that the higher potential risks of open-skull surgery are not worth the slight, if any, increase in success odds by going with MVD first.

"There are no easy answers," says Dr. Tew, "but fortunately there are multiple options."

Dealing with surgical complications

Any time the trigeminal nerve is injured – intentionally or not – ill effects can occur.

As surgeons have become more experienced with the five most common TN surgeries, they've been able to figure out why many complications occur and devise ways to limit them.

Monitoring the hearing nerve during an MVD, for example, has greatly reduced the odds of hearing problems in this procedure.

In radiofrequency lesioning, the use of a curved-tip electrode has allowed more precise targeting and sharply reduced the odds of anesthesia dolorosa and other troubling sensations.

In the balloon compression procedure, patients are now routinely fitted with an external pacemaker during surgery to virtually eliminate the chance of any dangerous heart-rate slowing during the needle insertion. Surgeons also have zeroed in on ideal balloon inflation rates and times to maximize results while minimizing problems. And Detroit neurosurgeon Dr. Jeffrey Brown has devised a way to monitor the pressure in the balloon as a way to maximize success rates.

And in radiosurgery procedures, surgeons have found the ideal radiation dose range to get good results while holding down the risk of troubling numbness.

As technology and technique improves, it's likely that complication rates will continue to drop.

Nonetheless, whenever you're opening someone's head or attempting to purposely injure a nerve, there's always going to be some risk of unwanted effects. Depending on which nerve fibers are injured and how much, the results can range from minor tingling to varying levels of numbness to constant, burning nerve pain.

London oral-pain specialist Dr. Joanna Zakrzewska says there has been little research in the area of post-surgery problems. She says data is scarce on questions such as how often these problems are temporary vs. permanent, how severe the problems are and how patients are coping with their complications.

"No studies have attempted to measure the quality of life or psychological status of patients at different points post-surgery," Dr. Zakrzewska says. For that reason, she developed a questionnaire in 2003 that she hopes doctors will begin using to measure both patient satisfaction and complications after the various surgeries.

She says she's found that in her patients, numbness and other annoying feelings often ease over time – most likely because of a combination of the nerve healing and patients adapting to the altered sensations. She says when you ask them, patients say they do not like these complications, but almost all say they far prefer numbness or tingling to the earlier pain.

In any event, there's little that doctors can do to undo pains and numbness that result from surgery. An MVD, for example, won't relieve burning pain caused by a radiofrequency procedure. Nor will radiosurgery ease numbness brought on by a balloon compression. Additional surgery may actually make nerve-injury problems worse.

Usually the best therapy is to try medicines such as tricyclic antidepressants and anticonvulsants – many of the same medications used to treat TN and related face pains initially. These often help alleviate bothersome complications.

If time and medicine don't help, some people find relief from local anesthetic creams and patches, from TENS units and from some of the other complementary and alternative medicine (CAM) therapies discussed in the next few chapters. There are also surgical procedures that can be done at the pain-processing center of the brain. Or as in the case of TN pain that just won't go away no matter what, there's always the last-resort option of disconnecting the nerve at its root.

We'll discuss these surgeries later in this chapter. But first, let's take a closer look at one of the most troublesome surgical complications – anesthesia dolorosa.

Pain and numbness both?

Anesthesia dolorosa is the seemingly impossible problem of dense numbness and severe pain at the same time. This is a fortunately rare result of trigeminal nerve injury, but it's a significant problem because once you get it, it's virtually impossible to fix.

Anesthesia dolorosa occurs when the trigeminal nerve is damaged in such a way that the sense of touch is diminished or eliminated while a malfunctioning sensation of pain is left intact. That's possible because different nerve fibers in the nerve perform different functions.

One theory is that the surgery has disrupted some of the nerve fibers carrying touch signals while causing only little or no damage to the fibers carrying pain signals.

Another theory is the surgical injury has prevented nerve fibers from overlapping as they should, and that's resulting in distorted signals being sent to the brain.

A third theory is that the pain is much like "phantom limb pain," only it's happened to an amputated trigeminal nerve branch instead of an arm or leg. The rationale is that the brain has been trained over a lifetime to read nerve signals from the face. Suddenly, TN surgery has stopped these nerve signals. As a result, the brain may deal with this loss of input by setting off pain alarms.

Anesthesia dolorosa may occur in 1 to 2 percent of radiofrequency-lesioning and glycerol-injection cases and maybe 1 in 1,000 balloon compressions. It's also a possibility in partial root sections (when nerve fibers are cut). It very rarely, if ever, happens in radiosurgery or MVD.

People with anesthesia dolorosa say this condition is a strange feeling of constant, burning pain in the same area of the face that's also numb. One West Virginia woman who has it says it feels like "hundreds of bees are stinging my face and lips."

Some say they get some sharp, shooting, electric-like jabs on top of the constant burning pain, and some report a feeling of pressure or heaviness as well.

Anesthesia dolorosa is normally diagnosed based on the symptoms. But irregularities also usually show up when thermograms are done on patients' faces. Thermograms are tests that measure minute temperature differences in various parts of the body.

Unlike TN, there are no two or three drugs widely regarded as effective for anesthesia dolorosa. So what happens is doctors try an array of drugs that cross over a variety of categories, including pain-killers, anticonvulsants, antidepressants, sedatives and narcotics, until they find one that seems to help. What helps one person may not help another.

Among the medications that sometimes help some people are amitriptyline (Elavil), nortriptyline (Pamelor), clonidine (Catapres) and paroxetine (Paxil), plus some of the same medications that help

TN – carbamazepine (Tegretol, Carbatrol), oxcarbazepine (Trileptal), gabapentin (Neurontin), topiramate (Topamax), phenytoin (Dilantin), baclofen (Lioresal), valproate (Depakote) and clonazepam (Klonopin).

Dr. Steven Graff-Radford, a face-pain specialist at Cedars Sinai Medical Center in Los Angeles, says he finds that carbamazepine usually knocks out the sharper pains while nortriptyline is his favorite for the more constant pain. He says he's also had success using gabapentin, topiramate and the muscle relaxant tizanidine (Zanaflex).

San Diego neurologist Dr. James Nelson says he treats anesthesia dolorosa patients with a combination of carbamazepine and one of the tricyclic antidepressants. If that doesn't help, he prescribes opioids for pain relief.

Some anesthesia dolorosa patients also find relief from local anesthetic injections (usually lidocaine), from topical hot-pepper creams (i.e. Capsazin-P or Zostrix) or from topical anesthetics such as EMLA, an anesthetic patch that's most commonly used to numb the skin before an intravenous line is inserted.

Others have found help from acupuncture (Chapter 16), biofeedback (Chapter 20) and TENS units (Chapter 15).

In some of the worst cases, patients have turned to operations that focus on the pain centers of the brain, such as motor cortex stimulation and the DREZ (dorsal root entry zone) procedure. More on these later in this chapter.

What isn't a good idea is to try even more destructive procedures on the trigeminal nerve itself. That usually only makes things worse.

Other avenues

If a surgery or two has failed, you've still got plenty of options. Repeating the same procedure or moving onto one of the other "big five" TN surgeries are just two of them.

Acupuncture, upper-cervical chiropractic, nutrition therapy and many other CAM therapies are all still options, if you've never tried them. Failed surgery doesn't mean there's now no chance one of these won't work for you or at least help somewhat.

Several other surgical procedures also are options. Some of these actually pre-date the big five procedures but were abandoned because the newer procedures proved to be more effective and longer lasting. Although they may be seldom used anymore, one of these older procedures may still turn out to be a good solution for you.

As medical science better understands the brain, surgeons also are looking into the newer field of stimulating or selectively disabling parts of the brain that process pain signals.

Let's start with a look at some of the older procedures.

"Peripheral" nerve treatments

Long before surgeons began operating on the trigeminal ganglion where the nerve's three main branches come together, the main surgery targets were the nerve's many small branches in the face.

These so-called *"peripheral"* branches are much easier to reach, and procedures on the branches usually can be done with the patient awake and under local anesthesia.

The basic idea of peripheral nerve procedures is much the same as the radiofrequency, glycerol and balloon surgeries — to cause enough selective damage to the branches to stop pain signals from getting through.

Signals can be stopped in three main ways. The branches can be injured mechanically (by cutting or removing them), injured thermally (by heat or cold) or injured chemically (by injecting them with alcohol, glycerol, phenol and other substances).

Depending on which part of the face is triggering the pain, specific branches can be injured while avoiding damage to branches that serve other parts of the face. Most of these procedures are done, when possible, through the mouth to avoid scarring of the face.

On the plus side, peripheral procedures can be done quickly and easily in a dental or oral-surgery office. General anesthesia is not needed. Serious and permanent complications are rare, and there have been no reports of death related to peripheral procedures.

Because these are the least invasive of the TN surgeries, they usually can be done on the elderly and those in poor health. The immediate results are good, albeit with a high likelihood of at least some numbness. If pain comes back, peripheral treatments can usually be repeated.

The down side is that the pain relief isn't very lasting. Nerve branches have the "bad" habit (from a TN point of view) of healing fairly quickly. When they heal, the numbness usually goes away, but the pain also usually comes back.

Dr. Zakrzewska says that in all of the peripheral procedures, the average time of pain relief is only 9 to 18 months. After four years, only about 10 percent of those who had peripheral treatments are still pain-free, she says.

For most people, that doesn't stack up very well compared to the other five surgeries. When Dr. Zakrzewska surveyed TN patients at a Trigeminal Neuralgia Association conference, most said they'd like to be able to expect at least five years of pain relief from any surgical procedure.

Besides the relative short-lasting effect of peripheral treatments, they aren't entirely painless even under local anesthesia. They also tend not to work as well in people who don't have distinct pain-trigger zones. And although peripheral treatments work quickly, in about half of the cases the relief isn't complete enough for patients to get off of their TN medications altogether.

At least some numbness (usually temporary) can be expected, and patients sometimes experience tingling or crawling sensations for varying times afterward. Some swelling or bruising also is common around the treatment site for a few days.

Complications are almost always confined to the treated branch. Other than occasional, temporary double vision and some rare, mild and temporary chewing difficulties, there's little chance of problems cropping up elsewhere in the face or head. Even numbness is normally confined just to the area of the face served by the injured branch.

Because the five newer TN surgeries give better and longer-lasting relief, peripheral procedures are done sparingly these days. Their main role is in people who are too old or sick to undergo other procedures, those who have failed other procedures and those willing to accept numbness and the high likelihood of only short-term relief in exchange for the limited invasiveness of the procedures.

Peripheral procedures are usually performed by oral or maxillofacial surgeons or dentists as opposed to neurosurgeons.

These procedures include:

- Neurectomies, which involve cutting and removing sections of nerves.
- Chemical injections, in which liquids such as alcohol, glycerol and phenol are injected into a nerve branch.
- Cryotherapy, in which a probe is used to freeze a nerve branch.
- Peripheral radiofrequency, in which an electrode is used to heat a nerve branch.

Let's take a closer look at them and their success rates.

Neurectomies

Surgeries that sever and/or remove nerve branches are among the earliest TN procedures, dating at least to the early 1700s.

In those days, though, surgeons didn't know the difference between trigeminal nerve branches and facial nerve branches. And so sometimes when they cut nerves out, the patient's face became paralyzed instead of pain-free.

Today, surgeons can zero in on the exact branches that are triggering TN pain and do away with them with a few quick cuts.

In this procedure, the surgeon numbs the area with a local anesthetic, exposes the branch underneath the skin, then dissects and removes the tiny section of nerve. By applying wax or similar sealants to the opening through which that dissected branch comes into the face, nerve regrowth can be prevented or at least slowed.

Of the peripheral treatments, neurectomies offer the best chance of longer relief. Success reports have been all over the board, ranging anywhere from 25 percent to 85 percent pain relief after one year. Dr. Zakrzewska says on average, she's found that pain relief from neurectomies lasts between two and three years.

The main drawback is that a neurectomy is guaranteed to create at least partial numbness. Occasionally, pain spreads to another branch of the nerve after a neurectomy stopped it in the first branch. One likely explanation is that the underlying cause of the pain is still at work – a blood vessel compressing the trigeminal nerve at its root near the brainstem. As increasing damage occurs there, additional nerve fibers are injured that spread pain to additional parts of the face.

Neurectomies can be repeated, but doctors have found that relief tends to be less lasting the second time around.

Chemical injections

All sorts of caustic and nerve-injuring chemicals have been injected into people's faces over the years in an effort to stop TN pain.

One of the most popular before the five newer surgeries came along was ethyl alcohol. This was the substance of choice from the early to mid-1900s.

Alcohol worked fairly well up front, but doctors quickly found that just about everyone got marked numbness from it, and nearly everyone got their pain back six months to five years later. Still, it was the best therapy of the time.

In one study of 1,500 alcohol-injection cases, the average pain relief turned out to be only between 8 and 16 months. Dr. Zakrzewska says that after just one year, only about 25 percent to 50 percent of alcohol-injected patients are pain-free.

Also a problem with alcohol is that it has been known to cause anesthesia dolorosa in up to 2 to 5 percent of the cases. Some patients also have had temporary inflamed corneas, temporary double vision and temporary chewing difficulties after alcohol treatments.

Alcohol also can scar the nerve, which may limit the effectiveness of other surgeries later, and it's more painful than cryotherapy (discussed below).

Two studies in the 1950s reported that about one-third of alcohol-injection patients were getting little or no relief from the treatment, even initially.

For all of those reasons, alcohol injections are seldom used anymore.

More recently, glycerol has been used instead of alcohol. This is the same thick, alcohol-like liquid that's used in glycerol injections into the Gasserian ganglion. Only in this case, nerve branches are injected instead of bathing the ganglion in this mildly nerve-corrosive liquid.

Glycerol doesn't seem to cause as many complications as alcohol, but it also doesn't work as well as when it's injected around the ganglion. One European study of 13 patients found that peripheral glycerol did not help two of the patients at all, and the rest got relief for 3 to 24 months. Half had at least some numbness.

Dr. Zakrzewska reports similar results in 22 patients. Five got no relief, and the rest had their pain back in one to 24 months. Only half of the patients reported complete relief in the first place. Numbness was common but mild.

A 2001 study reported in the Journal of Oral and Maxillofacial Surgery was the most optimistic, claiming 64 percent of patients were still pain-free after one year.

Phenol is another alcohol-like substance that's been occasionally used, often in a solution with glycerol. It's had about the same results as glycerol.

One 1999 study of 18 patients injected with 10 percent phenol in glycerol reported that after one year, 50 percent of the patients were pain-free.

Cryotherapy

A third peripheral treatment that's been used since the 1850s is cryotherapy, sometimes called *"cryoanalgesia."*

This technique uses a probe (made cold by nitrous oxide, liquid nitrogen or other refrigerant) to deliver sub-freezing temperatures to the nerve.

With the patient numbed by local anesthesia, the doctor first exposes the targeted branch of the nerve and then alternately freezes and thaws it. Two or three two-minute freeze-thaw cycles are typically used.

Using cold to treat pain actually is one of the earliest therapies, predating even Hippocrates. The earliest recorded TN cold treatment dates to 1850 when doctors used an ice-cold salt solution on the face with some success.

Other than swelling and pain around the incision immediately after the procedure, the main down side for patients is numbness. But Dr. Zakrzewska says the temporary numbness that results from cryotherapy is less bothersome to most people than the numbness of neurectomies and alcohol injections. Numbness typically lasts from six weeks to three months.

About 14 percent of cryotherapy patients have temporary chewing difficulties, and nearly 5 percent develop an infection, which usually resolves with antibiotics.

It's also not unusual for cryotherapy patients to report a somewhat different feeling of face pain or discomfort after their treatment. One 1993 British study of 145 patients found that one in three say they were left with a dull ache, a throbbing type of pain or a feeling of "pins and needles." Usually these sensations subside as the nerve heals.

Cryotherapy's pain-relieving effects are significantly less lasting than neurectomies. In the 145-patient British study, only 27 percent were pain-free after one year. Dr. Zakrzewska says that in her experience, pain typically returns in nine to 14 months. The treatment is repeatable, however.

Some suggest that better results might be possible by using colder temperatures (down around minus 180 degrees centigrade for at least one minute) and then quickly rewarming the tissue within one minute to avoid nerve damage.

Five German oral surgeons also reported in a 2002 paper in the Journal of Oral and Maxillofacial Surgery that a new cryoprobe can effectively freeze trigeminal nerve branches without having to cut into the skin and expose the branch.

This probe is inserted into the mouth and used to freeze selected portions of the lower and middle nerve branches. The German surgeons tried the new cryoprobe on 19 TN patients and found the results similar to the older cryotherapy method – all got relief for at least 6 months, but after that, 13 of the 19 had their pain back within the first year.

They conclude that at least the procedure is easier on the patient and all but eliminates the threat of infection. This procedure also is repeatable.

Peripheral radiofrequency

One other peripheral treatment being tried in a few clinics is a radiofrequency lesion delivered to the nerve's branches instead of the ganglion. This involves inserting an electrode against the nerve branch and heating it until it's disabled.

Though simpler and less risky than the ganglion radiofrequency procedure, peripheral radiofrequency also hasn't been nearly as effective. One 71-patient 1986 study by Drs. J.M. Gregg and E.W. Small found the average period of pain relief was only about 9 months and that 68 percent of the patients had their pain back within one year.

On the plus side, numbness seems to be less than with neurectomy and alcohol injections, and other than some bruising around the injection site, complications are low. It's also repeatable.

If all else fails...

For the rare, totally unremitting case that just isn't responding to anything else, a few other options remain.

One is severing the trigeminal nerve at its root. This was a common solution up until the 1960s whenever medicine and peripheral treatments weren't working.

In this procedure, the surgeon goes into the patient's head through a small opening behind the ear – the same entry as an MVD. But instead of seeking to put a pad between the trigeminal nerve and an offending blood vessel near where the nerve connects to the brainstem, the aim is to just snip the nerve at its root.

Snipping the nerve almost always leaves dense and permanent facial numbness, but it also "disconnects" the pain. It's like pulling the plug on all sensations on that side of the face. For those battling the worst and most stubborn cases of TN, even that usually comes as a welcome trade-off.

Because the sensory and motor portions of the nerve are distinct, it's possible for surgeons to completely cut the sensory portion without affecting the part of the nerve that controls chewing.

This procedure also does not cause the face to droop. Those muscles are controlled primarily by the separate facial nerve, which is not harmed.

A limiting factor is that patients have to be healthy enough to undergo the general anesthesia and rigors of this major surgery.

For the elderly and those in poor health, radiosurgery, the peripheral procedures and possibly one of the through-the-cheek surgeries are better options, if they haven't already been tried.

The DREZ procedure

Another surgery sometimes tried when all else fails is the so-called DREZ procedure. This is also major surgery that selectively injures the nucleus (origin) of the trigeminal nerve in the upper spinal cord.

DREZ stands for "dorsal root entry zone," and the procedure also is sometimes called "trigeminal tractotomy" or "trigeminal nucleotomy."

With the patient asleep, the surgeon makes an incision in the back of the neck, locates the nucleus of the nerve and then uses an electrode to heat the nerve tissue. A few surgeons use a laser to injure the nerve, and fewer still use a scalpel to cut nerve fibers. If all goes well, the damage will stop pain without causing dense numbness or injury to the nerve's motor function.

Patients are typically in the hospital for five to seven days.

The main drawback is that there are other nerves very close by, and sometimes this surgery injures those. Nearly 40 percent of patients have experienced arm- or leg-coordination difficulties, and there's also been occasional hearing loss and weakness in the arm or leg on one side.

Dr. John P. Gorecki, a neurosurgeon at Duke University Medical Center, says physical therapy usually resolves the movement problems, but many people "continue to report that their arm or leg just doesn't feel right."

In an effort to reduce complications, Dr. Gorecki says he and other surgeons have begun using electrodes to pre-test the function of nerve fibers before damaging them. "By identifying the places where the nerve seems most sensitive, we are able to get pain relief with fewer lesions," he says.

Dr. Gorecki says this testing has sharply cut complication rates. For example, only 10 percent of patients have coordination problems with pre-testing in comparison to the nearly 40 percent with those problems in earlier surgeries.

Success rates for the DREZ procedure have been improving in recent years. In the most recent study from Duke University, 67 percent of patients reported good to excellent results after one year, 11 percent had fair results and 22 percent got little or no relief. A few years earlier, only about half were getting good to excellent relief.

Pain relief from DREZ isn't always permanent either. As with other procedures, 20 to 30 percent of patients get pain back over time.

DREZ procedures seem to be slightly more effective earlier and less effective in people who have had pain for many years.

Because of the complications and limited success rate, DREZ obviously isn't a front-line treatment for TN. However, it does offer some measure of hope for the person who didn't get relief from any of the other procedures.

It's also a surgical option for those with troubling anesthesia dolorosa or persistent "atypical" TN (TN-2) that isn't helped by medication. And it's been used on a few occasions in patients who had TN caused by tumors but had persistent pain even after the tumor was removed.

"The DREZ procedure is useful for patients who fail other treatments for facial pain," says Dr. Gorecki, "but I would not advise it for those who simply have typical trigeminal neuralgia."

Deep brain stimulation

One other different approach for dealing with unremitting pain is to stimulate certain parts of the brain with constant, low amounts of electricity. Two techniques have been tried, and the aim of both is to help the brain's anti-pain system function more effectively.

The constant electrical stimulation either gives an alternate sensation that distracts the brain from focusing on pain in the face or possibly causes changes in the areas of the brain responsible for "reading" pain signals from the face.

Both procedures involve implanting electrodes into the brain. These electrodes are attached to an implanted, battery-operated stimulator device that produces the low-grade electric current.

The first technique is called *"deep brain stimulation,"* and it's an experimental treatment that's been under trial since the 1980s at several U.S. clinics.

In this procedure, surgeons insert a thin electrode through a small opening in the skull into the thalamus, a part of the brain where pain sensation occurs. The stimulation levels are tested and adjusted over a few days, and if significant improvement is found, the stimulator is implanted.

When it works, patients report a sense of warmth or mild buzzing in place of the painful sensations.

The main down side is that deep brain stimulation hasn't been terribly successful. The average success rate four years out is only 25 to 35 percent, although those figures have improved with experience in recent years.

Seizures can occur if the stimulation level is set too high, and as with any open surgery, infection also is possible. Strokes also are a rare but possible complication.

Motor cortex stimulation

More promising is a newer variation of deep brain stimulation called *"motor cortex stimulation."* This procedure places one or two small contact plates on the surface of the brain covering (the dura), over the cortex region that controls movement to the upper third of the face.

It's been found that stimulating this region with low-grade electrical current reduces activity in the thalamus, where pain is felt. As with deep brain stimulation, motor cortex stimulation is still an experimental procedure being trialed in only a few U.S. clinics.

Also as with deep brain stimulation, the electrodes are tested for a few days while stimulation levels are adjusted. If the stimulation is working, the stimulator device is implanted permanently.

In this case, levels are set high enough to help the pain but not so high as to cause muscle twitching. Seizures also can occur if levels are set too high.

Motor cortex stimulation usually doesn't stop pain altogether, but it's been giving a majority of patients at least 50 percent improvement. When used in patients with unrelenting neuropathic (nerve-injury) pain, worldwide reports are showing that nearly three out of four patients are experiencing at least 50 percent pain improvement two years after their stimulator was implanted.

Detroit neurosurgeon Dr. Jeffrey Brown, one American surgeon who has done motor cortex stimulation procedures, says the approach gives a potential solution to the kinds of pains that aren't well addressed by other procedures.

These include: neuropathic and deafferentation pains; severe "atypical" TN (TN-2) that hasn't responded to other treatments; pain related to strokes; severe post-herpetic neuralgia, and possibly painful numbnesses such as anesthesia dolorosa. (So far the success rate in anesthesia dolorosa patients is lower than neuropathic pains, with only about one in three getting significant relief.)

With computers now helping to guide electrode placement and other technical improvements, Dr. Brown believes success rates for the whole realm of brain stimulation will increase over time.

"This is not a new technique," he says. "What is new is that technology is now available to do it better, and more people around the world are doing it."

"My last visit turned out to provide the most pain relief I have had in eight years," said Bridget Kelly, a Wisconsin woman who had the motor cortex stimulation procedure done at the Cleveland Clinic in 2003. "This is saying a lot, given that I have tried over 15 medications, dental work and other treatments. I am no longer bed-ridden and am slowly regaining my life."

Kelly was diagnosed with both atypical facial pain and trigeminal neuropathy and was not a candidate for other surgeries because her constant, burning pain was apparently resulting from a degeneration of her nerve fibers. No medication helped.

She says motor cortex stimulation brought her a 50 percent improvement within the first two months.

"It's possible the effects will wear off or I could build up a resistance," she says, "but I am more optimistic than I have ever been."

CHAPTER 15

NOT SURGERY, NOT PILLS: THERAPIES BEYOND MAINSTREAM MEDICINE

"Some people say, 'No one is going to put a hole in my head and operate around my brain unless there's NO other treatment.'"
—Florida neurosurgeon Dr. Albert L. Rhoton Jr.

Let's face it. No one wants to have his skull opened or her nerves heated, irradiated or injected unless it's really necessary. And most people would rather get off anticonvulsant medications if there's a gentler, less-sedating way to control their pain.

That, in a nutshell, is a big part of the appeal of a whole range of non-surgery, non-medication therapies commonly lumped under the rather broad heading of "complementary and alternative medicine" (CAM) treatments. CAM therapies such as acupuncture, chiropractic, megavitamins, herbs and the like offer the lure of pain relief in a minimally invasive way.

This whole field, though, is filled with as many questions as answers – and a lot of sometimes bitter disagreement. On one hand, you may find practitioners and face-pain patients who tell of miraculous pain relief from CAM treatments. On the other hand, you'll find doctors and disillusioned patients who believe CAM is a hodgepodge of unproven gimmicks and sometimes even downright quackery.

It all can get pretty confusing when you encounter such diametrically opposing views of the exact same treatments. That's what we'll take a look at in this and the next three chapters on acupuncture, chiropractic and nutrition therapies.

Rising CAM trends?

There's been some evidence that Americans are becoming more interested in CAM therapies since the early 1990s. One often quoted report comes from Dr. David Eisenberg and six other researchers at Boston's Beth Israel Deaconess Medical Center.

They surveyed more than 2,000 people in 1997 and concluded that Americans paid more visits to alternative-medicine practitioners that year than to primary-care physicians.

The Boston researchers also found that:

- More than 42 percent of those surveyed used at least one of 16 types of CAM therapies in 1997 compared to just under 34 percent in 1991.
- Visits to CAM practitioners rose 27 percent between 1991 and 1997, with more of that increase coming from new CAM users as opposed to more visits by existing CAM users.
- CAM users paid more than $12 billion out-of-pocket for their CAM treatments in 1997, a number that exceeded out-of-pocket expenses for all U.S. hospitals.
- CAM therapies were most used to treat chronic conditions, such as back problems, anxiety, depression and headaches – conditions that mainstream medicine isn't terribly effective at "fixing."
- And, the CAM therapies that increased most in popularity were herbal medicine, massage, megavitamins, self-help groups, folk remedies, energy healing (such as Therapeutic Touch and magnets) and homeopathy (which uses low doses of mostly natural substances to promote healing).

Consumer Reports magazine also surveyed 46,000 of its readers for a May 2000 article called "The Mainstreaming of Alternative Medicine" and found that more than 40 percent of those people have tried CAM therapies. That number rose to more than half in the 35-49 age group.

Consumer Reports also found that mainstream medicine is becoming a bit more accepting of at least some CAM therapies. Of CAM users who told their doctors about their CAM treatments, 55 percent of the doctors expressed approval.

But despite these apparent trends (which not everyone accepts, by the way), *Consumer Reports* also found that mainstream medicine is still America's top treatment choice. "For nearly all medical conditions, readers said they got the best results from prescription drugs and from surgery, when it was recommended," the magazine reported. "Even among people who tried herbal therapies, prescription drugs won higher marks for all medical conditions."

Exactly what is CAM?

Before we get into details about particular CAM therapies and which ones might relieve TN pain, it helps to understand what these therapies are and how they differ from mainstream Western medicine.

Some definitions of CAM tell more about what it's *not* than what it is.

For example, some describe CAM therapies as those that, in general, are not taught in medical schools, not used in hospitals and not covered by insurance. Even the National Institutes of Health's National Center for Complementary and Alternative Medicine official CAM definition is: "A group of diverse medical and health-care systems, practices and products that are not presently considered to be part of conventional medicine."

NCCAM goes on to define complementary therapy as techniques that are used *together with* conventional medicine, such as how aromatherapy might be used to relax patients after a surgery.

It defines alternative medicine as treatments that are used *in place of* conventional medicine, such as using megavitamins to treat cancer instead of opting for surgery or radiation.

There's also a third term you may hear – *"integrative medicine."* NCCAM says this is a treatment plan that combines a mainstream medical practice with a CAM therapy that has at least some scientific backing.

NCCAM, the U.S. government's lead agency in researching and reporting on CAM therapies, breaks CAM down into five main categories:

1.) **Alternative medical systems,** which includes homeopathic and naturopathic medicines as well as non-Western medicines such as traditional Chinese medicine and India's Ayurveda system.

2.) **Mind-body interventions,** which includes techniques to enhance the mind's ability to affect body functions, such as hypnosis, prayer, meditation, mental healing, and art, music and dance therapies.

3.) **Biologically based therapies,** which use substances found in nature, such as herbs, vitamins and food supplements as well as natural but scientifically unproven agents such as shark cartilage or bee pollen.

4.) **Manipulative and body-based methods,** which involve specialized movements of the body, including chiropractic treatments, osteopathic medicine, craniosacral therapy and massage.

5.) **Energy therapies,** which involve applying energy fields that purportedly influence the body, such as magnets, Therapeutic Touch and Reiki.

CAM treatments can range from self-care (i.e. using over-the-counter creams, vitamins and food supplements) to group sessions (i.e. a yoga class or a seminar on meditation) to individual sessions by a professional (i.e. chiropractic adjustments or acupuncture treatments).

Many CAM treatments share some common traits, says Dr. B. Alex White, director of Kaiser Permanente's Oregon Center for Complementary and Alternative Medicine in Craniofacial Disorders.

"The Western approach is more standardized," he says. "We think of diseases with specific causes. Once you have a set of symptoms, we give a name to it... In CAM therapies, treatments tend to be more individualized and changes may be made throughout treatment."

Dr. White says CAM therapies also tend to:

- Address the patient's mental and spiritual issues as well as the physical problem.
- Mobilize the patient's capacity to heal.
- Focus on healing rather than curing.
- Place an emphasis on a strong rapport between the patient and practitioner.
- Offer a multi-faceted treatment program as opposed to a single modality.
- Effect more gradual changes that may have a bigger effect on the patient's peace, attitude and overall well-being than on the clinical symptoms.

"The philosophical approach of most alternative methods is that it is necessary to treat the whole person, not the disease," wrote neuralgian Wren Osborn on the Facial Neuralgia Resources web site (www.facial-neuralgia.org). "The belief generally is that disease is a result of an imbalance in the whole person, and restoring the balance allows the body to heal itself.

"This is in contrast to the traditional Western method of treating a specific disease with a specific remedy – usually a drug or surgical procedure," says Osborn, who has been helped by CAM therapies. "The alternative approach also recognizes the individuality of each person and often devises a specific remedy or approach for each person. Quite a contrast to the cookie-cutter approach of Western traditional medicine."

One other trait most CAM therapies have in common – there's little scientific research to document their safety and effectiveness.

"There are lots of hypothetical reasons why these things might work and anecdotal evidence galore," says Dr. Allen H. Neims, a pharmacology professor and director of the University of Florida's Center for Spirituality and Health. "But often there's meager evidence, at least in the Western sense of the word."

Most of the support for CAM therapies comes from patient testimonials, practitioner claims and case studies that typically don't compare treated patients to similar patients who got no treatment or another type of treatment.

That doesn't necessarily mean CAM treatments don't work or aren't worth exploring, as people who are helped by them will quickly tell you.

As Osborn puts it, "An individual has to take charge, read, think and experiment in order to reach optimal health. And why settle for less? That doesn't mean that Western medicine should be rejected, just judged with a healthy dose of skepticism. But it also means studying non-traditional approaches with an open mind, while retaining the healthy dose of skepticism."

We'll discuss these issues in more detail below. But first, let's look at who's using CAM and why.

CAM's roots

The boundary of where mainstream medicine ends and CAM begins is a murky one. The lines tend to change over time depending on factors such as new research and our changing values and opinions.

Through the middle 1800s, conventional American medicine *was* very much like today's homeopaths and naturopaths. If you got sick in those days, the doctor would come by with his black bag of herbs and oils, listen carefully to your description of the ailment and then custom-concoct a treatment.

That began to change in the later 1800s when researchers discovered germs' role in disease and began to develop antiseptic techniques and better anesthesia and surgery. William Osler's 1892 *"The Principles and Practice of Medicine"* laid the foundation for our scientific- and research-based medical system.

As new drugs and improved surgeries began solving one acute illness after another during the 20th century, many older therapies fell by the wayside.

"Although most of the other health-care systems and their therapies did not disappear, they were considered by most of the public and the mainstream medical community to be unscientific relics of the past," the White House Commission on Complementary and Alternative Medicine Policy wrote in a March 2002 paper.

Ironically, mainstream medicine's success seems to be a factor in our recent renewed interest in CAM therapies.

Improvements in health care sharply increased Americans' life expectancy, which has led to a burgeoning field of chronic and hard-to-treat conditions related to aging. Increasingly, Americans are seeking medical care for problems such as arthritis, chronic back pain, heart ailments and cancer as opposed to one-time widespread acute threats such as smallpox, polio, tuberculosis and assorted infections.

Why people are interested in CAM

"Fixing" chronic conditions like back pain and arthritis has proved more difficult for mainstream medicine than curing acute illnesses. Not surprisingly, the main reason people give for seeking out CAM therapies is that they either weren't helped by conventional methods or they believe CAM therapies will work better.

Another big chunk of CAM users say they sought alternatives because they didn't like the side effects of conventional medicines. In the case of TN, many say they don't like the medications but also don't like the possibility of facial numbness or some of the other potential complications of surgery.

Still others complain about the lack of time their doctors give them. Two common lines heard at TN support group meetings are: "All my doctor wanted to do was give me some pills and get on to the next patient," and "He didn't explain anything to me."

Fragmented care – seeing one specialist for this and another for that – is a fourth complaint that drives some to a CAM practitioner. Most patients prefer someone who views them as a person in pain rather than as a walking collection of symptoms to be sorted into the right box.

It's not just dissatisfaction with mainstream medicine that's fueling CAM's apparent growth. CAM therapies offer a variety of features that many people find appealing.

Stanford University researcher Dr. John A. Astin got a surprising answer when he surveyed 1,035 Americans in 1998 on why people seek out CAM therapies.

"The majority of alternative-medicine users appear to be doing so not so much as a result of being dissatisfied with conventional medicine," Dr. Astin concluded, "but largely because they find these health-care alternatives to be more congruent with their own values, beliefs and philosophical orientations toward health and life."

CAM users often say they like being treated as a "whole person" trying to cope with the mental, emotional and spiritual issues of chronic pain as well as the physical issue. In particular, CAM users say they like CAM practitioners who listen to them, develop a caring relationship and give them a say in their own treatment decisions. Even if the therapy doesn't help the pain, at least they may end up with more peace of mind, an improved outlook or a feeling that they've at least played a role in trying to find a solution.

Dr. Neims, who has studied and written about CAM's role in medicine, believes this kind of rapport may be as important – maybe even more so – than the treatment itself.

He says that whether a practitioner is using a homeopathic medicine, an herb or a magnet, "these therapies do help some people. We just don't know whether it's their magnet or their voice."

Whether you call that "power of suggestion," a "placebo effect" or something else, healing seems to be aided when both the practitioner and patient firmly believe a treatment works, Dr. Neims says.

NCCAM and the White House Commission on CAM Policy say there are other reasons for CAM's attractiveness:

- The appeal of tapping the body's own healing abilities, which is a tenet of many CAM therapies.
- Alluring testimonials from people who say they've had impressive results.
- Individualized treatment plans instead of a perceived "cookie-cutter" approach.
- Treatments that are "natural" or gentler than mainstream therapies.

NCCAM also attributes part of the renewed interest to widespread advertising of and greater media attention to CAM approaches.

And Dr. Neims says there's another reason – some of these treatments really *do* help some of the time.

Who's using CAM today

The overwhelming majority of CAM's growth seems to be on the complementary side as opposed to the alternative side. Dr. Astin's Stanford research found that less 5 percent of CAM users had completely ditched mainstream medicine in favor of an alternate approach.

Most are using a CAM treatment in addition to a more conventional therapy, for example, using hot-pepper cream or getting chiropractic adjustments in addition to taking carbamazepine tablets.

Dr. Astin also found that those with back pain and neck pain are most likely to seek CAM therapy and that CAM users tend to have higher-than-average education, poorer-than-average overall health and a "holistic" orientation toward health. Many users also tend to have had a transformational experience that changed their view of the world, he found.

The *Consumer Reports* survey found the most likely CAM users to be people in severe pain (including those back- and neck-pain sufferers) and those suffering from stress-related ailments (anxiety, depression, insomnia, etc.)

People's varying outlooks and goals also play a key role in who's more likely to try CAM methods, says Dr. Neims.

"Many people who seek therapy, especially alternative or complementary therapy, are seeking gentle yet effective treatments with minimal adverse actions," he says. "More powerful is not necessarily preferred if the adverse effects are also increased."

In TN, the majority of people who try CAM are those who have failed at least one of the more conventional approaches. This includes those who were allergic to the front-line medications, those who didn't get good relief from medication, those who had troubling side effects from medicine and those who have failed one or more of the surgeries. However, a few are using CAM approaches as their first or main treatment.

Those with so-called "atypical" TN (TN-2), nerve-injury pains (i.e. neuropathic and deafferentation cases) and mixed face pains that stray outside the TN umbrella are others who are more likely to use CAM therapies.

In many cases, CAM users are using more than one CAM approach at a time. It's not unusual for patients to experiment with a variety of therapies until they find one or a combination that works best.

Most of these therapies do not preclude others. For example, one patient may find relief through a combination of acupuncture and herbal therapy. Another may be helped more by a combination of upper-cervical chiropractic and dietary changes. It's always a good idea, though, to check with your physicians and CAM practitioners before adding new therapies.

How to determine if CAM is right for you

Some people are more likely than others to be comfortable trying CAM therapies. "Probably the most important first step in choosing the best path is to reflect about who you are as a person: body, mind and spirit, and as a member of a family and community," says Dr. Allen Neims.

He offers the following two sets of questions as some of the points that might help you decide whether CAM is right for you:

Questions about yourself:
- Are you the sort of person who tends to distrust modern science, or to almost worship it?
- Do you need to have scientific evidence before you believe something? If so, how much and what kind? What do you accept just on "faith?"
- Do you tend to believe or disbelieve the things family members, neighbors or even strangers tell you?
- How much do you believe in "natural cures," "balance leads to healing" and "energy that flows about the body and between people?" Some people are open to these concepts, others discount them completely.
- What do you believe caused your illness? Different therapies might make more or less sense depending on your thoughts here.
- What do you fear about your illness? How do different therapies and therapists address them? It may be that some of the fears are unfounded.
- What do you fear and distrust about modern medicine? Some of these may be unfounded, too, but if not, what therapies avoid those fears and distrusts?
- How is your family and community life being impacted? If they're largely unaffected, you may be more willing to try low-impact therapies even if the prospect of helping is lower.
- How patient or impatient are you? If you're hurting badly or impatient to "get back to normal," you may be more inclined to go for a higher-impact therapy even if it means more risk of unwanted effects.
- How compliant are you? If you have a hard time sticking to something over a period of time, you may be better off with a once-and-done or short-term therapy as opposed to long-term therapy.

Questions about therapists:
- What are you looking for from your doctor or therapist? Do you want a partner or do you want someone to tell you what to do?
- Would you be more pleased with a confident therapist who expressed no doubts about the value of his or her approach or would you prefer a cautious person?
- Do you want someone in a white coat and a simple office with plain walls or someone in flowing robes, nice music and relaxing atmospheres?
- How much time and money are you willing to devote to therapy?
- Do you need something covered by insurance?

The issue of evidence

Before we go too much farther down CAM road, a few cautions are in order.

First, as we mentioned earlier, the evidence behind most CAM treatments is largely anecdotal. Most of these treatments have undergone little, if any, scientific testing for their effectiveness in helping TN – or other conditions, for that matter.

Here's what the 2002 White House Commission on CAM Policy report had to say: "Most CAM therapies that are currently being used by consumers have not been studied adequately in regard to either efficacy or safety. Even when evidence indicates that a particular CAM approach or modality is safe and effective for a particular condition, new safety concerns may arise when it is used in conjunction with conventional medications, which is the way most consumers use CAM."

Dr. Stephen Barrett, a Pennsylvania psychiatrist who runs a consumer-health advocacy service called QuackWatch (www.quackwatch.org), is an even harsher critic of this dearth of evidence.

"Under the rules of science, people who make the claims bear the burden of proof," he says. "It is their responsibility to conduct suitable studies and report them in sufficient detail to permit evaluation and confirmation by others."

Dr. Barrett says anecdotal evidence is notoriously unreliable. "We all tend to believe what others tell us about personal experiences," he says. "But separating cause and effect from coincidence can be difficult… That's why testimonial evidence is forbidden in scientific articles, is usually inadmissible in court and is not used to evaluate whether or not drugs should be legally marketable. Imagine what would happen if the FDA decided that clinical trials were too expensive and therefore drug approval would be based on testimonial letters or interviews with a few patients."

He says CAM practitioners too often "regard personal experience, subjective judgment and emotional satisfaction as preferable to objectivity and hard evidence."

Dr. Neims agrees there's a difference between having success with a therapy in your case vs. projecting it to work for others.

"Although I believe strongly in scientific evidence and clinical trials," he says, "I also believe that for an individual patient, how he or she feels and functions is most important. It is still valid for me to love a book even if 99 percent of people derived nothing from it. For my well-being, my own experience is important. But for my therapist or me to state publicly that this thing works – other than for me – demands clinical trials."

A big part of the federal government's NCCAM office is to evaluate and report on the safety and effectiveness of CAM therapy. So far, only a few have produced compelling evidence. Among them:

- Acupuncture has been shown to help nausea, acute dental pain, headaches, temporomandibular joint dysfunctions, fibromyalgia and depression.
- St. John's wort is helpful in treating mild to moderate depression.
- Herbal and glucosamine therapy is helpful in treating arthritis.
- And meditation and guided imagery are effective in managing pain and relieving stress and anxiety.

Ongoing reports about other therapies can be found on NCCAM's web site at www.nccam.nih.gov. The Cochrane Library is another good resource for CAM research. Its web site is www.cochrane.org. For links to specific associations and organizations involved in various CAM therapies, try NIH's Directory of Information Resources Online at http://dirline.nlm.nih.gov.

The 2000 *Consumer Reports* survey also attempted to gauge CAM's effectiveness by asking its CAM-using readers to rate what therapies worked best for them in 10 different disorders. Prescription drugs and surgery topped the list in most cases, although some CAM therapies also scored very well. On the other hand, other CAM therapies turned out to be of very little help to most.

In treating arthritis, for example, *Consumer Reports'* readers ranked prescription pain-killers, exercise, megavitamins, massage and physical therapy as the top five treatments. Acupuncture, ginkgo and magnet therapy brought up the bottom, with more than half of the people who reported using those three therapies saying they gave little or no relief.

In back pain, the readers ranked massage, chiropractic treatment and exercise as their three most effective treatments with glucosamine, magnet therapy and garlic bringing up the rear.

With chronic headaches, the readers ranked prescription drugs, massage and chiropractic treatment as their top three and meditation, dietary changes and physical therapy as their bottom three.

TN and related face pains were not included in the magazine's survey.

Why there's little research

CAM practitioners say it's difficult to do research for a variety of reasons. One is that treatments often vary from patient to patient, making it hard to consistently measure what's essentially a moving target.

Even bigger variations crop up between different practitioners or between different brands or types of products. Two examples:

1.) A sub-specialty of chiropractic called upper-cervical chiropractors say their techniques are much more effective at helping TN than standard chiropractic. However, even in that sub-specialty, there are at least 10 different approaches. Depending on which type a particular patient happens to pick, the treatments and results could differ markedly.

2.) As you'll read later in the section on magnet therapy, sometimes patients report no help at all from one type of magnet. Then they'll try another brand or size or type and get much better relief.

With so many techniques, variations, sub-specialties and different brands floating around, it could quickly become very confusing even if someone managed to conduct – and pay for – clear, unbiased studies.

CAM therapies also often employ a variety of modalities used at the same time as opposed to just one easily measurable technique. As Dr. Neims points out, sometimes with CAM it's the "whole" that produces the results, not any of the particular parts. He equates this to how a mother can quickly end the suffering of a child who has just scraped a knee even though she did nothing clinically therapeutic – other than give a hug and kiss and apply a "magic" bandage.

Dr. Neims says he has offered to help CAM therapists set up scientific studies to prove whether their particular medicine, product or technique works or not. "The therapists almost always refuse to agree to the notion that a negative result would be evidence that their therapy doesn't work," he says.

Dr. Neims says CAM therapists often tell him they already know the treatment works from patient experience and that they don't need studies to prove it. He says he suspects that as with the mother relieving her child's scraped-knee pain, CAM treatments may not work as well when the product is split apart from the overall therapy session.

"The less a human has to do with a therapy, the easier it is to study," Dr. Neims says. "The more humans are involved, it becomes harder to control that and double-blind that."

Further confounding hard evidence is that many CAM therapies can't be measured. An example is acupuncture. It seems to work for TN at least some of the time, but we have no technology to measure whether the needles actually unblock the body's "Qi" energy that is the underlying premise for the whole therapy.

What that leaves, for the most part, is individual testimonials and case reports from practitioners.

A particular problem with anecdotal evidence in the case of TN is that it's difficult to tell whether the therapy in question really caused relief or whether the pain coincidentally went away on its own. After all, a hallmark of TN is how it suddenly comes and goes as if it has a mind of its own.

"When someone feels better after having used a product or procedure," says Dr. Barrett, "it is natural to credit whatever was done. This is unwise, however, because most ailments resolve by themselves and those that persist can have variable symptoms. Even serious conditions can have sufficient day-to-day variation to enable useless methods to gain large followings."

One way to prove or disprove a therapy's success is to try it repeatedly. If it works the second or third or fourth time the pain comes back, then the cloud of coincidence can be removed.

A few other caveats

That brings us to a second caveat. Even when a CAM therapy helps TN, much of the time the relief is short-lived, say TN support-group leaders who often hear about their members' CAM experiences. Soon after the cream is stopped or the alternative therapy ends, they say, the pain tends to return. Many times it returns anyway even when the treatment continues.

On the other hand, there *are* people who have found long-lasting TN relief from CAM therapies. But because hardly any of the few CAM studies do follow-ups over time, it's been impossible to gauge the rate of long-term successes and compare these successes from one therapy to another.

Third, CAM treatments often aren't as widely or as completely effective as the mainstream TN treatments.

It's not unusual to hear one person say one treatment helped a lot while another says it was useless. Sometimes there are more people who aren't helped than those who are. The only way to know for sure if it'll help you is to try it and see.

Unlike surgeries and even medications that often are able to knock out all or most TN pain, CAM therapies tend to bring improvements more so than complete relief. Once again, trying the therapy is the only way you'll know how much it helps your particular pain.

A fourth potential drawback is that it may be difficult to find a practitioner for a particular therapy in your area. You may end up traveling a long distance to find someone who's trained and skilled in the technique you'd like to try.

Even when a practitioner is found, insurance often does not cover the cost. Thus much of CAM's cost is paid for out-of-pocket by patients.

Worth trying?

Some medical doctors are adamantly opposed to most CAM therapies, and they'll come right out and say you're wasting your time and money on them. "Most of these practices have no scientific basis," Dr. Barrett says.

His QuackWatch group and the Massachusetts-based National Council Against Health Fraud (www.ncahf.org) have a variety of concerns about CAM. Among them:

1.) Companies and practitioners often make exaggerated or unproven claims.
2.) Practitioner training is spotty and sometimes very limited.
3.) Government oversight of herbal products and other natural products is limited, which has allowed poor quality and sometimes adulterated products. For example, when *Consumer Reports* tested a dozen brands each of echinacea and ginkgo for a 1999 article, it found wide variations in the amount of those herbs among different brands.
4.) The largely anecdotal evidence behind most therapies gives no idea how many failures might occur for each success.

Doctors' greatest concern, though, is the possibility that CAM therapies could be harmful.

They point out that although herbs, vitamins and minerals may be "natural" and seemingly harmless, that's not always the case. Taken at high doses, some vitamins can build up to toxic levels in the body and others can lead to problems such as kidney stones.

Like prescription medicines (about a third of which are plant-based), herbs also can interact with other agents. Some thin the blood (which can pose a problem when overdone or taken near surgery), some lower blood sugar and some can increase the strength of anesthetics. Some herbs can even kill, as was the case with the weight-loss herb ephedra that the U.S. Food and Drug Administration banned in early 2004 after it was linked to more than 100 deaths.

"Natural or not, some supplements are proving to have drug-like effects in the body," says Ronni Sandroff, *Consumer Reports* health editor during the magazine's 2000 survey on alternative medicine. "They can cause side effects and interfere with prescription drugs. There's an urgent need for more research and regulation to help consumers make the best use of all forms of alternative medicine."

Doctors are particularly concerned because many – if not most – of their CAM-using patients do not tell them about what supplements or other CAM therapies they're trying. A 1998 Journal of the American Medical Association article put that number at 60 percent. *Consumer Reports'* survey done two years later found that 40 percent don't tell their doctors about their CAM treatments.

Some TN surgeons have an additional concern about CAM therapies even if they don't do direct harm – the potential drop in success rates if surgery is eventually done. They argue that the best surgical results come in the first seven to eight years after a person's TN begins. After that time, they say, success rates start to drop off, presumably because a compressing blood vessel does enough cumulative damage to permanently injure the trigeminal nerve. By spending months or years trying various CAM therapies, they argue, precious time has been shaved off the surgical clock.

Dr. Marcia Angell and Dr. Jerome P. Kassirer summed up mainstream medicine's concerns in an editorial in the Sept. 17, 1998, edition of the New England Journal of Medicine: "There cannot be two kinds of medicine – conventional and alternative. There is only medicine that has been adequately tested and medicine that has not, medicine that works and medicine that may or may not work. Once a treatment has been tested rigorously, it no longer matters whether it was considered alternative at the outset. If it is found to be reasonably safe and effective, it will be accepted. But assertions, speculation and testimonials do not substitute for evidence."

Others take the more middle-of-the-road view of Florida neurosurgeon Dr. Albert L. Rhoton Jr., who says, "Most of these (alternatives) are low-risk forms of therapy with some modest expense. I don't try to discourage patients from trying them."

He takes the approach that so long as the therapy isn't harmful, patients should feel free to try something they believe might help.

After all, if an alternative therapy isn't working, you're going to be the first to know... and you're probably going to be highly motivated to move on to the next option.

Even if none of the alternatives work, going through the process can help in the ultimate decision to try one of the more invasive treatments. You may feel more comfortable about a surgical decision, for example, knowing you haven't overlooked some less-invasive option that *might've* worked.

"Whatever label we apply to a therapy," says Dr. Neims, "we should not let that label evoke a knee-jerk judgment, pro or con. This criticism goes both ways. It is as foolish for an alternative medical practitioner to label all drugs and operations as poisons and butchery as it is for a physician or scientist to conclude that all complementary or alternative therapies are snake oil or quackery."

A CLOSER LOOK AT SOME CAM
AND OTHER OPTIONS...

The following information — like all the information in this book – is not intended as specific medical advice. You should always discuss any treatment with a trusted medical professional before trying it – even if the treatment seems harmless or involves only over-the-counter medications or vitamins.

The alternatives below and in the next three chapters are not the only ones TN sufferers have tried, but they are among the more common ones.

Not all fall under the CAM umbrella either. Some of the therapies fit into the Western understanding of the body and are even used sometimes in conventional medicine. Others are based on different approaches altogether. Still others fall somewhere in between.

Hot-pepper creams

One type of over-the-counter medication that some TN sufferers say helps is hot-pepper cream. The active ingredient in these creams is *"capsaicin"* (kap-say'-eh-sin), the chemical that makes hot peppers hot. Capsaicin creams are sold in tubes under such brand names as Zostrix, Axsain, ArthiCare, Capzasin-P and Dolorac.

Topical creams that give a burning sensation have been used for muscle pain and joint stiffness for decades. Most contain menthol, camphor and/or eucalyptus, which are counter-irritants that distract the brain's attention and thereby mask the pain.

Capsaicin relieves pain in a different way. It works by depleting the area of the neurochemicals needed to transmit pain signals. That's why the cream burns at first but then gives relief as the pain-signaling nerve fibers basically "wear out." It's also why the cream needs to be reapplied at regular intervals – to prevent the fibers from recharging themselves.

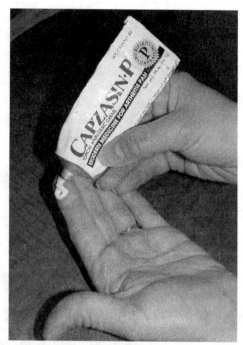

Capsaicin creams are marketed largely for arthritis sufferers, but they're also used to treat other inflammations, plus shingles, itching disorders and diabetic neuropathy, a burning and/or numbing nerve pain that often occurs in diabetics. It's been used with at least some success in treating TN.

Although some have had very good relief from capsaicin cream, others have found only partial relief or no relief at all. It also hasn't proved to be reliable effective over the long run. Pain usually comes back soon after the cream is stopped.

Capsaicin cream is available over-the-counter in a variety of brands and strengths.

(Photo by George Weigel)

In a 1991 study at the Institute of Medical Pathology in Rome, 12 patients got one gram of capsaicin cream (.05 percent strength) three times a day for several days. All had been off all medication for at least 10 days prior to the test.

Half of those people got complete relief and another four reported partial relief ranging from a 60 percent to an 80 percent reduction in pain. Two reported no benefit.

In a one-year follow-up of the 10 patients who got full or partial relief, six of those either remained pain-free or at least had pain that didn't worsen. Pain recurred in the remaining four, but three of those four got relief from a second round of capsaicin treatment.

The Italian researchers concluded that because the cream's effect was repeatable, it was unlikely that the patients got relief because of coincidental remissions.

TN support group members in Australia had similar results. Twenty-one members tried capsaicin cream, and 10 got complete relief, five others got partial relief and the remaining six were not helped at all. Most got at least 6-12 months of relief, although pain occasionally broke through and required some low dose of medication. One member got pain relief for more than two years.

Australia TN support group leader Irene Wood said the best results are with .075 percent strength capsaicin used four to five times a day without fail – even after pain has subsided. She said only small amounts are needed ("No bigger than a small pea"), and the cream is best applied to the trigger zones.

"Most noticed a significant improvement *only* after four to six weeks of persistent, consistent application," Wood says. "Do not expect an overnight miracle."

Wood said those who gave up on capsaicin said it was troublesome to keep to the four- to five-times-a-day routine. Others said the cream was too hot when worn outside in the sun, and one said she stopped it after her grandchild kissed her capsaicin-creamed cheek and ended up with burning lips.

A small 1994 study of five TN patients in British Columbia, Canada, and Washington state was less optimistic. Researchers found that only one patient out of five got significant relief from Zostrix cream, three had little or no improvement and one went into remission without using the cream. Those researchers concluded that hot-pepper cream seems to be more effective in diabetic neuropathy and other types of facial nerve pain than in treating TN.

Most capsaicin-cream labels advise applying the cream to painful areas three or four times a day for several days or until the pain is gone. If results aren't apparent within a month, it's probably not going to work.

The cream may redden the skin and burn, but users often get used to the sensation after the first few applications.

The main drawback is that it can cause a distressing burning sensation if the cream gets in your eyes, in a cut or in other tender areas. For that reason, capsaicin cream should be applied carefully and with gloved hands. Also, wash your hands well after using it. (A solution of vinegar and water may help.) Contact lens-wearers need to be especially aware of this precaution.

Otherwise, capsaicin creams have none of the side effects common to oral, system-wide TN pills. It can be bought in most drugstores without a prescription, and it's approved for pain relief by the U.S. Food and Drug Administration.

Hot-pepper cream has helped "atypical" TN (TN-2) and post-herpetic neuralgia as well as classic TN. It's also helpful as a stopgap measure (i.e. while trying to build up to a therapeutic dose of medication or waiting for surgery), and it can be used in conjunction with medication or other CAM therapies.

Capsaicin candies and lollipops also are made that might be helpful to neuralgians whose TN trigger points are the gums or inside the cheeks.

Local anesthetics

One quick and logical way to deal with pain is to numb it – either by numbing the painful area directly or numbing the area that's triggering the pain.

This can be done in a variety of ways, including creams, patches, injections, eyedrops and even anesthetic gums and lollipops.

Local anesthetics such as procaine (Novocain), lidocaine (Xylocaine) and bupivacaine (Marcaine) have long been used by dentists and oral surgeons to temporarily numb the teeth and gums of patients during dental procedures. Hospitals often use EMLA cream to numb the skin before starting an intravenous line. And eye doctors usually use anesthetic eyedrops to numb the cornea before checking for glaucoma.

In the case of face pain, anesthetics offer a few benefits. For one thing, they work pretty quickly. For another, they don't carry troubling side effects. The big problem is that they don't work for very long. And once the feeling comes back, the pain usually returns in short order.

For that reason, local anesthetics are mainly used to get people out of acute pain attacks until longer-term solutions can be put into effect. Because they're usually administered by doctors, this approach doesn't make good practical sense in the long run.

Doctors report that sometimes local anesthetics have a lingering effect, especially when a series of injections are done over a short period of time. Even after the numbness wears off, the pain may not return for weeks or months.

In the 1980s, a European study was published reporting that 16 of 20 TN patients got relief for more than two years after a series of lidocaine and streptomycin sulfate injections. The patients in the study got one injection of 2 percent lidocaine and 1 gram of streptomycin (an antibiotic drug) next to the trigeminal nerve each month for five months. No side effects were reported, and the patients had no loss of sensation after the local anesthetic wore off.

Nebraska dentist Dr. Gerald D. Murphy, who specializes in orofacial pain, reports that he has had good success by injecting Marcaine in patients' trigger zones. He says one or two injections are sometimes enough to break the TN pain cycle for up to several months.

San Diego dentist Dr. Bradley Eli says he also has been able to control face pain by giving weekly injections of local anesthetic with a small amount of steroids.

Some doctors have theorized that the reason these drugs control pain after the numbness wears off might be because they block the transfer of sodium in nerve cell membranes.

Los Angeles facial-pain specialists Dr. Steven B. Graff-Radford and Dr. Geber T. Bittar attempted to replicate the European lidocaine results in a double-blind study of 20 of their patients a few years later but without success.

"Unfortunately, we didn't get any relief," Dr. Graff-Radford reports. Not only did no patients get relief, he adds, they had marked swelling of the face soon after the injections.

Cincinnati neurosurgeon Dr. John M. Tew Jr. says he considers local-anesthetic injections to be of temporary help only. "These solutions are toxic to the nerve and destroy some of its fibers to relieve pain," he says. "However, the fibers regenerate and pain recurs. In addition, these injections cause facial numbness, which in some cases may be bothersome to the patient."

There also have been a few reports of patients getting at least some temporary relief from another "caine" drug – the eye anesthetic proparacaine (Ak-Taine, Alcaine, Ocu-Caine, Ophthaine or Spectro-Caine).

Dr. Mitchell Zavon of Lewiston, N.Y., reported in a 1991 letter to the Journal of the American Medical Association that his own TN pain was relieved by two drops of this solution in his eyes. He subsequently told the Chronic Pain Letter that he was able to help nine other TN patients with the anesthetic eye drops.

A group of European doctors also reported in 1992 that 15 of 25 patients they treated with proparacaine eye drops also got at least some relief from just a single application.

However, when Pittsburgh neurosurgeon Dr. Douglas Kondziolka conducted a double-blind trial on 47 patients in 1992, he found the drops were of no benefit in either the severity or frequency of TN attacks.

As with injections, proparacaine eyedrops seem to be of most value as a possible way to temporarily stop an acute pain attack. In almost all cases, pain returns in less than two weeks. Repeated use may begin to cause eye injury.

Some patients also have tried using lidocaine in cream or spray form.

Rather than being injected, lidocaine cream is rubbed on the trigger zone or painful area several times a day. Although there have been no studies, lidocaine cream reportedly hasn't been very effective in classic TN cases but occasionally has been of some help to those with post-herpetic neuralgia and atypical TN.

Lidocaine spray is sprayed up the nostrils to relieve nose or sinus pain. In the case of TN, it may be somewhat helpful if a key trigger point is the nose.

Lidocaine or benzocaine gels and ointments also may be temporary helps when TN trigger points are inside the mouth. Gels can be bought over the counter and rubbed on gums or inside the cheek.

None of these are viewed as long-term solutions.

Botox injections

Most people know the botulinum toxin or *"Botox"* either as the "food-poison germ" or the new cosmetic treatment that eliminates skin wrinkles. But it's being used and studied for far more than wrinkles, including migraines and face pain.

Botox was first approved by the FDA in 1989 to control eye-muscle disorders. This agent is actually a purified form of the botulinum toxin, which is produced by the same bacteria that cause botulism. Botox injections contain only minute quantities of the toxin and no actual bacteria.

Its main effect is in paralyzing muscle, and so it was first used to treat muscle and movement disorders, such as involuntary spasms, torticollis (uncontrolled twisting of the neck), writer's cramp (involuntary finger contractions) and muscle stiffness related to strokes and multiple sclerosis.

However, the way it affects muscles is by preventing the release of a nerve-impulse chemical (acetylcholine) that causes muscles to contract. In recent years, Botox has been tried in a variety of nerve, muscle and other disorders, ranging from migraines to low back pain to cerebral palsy.

So far only one published study has looked at Botox's effectiveness in face pain, and the results were fairly good in the short term.

Dr. Gary E. Borodic and Dr. Martin A. Acquadro at Massachusetts General Hospital in Boston treated 44 face-pain patients with anywhere from one to four Botox injections. Eleven of those 44 were classic TN patients, and the others had temporomandibular joint pain, post-surgical face pain or headaches.

After following the patients for 6 weeks, Drs. Borodic and Acquadro found that 75 percent of the patients – including eight of the 11 TN patients – got at least a 50 percent reduction in the frequency and severity of their pain.

Side effects were temporary muscle weakness in the injected area and some asymmetry in facial expression. Both effects wore off in a few weeks. But so did the pain relief in anywhere from five to 12 weeks.

Botox injections can be repeated, but so far there are no long-term studies to determine if face-pain patients can get lasting relief by going back for Botox injections every two to three months.

Those with muscle disorders who have used Botox for years have found that sometimes a resistance is built up, and the agent doesn't work as well as time goes along. However, Drs. Borodic and Acquadro used pain-relief doses of between 25 and 75 units of Botox, which is about a quarter of the dose used for treating torticollis. They suggest that resistance is much less likely to occur at this lower level.

So far it appears that Botox may at least be useful in some cases as a temporary measure, functioning much like an extended-action local anesthetic. Although it doesn't cause numbness, most people notice changes in how they can move their face.

Wrote Drs. Borodic and Acquadro: "Although occasionally annoying, patients generally found these complications tolerable, considering the gravity of the affliction for which treatment was being sought, particularly for trigeminal neuralgia."

In other words, the majority of TN patients said it was worth putting up with some crooked smiles for a few weeks to get some relief from their pain.

Most any type of doctor is able to administer Botox injections, although neurologists, anesthesiologists and plastic surgeons are most likely to have experience with it.

Dr. Graff-Radford says Botox may turn out to play a useful role in face pain, but for now, it's too early to tell. "There's still a lot of work to do before we can clearly utilize Botox in a general sense."

TENS units

A transcutaneous electrical nerve stimulation (TENS) unit is a small, battery-operated box that generates pulses of electricity aimed at interfering with or "jamming" nerves' pain signals to the brain.

TENS units are FDA-approved, physician-prescribed devices that are often used for temporary pain relief following surgeries and injuries. But they're also sometimes used for more chronic conditions, such as arthritis, back pain, shingles, nerve injuries, headaches, multiple sclerosis pain and bursitis.

The units come with several electrodes that are attached to the skin of painful areas by adhesive pads. The unit puts out regular, low-grade pulses of electricity that can be adjusted in intensity and speed. People who use them describe the feeling as a mild tingling sensation.

Some people wear their units for only 30-60 minutes a day, but others wear them for several hours at a time.

Results have been mixed when it comes to their effectiveness in treating TN and related face pains. The Chronic Pain Letter summed it up well in a 1990 article on TENS units: "There are people with pain problems who would not be without their TENS units. Others will tell you that they donated the device to the nearest tag sale after a brief trial period."

Often the effectiveness of TENS falls somewhere between those two extremes.

One study at the University of Colorado Medical Center found that TENS units help about half the people who use them get 50 percent or better pain relief. Other studies have found that the effectiveness tends to lessen with time to the point where only 30 percent of the users report good pain relief after one year of using the device.

Dr. Murphy, the Nebraska oral-pain specialist, says that can happen because the body adjusts to the TENS stimulations, a process known as *"sensory adaptation."* He says doctors can head that off by varying the modulation of the TENS unit. Another alternative is to switch to a different brand of unit.

Dr. Murphy reports that he's been having success in about 65 to 70 percent of the TN patients on which he's tried TENS. Patients typically attach the electrodes to their pain trigger points for several hours in the evening or overnight.

"The idea is to break the pain cycle," says Dr. Murphy. "If it's effective, usually you're going to know within an hour."

He says the electrical impulses from the TENS unit act as "new information" to the central nervous system, superseding the pain signals. If these artificial impulses interrupt the pain signals long enough, he adds, it may be enough to end the entire cycle of TN attacks. As the attacks subside, wear time can be decreased and eventually stopped.

Besides being potentially useful against the sharp stabs of classic TN, TENS units also sometimes help those with "atypical" TN (TN-2), postherpetic neuralgia and nerve-injury pains.

Dr. Murphy points out there are no serious side effects with TENS, and the unit can be used each time a new cycle of pain starts. Those with cardiac conditions or pacemakers and pregnant women may be given special precautions.

TENS units are used in a variety of medical specialties, including neurology, physical therapy, psychiatry, oral surgery and dentistry. They usually cost under $50 and are typically covered by insurance.

Magnet therapy

The use of magnetics in treating illness dates back to at least 200 B.C. when the Chinese used magnetic stones to treat a variety of conditions. Chinese healers placed these stones on acupuncture points and believed the magnetic charges worked by restoring the natural flow of the body's energy.

Swiss holistic healer Holger Hannemann gave a similar explanation in his 1990 book, *"Magnet Therapy: Balancing Your Body's Energy Flow for Self-Healing"* (Sterling Publishing Co. Inc.) "It is the task of magnet therapy to remove the blockages that get in the way of normal functioning," he wrote.

More recently, companies that manufacture medical magnets claim that magnets help by stimulating the body's ions, which in turn improves oxygen uptake in the cells. Ions are electrically charged particles that give the cells in our body a weak, natural electrical current.

Magnets of any type can have an effect on the body's electrically charged cells. The original magnets used for healing were metal or "static" magnets that produced one, constant charge. In the 1700s, French scientists developed a machine that could generate electromagnetic fields that put out wave-like charges called *"pulsed electric magnetic fields."*

Both types have long been used to treat all sorts of disorders. Magnet therapy became especially popular in the United States starting in the 1980s when a wave of companies began marketing all sorts of magnet wraps, mattresses, shoe inserts, bracelets and the like.

Testimonials implied that the devices could help everything from sleep problems to high blood pressure to cancer. Several of these companies ended up paying fines for making health claims that couldn't be backed up.

The magnets themselves are not illegal, and they can be used for any health condition a consumer wants to use them for. However, magnets are not FDA-approved medical devices, and therefore companies can't market them to treat specific illnesses without having evidence to verify the claims.

What fueled a lot of the marketing was a 1987 pilot study at Baylor University that tested magnets on 50 patients with knee pain. More than half of these patients wore static magnets for 45 minutes and the rest got sham magnets. Pain improved in both groups, but the relief ratings were higher for the magnet group.

Although it was a brief, limited study with no follow up, the magnet industry used the study widely in its advertising as proof that magnets really do heal. Ads also usually point out that magnets are natural, drug-free, safe, durable and non-invasive.

Some people who have tried magnets for face pain say they get at least some relief by sleeping with pea-sized magnets attached to their face. Others, though, have reported little or no help.

In a 2000 survey of its readers, *Consumer Reports* magazine found that magnets were among the least effective therapies for 10 different disorders. For arthritis, magnets ranked 14th out of 14 therapies its readers tried, and for back pain, magnets ranked 13th out of 14 therapies.

The New York College of Podiatric Medicine found magnets to be of no more help than sham magnets in a four-week study it conducted in 1997 using magnetic sole inserts in the shoes of 34 foot-pain patients.

The Veterans Administration Medical Center in Prescott, Ariz., also conducted a study in 2000 in which it found real magnets did no better than sham magnets in helping 20 patients with back pain.

"There is no scientific basis to conclude that small, static magnets can relieve pain or influence the course of any disease," says Dr. Barrett of QuackWatch.

On the other hand, there has been research showing that pulsed electromagnetic fields (PEMFs) can stimulate healing of bone fractures. The FDA approved the use of these fields for that purpose in the 1980s.

Although PEMFs still are not in widespread use in bone breaks, recent studies have found they may be somewhat helpful in the broader fields of arthritis, migraines and neck pain. About half of the patients who have used PEMFs for those problems have reported improvements in either pain or movement. No studies have yet been done on face pain or dental pain.

Dr. William Pawluk, an assistant professor at Johns Hopkins Medical School, believes PEMFs have the potential to help a variety of disorders with virtually no risks or side effects.

"Even the strongest magnetic fields generated by MRI machines have been found to be safe, except for very limited circumstances," he wrote in an article for the Natural Health Web web site (www.naturalhealthweb.com).

Dr. Pawluk, who is also a consultant for a company that markets one PEMF system, says some of the newest PEMFs stimulate muscles and nerves. High-frequency units are available that can help decrease pain and swelling, he adds.

"More and more medical care will include medical magnetic fields in all sorts of applications to heal the body," he predicts. "They will be used in conjunction with conventional medicine and other complementary health techniques."

Patients do not need a physician's prescription to buy PEMFs. They are much more expensive than static magnets, however, often running more than $2,000. They are not normally covered by insurance.

One TN patient who has tried both types of magnets says he's had much better and longer-lasting pain relief with a PEMF system.

"I did not get great results using static magnets," says Carlo Javier of New Jersey. "Although I got some comfort and great relaxation and sleep with static magnets, my body became immune to them a few days later."

Javier was using a static magnetic mattress mat and pillow liner but found they apparently weren't strong enough and didn't change polarity. He then bought a more expensive PEMF system that he uses twice a day for 8 minutes at a time.

"Its magnetic field reaches up to three feet and penetrates my entire body," Javier says. "It also changes polarity every two minutes." He believes that and the 10 changeable magnetic intensities will prevent him from becoming "immune" to the effects of the PEMF system.

One other case study from Ecuador told about a man who also got relief from his TN using PEMF – at least after a few weeks. However, it's unknown how widespread PEMF's success might be in treating TN and related face pains and also how lasting any relief might be.

As the Chronic Pain Letter pointed out about TENS units, maybe you'll find great relief from magnet therapy. Or maybe you'll have a new $2,000 item for the next tag sale.

No magnets – static or PEMF – should be used without medical advice in patients who have cardiac pacemakers or defibrillators.

Low-intensity laser therapy

Lasers are devices that emit single, highly focused wavelengths of light. They can emit light that's visible but also light (or more accurately, radiation) that's *not* visible.

Its roots go back to the late 1960s when Hungarian surgeon Dr. Endre Mester began researching the possible use of lasers in treating cancer. In experimenting with different laser intensities on rats, Dr. Mester found that low intensities of this light stimulated rat hair growth while high levels inhibited it.

Eventually researchers found that even higher levels of laser radiation could be used to injure tissue. That ultimately led to surgical lasers that allow surgeons to cut, coagulate or even evaporate tissue without using a scalpel.

Another lesser-known use of lasers has been at the opposite end of the treatment spectrum – using low-intensity light to stimulate healing. Just as Dr. Mester found that low-intensity light could stimulate hair to regrow faster on rats, other doctors soon learned that low-intensity laser therapy (LILT) could speed the healing of wounds.

Since then, LILT has been studied for a variety of other uses, including carpal tunnel syndrome, tendinitis, arthritis, migraines and inflammatory conditions. In face pain, there have been a few early studies showing that LILT can give 60 to 70 percent relief in post-herpetic neuralgia. It also may help TN and temporomandibular joint disorders.

In a pair of studies dating to the 1980s at The Pain Institute in Los Angeles and the Walker Institute in Pacific Palisades, Calif., patients with TN, post-herpetic neuralgia, sciatica and arthritis were treated with low-power helium-neon lasers. The doses were low enough to avoid creating nerve damage.

The results found that about three-quarters of these patients got at least short-term relief from several treatments.

In 1996, researchers at Odense University Hospital in Denmark used LILT on 30 patients. Sixteen of them were treated with actual lasers, while 14 got treatments with non-laser probe. Both groups got weekly treatments for five weeks.

At the end of the five weeks, only one of the 14 non-laser patients was pain-free, four reported less pain and the remaining nine reported no improvement. However, 10 of the 16 laser-treated patients were pain free after five weeks, two reported less pain and four reported no improvement. One year later, six of the 16 laser-treated patients were still pain-free.

LILT therapy has been used more often in treating TMD and other joint pains, and the FDA recently approved the marketing of a home device for light therapy of the joints.

Its unknown exactly how lasers might be able to affect such a wide range of conditions, but researchers speculate it's related to photochemical changes the lasers cause in the body's cells. It's also thought that lasers may change the metabolism of serotonin, a body chemical that's involved in pain transmission.

Prof. Paul F. Bradley at London's University College Hospital says research has found that LILT:

- Desensitizes the firing of some nerve cells by changing the way sodium, potassium and calcium move across cell membranes.
- Stimulates the production of enzymes involved in pain.
- Elevates the body's endorphin levels. Endorphins are body chemicals that mute the perception of pain.

What's not known is exactly what light wavelengths, light intensities and treatment times will give the best results in the various conditions. Skin color, age of the patient and body type are just a few of the variables that can affect results.

It's also unknown how widespread pain relief might be in larger groups of people, how lasting the relief will be and whether treatments are repeatable if pain comes back.

At the levels used in these early LILT treatments, no patients have reported any troubling side effects or complications.

Treatments are painless and can be done by any type of physician trained in the use of lasers, including vascular surgeons, neurosurgeons and plastic surgeons. Although LILT isn't widely used for pain, some insurance plans cover it.

Massage

You'd think massage would be one of the last things anyone with TN would want done to them, considering how even a light touch can set off waves of pain. However, the deeper pressure and sensation from massage activates different nerve endings than the light-touch endings that more commonly trigger TN pain.

There are two approaches to using massage in treating face pain.

The first is directly rubbing the face. Some neuralgians say this can either prevent attacks or help shorten attacks once they've been triggered.

The most likely explanation for why that might help is by distracting the brain's attention away from the misguided pain signals. By adding the stimulus of deeply rubbing the face, those signals compete with the pain signals also vying for the brain's attention.

The second approach is using massage of the back, neck and other parts of the body as a way to generally relax tension.

Massage has been used for that purpose for centuries. Egyptian tomb paintings even show people being massaged, so this therapy is arguably the world's oldest medical treatment.

Massage today is most often used for treating stress-related ailments, such as insomnia, headaches, tight muscles, stiff necks, digestive disorders and high blood pressure. It's also been helpful in some pains, particularly those related to muscles and joints.

While it's unlikely to have a major impact on TN, massage may help take some of the edge off pain attacks. Besides reducing stress and tension that can increase the perception of pain, massage is thought to stimulate the production of endorphins – the body's natural pain-killing chemicals.

Numerous clinical studies have found massage helpful for a variety of problems, but it's usually not covered by insurance. It's not only offered by licensed massage therapists, but it's also a component used in many other therapies, including osteopathy, chiropractic, India's Ayurveda system, reflexology and Rolfing.

Even simple self-massages or a few minutes of back or neck massage by a friend or family member may be somewhat helpful.

The only downside for a neuralgian is the possibility that the initial touch could set off an attack. Otherwise, there's virtually no risk of it being harmful. Doctors generally approve of the technique.

Herbal therapy and aromatherapy

In the days before pharmacy counters and mega-drugstores, herbs were the only medicines. Most people grew their own healing herbs, and even apothecaries stocked medicines made from dried roots, leaf extracts and the like.

As the Industrial Revolution swept the country, medicines soon became neatly bottled pills and capsules manufactured by large pharmaceutical companies using formulas crafted out of lab-isolated ingredients. Partly because of cost and partly because of unwanted side effects and interactions, many health-care consumers have begun turning back to some of the herbal or "natural" remedies of yesteryear.

Fueling the herbal revival, at least in part, have been several studies backing the effectiveness of some herbs for some health problems.

Feverfew for migraines, saw palmetto for prostate enlargement and St. John's wort for mild depression are three examples of herbs that have been scientifically demonstrated to be at least mildly useful.

Herbal backers say we're likely to continue to find that many of the old-fashioned "wives' tales" turn out to have scientific backing when they're put to the test. Those tests may come more often now that some of the pharmaceutical giants like SmithKline Beecham and Warner-Lambert are grazing into the herbal field.

At the same time, there's the concern that consumers will get swept up in "herbalmania" and expect more from herbs than they can really deliver.

As the *Consumer Reports on Health* newsletter (October 1998) put it, the upgraded image of herbal remedies may spur a misconception that "glorifies herbs, overstates their benefits and obscures their possible risks."

"While some studies have suggested that certain herbs may be beneficial, romanticizing all 'natural' remedies and ignoring their potential risks can lead to disappointing – or dangerous – results," the newsletter states. "Herbs can cause allergic reactions, side effects and drug interactions, especially if you take too much of the herb or use it for too long. And because herbal remedies are virtually unregulated, you can't rely on their potency or purity – or on the claims made on the label."

An example of that is the herb ephedra (ma huang), which was long used as a non-prescription weight-loss agent. The U.S. Food and Drug Administration banned it in 2004 after linking more than 100 deaths to it. The FDA in 2002 also issued a warning about rare but possible severe liver damage associated with the use of the herb kava *(Piper methysticum)*.

Analyses of some herbal remedies also have found the pills to be lacking the effective plant parts, varying widely in potency and sometimes even containing pesticides and toxic chemicals from the fields. And while testing has found benefits to some herbs, others (such as alfalfa, goldenseal, pennyroyal and yucca) could not be shown to be useful for their claimed healing properties.

In the case of TN, several herbs have been used for centuries as "nervines" to settle or calm the nervous system. But because none of them has been tested for TN, there is no scientific data to show which one or ones are effective or what dose might work.

Most of the herbal healing books on the market do not list specific suggestions for TN.

One neuralgia remedy listed in *"The Encyclopedia of Medicinal Plants"* by Andrew Chevallier (DK Publishing Inc., 1996) involves rubbing St. John's wort *(Hypericum perforatum)* infused oil on the painful area several times a day. Chevallier also suggests adding 20 drops each of clove and lavender essential oil to 50 ml of St. John's wort infused oil and applying that every two to three hours to the painful area.

Chevallier lists peppermint as another herb that can help nerve pain. He suggests infusing 25 grams of peppermint *(Mentha piperita)* in 75 ml of warm water and soaking it against the painful area as needed.

"The Complete Home Healer" by Angela Smyth (HarperCollins, 1994) suggests two herbal approaches for neuralgia. One is an aromatherapy mixture of two drops each of lavender oil and basil oil added to baths and inhalations. (Aromatherapy involves breathing vapors given off by herbs.)

Smyth's other suggestion is a pair of herbal drinks. One involves pouring one cup of boiling water over two teaspoons of dried St. John's wort, infusing for 10 minutes and drinking it. Smyth suggests three cups per day. The other drink is made by pouring one cup of boiling water over two teaspoons of valerian root *(Valeriana officinalis)*, infusing for 15 minutes and drinking as needed.

Michael Castleman suggests that same valerian tea in his book *"The Healing Herbs"* (Bantam Books, 1995) under treatments for epilepsy. Castleman also suggests a valerian tincture of one-half to one teaspoon per day to quiet seizures. (You'll recall that the same anticonvulsant drugs that work for epilepsy are also prescribed for TN.)

In his book *"The Green Pharmacy"* (St. Martin's Paperbacks, 1997), Dr. James A. Duke lists 13 herbs or spices for pain in general. These are: cloves, hot peppers *(Capsicum frutescens)*, willow *(Salix alba)*, evening primrose *(Oenothera biennis)*, ginger *(Zingiber officinale)*, lavender *(Lavandula officinalis)*, kava *(Piper methysticum)*, mountain mint *(Pycnanthemum pilosum)*, peppermint *(Mentha piperita)*, sunflowers *(Helianthus)*, turmeric *(Curcuma longa)*, eucalyptus *(Eucalyptus globulus)* and rosemary *(Rosemarinus offinalis)*. (Note: kava has been associated with rare but possible severe liver damage.)

Several other herbalists say chamomile *(Chamomilla)*, hops *(Humulus lupulus)*, skullcap *(Scutellaria lateriflora)* and passion flower *(Passiflora incarnata)* teas are other nerve-calming remedies.

Remember, use herbal products only as directed on the labels *and* only after consulting with your doctor or pharmacist to make sure they won't adversely interact with any other medications you might be taking.

It's unlikely that any single herbal remedy will knock out TN pain completely, but sometimes people report some relief when herbal therapy is used in conjunction with other therapies.

More information on herbal medicine is available through the Herb Research Foundation, 1007 Pearl St., Suite 200, Boulder, CO 80302. Its phone is 303-449-2265 and its web site is www.herbs.org.

Two organizations that may be able to help locate practitioners who practice herbal medicine in your area are:

- The American Association of Naturopathic Physicians,
  8201 Greensboro Drive, Suite 300, McLean, VA 22102
  703-610-9037
  www.naturopathic.org.
- And, the American Herbalists Guild,
  1931 Gaddis Road, Canton, GA 30115
  770-751-6021
  www.americanherbalistsguild.com.

Craniosacral therapy

This therapy has elements of chiropractic and osteopathic medicine with a touch of physical therapy. Its roots go back to the 1920s and 1930s in a variant of chiropractic called *"craniopathy"* and a type of osteopathy originally called *"cranial osteopathy."*

The underlying premise of what became craniosacral therapy in the 1970s involves a controversial pulse put out by the body's craniosacral system. The "cranio" refers to the head, and the "sacral" refers to the base of the spine. Therefore, the craniosacral system includes the spinal cord, the bones of the skull and spine, the coverings of those areas and the cerebrospinal fluid that flows through these areas.

Cerebrospinal fluid is a clear liquid that provides nutrients to and removes waste from the craniosacral system. It also provides cushioning and shock absorption that help protect the brain and spinal cord from trauma.

Craniosacral practitioners contend that this fluid pulses at a rate of 6 to 16 times per minute, independent of breathing and blood flow. In other words, it's a separate pulse from the one we think of when the nurse puts his or her finger tips on our wrist to see how fast our heart is pumping.

Craniosacral practitioners say they can manually feel the craniosacral pulse and that its existence can be verified by instruments such as MRI, encephalograms and myelograms.

They also say that skull bones move minutely in response to the changes in the pulse pressure and that anything that misaligns these bones (a car accident or fall, for example) can impede the pulse and lead to all sorts of maladies, including face pain.

What craniosacral practitioners attempt to do is figure out what is impeding the pulse and then make corrections to slowly restore it to balance. This can range from light finger taps on certain parts of the skull to gentle pressure on bones or muscles to suggestions of how the patient should change posture, walking and other habits.

Treatments are usually done on a massage table while fully clothed and typically last 45 minutes to an hour.

In TN and related pain, all the evidence has been anecdotal. No studies have been done to demonstrate how many people are helped, to what degree or how long-lasting any relief is.

One neuralgian who tried this therapy was Kate Borland of Virginia. "The treatments were gentle, safe and gave me a year of nearly pain-free existence," she says. However, the therapy stopped working soon after that, and Borland went on to have sinus surgery for a related face pain and upper-cervical chiropractic treatment.

Craniosacral practitioners may include physical therapists, chiropractors, osteopaths, physicians, nurses and even some dentists.

Most physicians discount the entire underlying premise of craniosacral therapy, saying there is no craniosacral pulse, that it isn't something that has been verified by instruments and that any manipulations that help would have nothing to do with any pulse impediments.

One of the most comprehensive medical reviews of craniosacral therapy came in 1999 when the British Columbia Office of Health Technology Assessment concluded that the whole underlying theory is invalid and that there is no evidence that practitioners can measure what they say they're measuring.

Doctors also caution that patients could be harmed by this therapy or at least be deprived of more effective therapy. Examples: A group of parents in Crescent City, Calif., won a $565,000 judgment against one craniosacral practitioner who allegedly traumatized children with forceful manipulations while another California practitioner was put on probation by that state's Osteopathic Medical Board for treating two infants with cranial manipulation instead of what the board deemed to be appropriate treatment.

Nonetheless, craniosacral practitioners claim this therapy is a very safe, low-impact, low-risk treatment that has a track record of helping many people in a variety of disorders.

It's usually not covered by insurance, and treatments may cost anywhere from $40 to $200, according to the Florida-based International Association of Healthcare Practitioners, an organization of craniosacral practitioners.

IAHP also offers patients help in locating practitioners in their area.

Its address is 11211 Prosperity Farms Road, Suite D-325, Palm Beach Gardens, FL 33410-3487, its web site is www.iahp.com, and its phone numbers are 1-800-311-9204 and 561-622-4771.

Therapeutic Touch/Healing Touch

These are both concepts based on what has long been known as the "laying on of hands." Practitioners usually do their healing via focused touching after a brief exam, but sometimes the hands are merely held or moved near the patient.

Therapeutic Touch was developed in the 1970s by Dora Kunz and Dr. Dolores Krieger, a registered nurse and faculty member at New York University. The premise is that healing takes place because the practitioner transfers energy to the patient.

In a typical treatment, the practitioner uses his or her hands to detect energy levels emanating from the patient. Hand movements are then used to sweep away negative energy, and then the practitioner makes hand contact with the patient to transfer positive or excess energy to the patient.

Healing Touch is a similar therapy developed in the 1990s that bases energy assessments on the body's seven main energy centers (or *"chakras"*) as identified by the Indian chakra system.

Jacquelyn J. Phillips, Healing Touch practitioner with the Center for Healing Intervention in Accomac, Va., demonstrated the technique on a volunteer at the 2000 Trigeminal Neuralgia Association conference in Pittsburgh.

She first dangled a pendulum over each of the volunteer's chakras, made several assessments based on how the pendulum moved and then placed her hands on the woman's shoulder and hip to transfer energy.

Phillips also demonstrated a "pain drain" by holding her left hand near the volunteer's cheek with her right hand pointed at the floor.

Phillips said she helped two of three of her patients with TN reduce their pain levels and medication with regular Healing Touch sessions. The third gave up after two sessions and went on to have surgery.

Many of the practitioners of these two therapies are nurses. Some do their treatments in hospitals and clinics, others in free-standing practices with CAM practitioners in such fields as acupuncture, massage and Reiki. Either way, it's seldom covered by insurance.

Practitioners point to numerous patient surveys that claim these therapies are especially helpful in anxiety, stress and relaxation but also in reducing pains of various sorts, including cancer pain, abdominal pain and surgical pain.

Critics say if these work at all, it's because of the comforting aspects of the therapy, not any transfer of energy.

In a 1998 study that aimed to either prove or disprove practitioners' ability to sense patients' energy fields, nurse Linda Rosa recruited 21 Therapeutic Touch practitioners to participate in a blinded experiment.

She placed the practitioners behind a cardboard screen with their hands extended on the other side. Rosa's daughter then randomly put her hand above one of the practitioner's hands, and the practitioner had to determine which hand it was. Each practitioner was tested between 10 and 20 times.

In the end, the practitioners determined the correct hand only 44 percent of the time, which is less than the expected 50 percent from pure chance.

Some practitioners called the study unfair and unscientific, but the Journal of the American Medical Association, which published the study, concluded that patients should "refuse to pay for this procedure until or unless additional honest experimentation demonstrates an actual effect."

The James Randi Foundation also has had a standing $1 million offer since 1996 for any practitioner who can demonstrate an ability to detect a human energy field under the kind of blind test Rosa used. Only one person attempted the test and failed.

"It is safe to assume that any reactions to the procedure are psychological responses to the 'laying on of hands,'" concludes Dr. Barrett of Quackwatch.

More information on Therapeutic Touch is available by writing: Nurse Healers – Professional Associates International, 3760 S. Highland Drive, Suite 429, Salt Lake City, UT 84106. Or visit online at www.therapeutic-touch.org or call 801-273-3399.

More information on Healing Touch is available by writing: Healing Touch International, 445 Union Blvd., Suite 105, Lakewood, CO 80228. Or visit online at www.healingtouch.net or call 303-989-7982.

A QUICK LOOK AT OTHER *CAM* THERAPIES

The following are only occasionally used in treating trigeminal neuralgia and related face pain. None are likely to give complete relief, but some may "take the edge off" pain or help with coping. When used, these are most often done in conjunction with other therapies, including conventional and other CAM approaches.

Therapy	What it is:	Evidence of Effectiveness	Medical Opinion
Ayurveda	India-based holistic healing system that includes diet, yoga and breathing exercises	++	++
Homeopathy	Healing system based on premise that "like cures like" – i.e. an agent that causes symptoms can treat those same symptoms at diluted levels	+++	+++
Hyperbaric oxygen therapy	Treatments of pure oxygen in hyperbaric chamber, designed to saturate cells with oxygen and promote healing	+ (for pain)	+ (for pain)
Naturopathy	Holistic system that promotes healthy lifestyles to prevent illness, including dietary changes, exercise, relaxation techniques and herbal remedies to treat symptoms	+++	+++
Qigong	Combination of deep breathing, meditation/visualization and gentle, repeated movements designed to improve energy flow, often used with acupuncture	+	+++
Reiki	Form of Japanese spiritual healing using gentle touch and transfer of healing energy	+	+
Rolfing	Deep massage and muscle manipulation aimed at restoring body's natural symmetry	++	++
Shiatsu	Japanese massage technique that focuses on acupuncture pressure points to stimulate energy flow	+	+++
Yoga	Gentle exercises combined with breathing and relaxation techniques	+++	++++

Information and ratings (except for hyperbaric oxygen therapy) from the "Encyclopedia of Healing Therapies" by Anne Woodham and Dr. David Peters (Dorling Kindersley, 1997)

See rating guide for this chart on next page...

...Rating guide for chart on previous page

RATING GUIDE:

Evidence of Effectiveness:
+ *Primarily anecdotal evidence or inconclusive*
++ *Some published research but limited conclusive evidence*
+++ *Good scientific trials with positive results*

Medical Opinion:
+ *Most doctors unconvinced it helps or some concern it could hurt*
++ *Doctors divided over efficacy*
+++ *Doctors concede it may help some people*
++++ *Doctors generally well disposed toward the therapy*

TIPS ON CAM SHOPPING

Some points to ponder when considering an alternative or complementary treatment:

• **Do your homework.** Popular magazines and health publications often cover CAM topics, and whole books have been written on many CAM topics.Check the periodicals index at the library and visit a bookstore. Health-food stores also often have CAM literature.

Keep in mind that much of the popular literature is written by or based on information from advocates of these therapies. This information may stem mostly from personal experience rather than controlled scientific studies.

The U.S. government's lead resource on CAM is the National Center for Complementary and Alternative Medicine, an arm of the National Institutes of Health. Its web site is www.nccam.nih.gov and its toll-free phone is 1-888-644-6226. Or write: NCCAM Clearinghouse, P.O. Box 8218, Silver Spring, MD 20907-8218.

For a counter-balance on CAM from conventional medicine, visit Quackwatch at www.quackwatch.org or the National Council Against Health Fraud at www.ncahf.org.

• **Research prospective practitioners.** Your state's professional-licensing agency can tell you if a practitioner is licensed or certified (if it's required) and possibly if there have been any complaints. Many states license acupuncturists, chiropractors, homeopaths, clinical herbalists and massage therapists.

Professional organizations also may be able to tell you if a practitioner is a member or is professionally accredited. That doesn't guarantee expertise, but at least it may indicate the practitioner has at least basic training. These organizations also may offer referral services. (See Chapter 24 for contact information on some of them.)

Ask your practitioner about his or her own training, accreditation and experience.

Continued on next page...

...Tips on CAM shopping continued

• **Get first-hand referrals.** Ask your practitioner for patient references and talk to these people, preferably before starting treatment. Seek out support groups and others with face pain and find out their experiences with local CAM practitioners.

Don't overlook asking around the community – friends, co-workers, health-care workers, the local health-food store, etc. You're bound to come up with at least some input that might help if you ask enough people.

• **Get details about the proposed therapy.** Exactly what is to be done? How long will the treatments likely be needed? Will there be side effects? Will the therapy conflict with any other measures you're using or considering?

Don't be swayed by jargon. Keep in mind that just because something sounds scientific doesn't mean it's true. If you don't understand something, ask. If it still doesn't make sense or seem reasonable, either do more research or go elsewhere.

• **Find out about safety and effectiveness.** Are there any risks? What are they and how common are they? What's the track record of success?

Get your own practitioner's views and ask for literature written by others – or where else you can get solid information on these issues.

• **Get a prognosis.** Ask the therapist about how long it should take to see results. Ask what kind of results you should expect and how and when you'll both be able to tell whether the therapy is working or not. It may help to keep a diary to evaluate your progress.

• **Ask about cost.** How much is the therapy? How often will you need it? Will anything else need to be purchased? Will insurance cover any of it?

• **Keep your primary-care doctor informed.** Even if your CAM therapy involves only herbal or over-the-counter preparations, let your doctor know the specifics. These may pose potential problems for other conditions you may have or other medications you may be taking.

• **Evaluate the first session.** Did the CAM practitioner answer all your questions? Did he/she respond in a way that satisfied you and made sense to you? Were you comfortable with the practitioner? Did he/she seem knowledgeable about face pain? Does the treatment plan seem reasonable and acceptable?

— *Sources: NCCAM, Consumer Reports, Dr. Allen Neims*

CHAPTER 16

ACUPUNCTURE FOR FACE PAIN

"Some 160 generations of Chinese can't all have been wrong. Has there ever been a longer clinical trial in history?"
—Rick Weiss, writing on acupuncture in Health magazine, 1995

Another non-surgical treatment for trigeminal neuralgia is the practice of acupuncture. This method of pain relief and disease prevention is a prime tenet of Chinese medicine, which originated some 5,000 years ago.

Although acupuncture has long been used in China, Japan, Korea and other Asian nations, it's only been used in the United States for about 150 years, according to the American Association of Acupuncture and Oriental Medicine. However, it's only become well known here since the 1970s. So in essence, acupuncture is an ancient therapy that's still in its infancy to Americans.

TN is one of the medical conditions that the World Health Organization, the medical arm of the United Nations, lists as being treatable by acupuncture. In Asia, the combination of acupuncture and herbal therapy is a front-line approach to treating all sorts of face pain.

The heart of acupuncture is the insertion of long, slender needles into various areas of the skin. Patients typically say they feel a "pricking" sensation when the needle is first inserted – something akin to a mosquito bite. Most say it's not as painful as the more piercing pain of a hypodermic needle injection.

Once the needles are in, some people say they feel nothing. Others say they can feel a mild tingling, and a few describe sensations such as cramping or "heaviness."

Acupuncture needles are typically inserted one quarter of an inch to one inch and left in place for 20 to 30 minutes. Sometimes they're stimulated with light amounts of electricity.

While at least a few needles are typically placed in the face when treating TN, others may be inserted in seemingly unrelated locations, such as the hands or feet.

The needle sites and number of needles used may vary from patient to patient and acupuncturist to acupuncturist. "Acupuncture is an art," is how Florida dentist and acupuncturist Dr. Chun-In Jerry Lin explains it. "It depends on the acupuncturist's skill and experience. We could use as many as 100 (placement) points."

Besides just inserting needles, acupuncturists also sometimes employ such techniques as heat therapy, massage, skeletal manipulation and lifestyle advice, including nutrition tips, exercise, herbal and vitamin supplements and stress-reduction techniques.

Understanding acupuncture

To understand acupuncture, forget everything you think you know about how the body works. Chinese medicine is based on an entirely different concept.

Chinese medicine revolves around what it calls *"Qi"* (pronounced "chee"), which is considered the basic substance of the universe. It's often translated as "vital energy" in English.

Qi energy is thought to flow throughout the body through a network of 12 main channels or "meridians," each of which is connected to a particular organ. These meridians branch out into numerous other smaller channels.

If any of these channels is impeded, the normal "circuit" is not being completed and symptoms may result. The job of the acupuncturist is to locate the impeded channels and free them at various acupuncture points so the body can return to a balanced state.

"These points are like valves into the meridians," says Pennsylvania acupuncturist Leada Lentz. "An acupuncture treatment is like adjusting a valve, depending on where you place a needle, for how long and how much the needle is manipulated or twisted."

The Chinese even have a saying: "There is no pain if there is free flow; if there is pain, there is no free flow."

Acupuncturists locate impediments in a variety of ways – and much of it may seem to have little to do with the trigeminal nerve.

"If you come to me as a patient," says Lentz, who is also trained as a registered nurse, "first you have to let go of the term 'trigeminal neuralgia.' You can't think only in terms of a problem with that particular nerve. What is important to me is where it hurts, what you feel like, what makes it hurt, what makes it better and so on."

Acupuncturists also use other clues to zero in on the problem meridians, such as examining the tongue, checking one of six "energy pulses" in each wrist, observing how the person looks and sounds, and finding out about the person's lifestyle habits.

By putting it all together, the acupuncturist arrives at what the Chinese call a "pattern of disharmony." Based on that determination, the acupuncturist then decides which specific points on the body should get needles.

The insertion of the needles is thought to free the flow of Qi, allowing this energy to flow from areas where it's excessive and into areas that are low in it.

Lentz likens this difference in thinking between Western and Chinese approaches to two different ways of cleaning out a gutter full of leaves. She says the Western approach would be to go directly into a clogged area and pull out a wad of leaves while the Chinese approach is more akin to placing a hose at the end of the gutter and washing the whole thing out.

"Chinese medicine is not about curing," Lentz says. "It's about figuring out what is out of balance in this tremendous collection of body, mind and spirit and then restoring that balance... Chinese medicine is about letting the body heal itself."

Not always needles

Originally, Chinese healers used 365 potential acupuncture points – one for each day of the year. Now there are some 2,000 different points that acupuncturists might use to treat various conditions.

Although inserting needles is the most common way these acupuncture points are stimulated, it's not the only way. These same points can be stimulated by pressing them ("acupressure"), by heating them with laser beams ("laserpuncture") or even stimulating them with magnets (as discussed in Chapter 14).

Shelly Wilson, a TN support group leader in Dallas, got relief from her dual-sided atypical TN by using a small metal roller on an acupuncture point on the back of her middle fingers.

This approach was developed by Dr. Yoshiaki Omura, president of the International College of Acupuncture and Electro-Therapeutics, and also includes drinking cilantro tea and taking fish-oil capsules. Dr. Omura claims the cilantro (a herb also known as "Chinese parsley") helps rid the body of excess heavy metals, while the fish oil helps fight viruses.

Dr. Omura also suggests not wearing jewelry and avoiding sugar, garlic, onions, caffeine, Vitamin C and chocolate.

By using the roller, drinking four cups of cilantro tea a day and following the other guidelines, Wilson says she was out of pain and off medications in about three weeks. "Omura's protocol has left me pain-free and medication-free since April 2002," she says. "I haven't taken the cilantro or fish oil for several months now."

Dr. Allen Sprinkle, the Texas dentist who told Wilson about the program, reports that about 20 of his face-pain patients have tried this program, and it has helped about half.

Finding a balance

Qi can become unbalanced for a variety of reasons, including emotional factors, lifestyle changes, injuries and changes in the environment around us. When the body can't adjust quickly enough to changing conditions, symptoms result.

That's why Chinese medicine practitioners tend to spend time probing for these underlying causes of imbalance. They believe that mind and body are intertwined and that no single part of the body can be affected without it affecting the body as a whole.

While Western medicine may prescribe one treatment, Chinese practitioners often suggest a multi-pronged treatment plan that includes more than just acupuncture sessions.

For face pain, for example, Chinese practitioners may recommend herbal supplements in addition to acupuncture sessions, as in Dr. Omura's program.

They also may recommend lifestyle and dietary changes and may suggest Qigong therapy, which involves a combination of deep breathing, concentration and relaxation techniques.

Most of this runs counter to Western medicine, which doesn't even recognize Qi, the channels it flows through or the six pulses that acupuncturists use to measure imbalances.

Yet acupuncture somehow and at least sometimes seems to help a wide variety of disorders, ranging from pain to high blood pressure to muscle disorders and even behavior-related problems (i.e. overeating, smoking, drug dependence).

Why else might acupuncture work?

Western doctors suggest the needles have nothing to do with Qi but a lot to do with stimulating the body's immune system, which is responsible for preventing and fighting off viral-, fungal- and bacteria-related disorders.

In the case of pain, doctors say the needles also cause the body to release its own natural pain-relieving brain chemicals called "endorphins" and possibly impede pain impulses from reaching the spinal cord and brain.

Still others suggest that the needles are primarily a distraction technique in which the brain refocuses from the original pain onto the sudden pinpricks from all of the needles.

Then there's the so-called "placebo effect" – the contention that if the practitioner and patient really believe a therapy is going to work, the power of suggestion alone is enough to cause a perception of pain relief.

The National Council Against Health Fraud, for example, contends that any positive effects of acupuncture are due to a combination of expectation, suggestion, psychological conditioning and the distracting counter-irritation from the needles.

Acupuncturists counter that by arguing that acupuncture often works in animals.

However it may work, acupuncture usually takes at least five to eight sessions to begin relieving face pain. Although some people get quicker results – a few after as little as one treatment – the norm seems to be somewhere between 10 and 20 treatments for complete or significant relief.

For acute pains, acupuncturists may suggest two or more treatments a week at first. For more chronic pains, weekly sessions may be done over several months. Once pain is under control, acupuncturists typically suggest "maintenance" treatments about four times a year.

Dr. Lin says that if acupuncture is going to work, you should notice at least some improvement within 10 treatments. "If after 10 treatments you don't feel any different," he says, "the chances are very low that acupuncture is going to help you... If you have any response, better or worse, that's good. If you have no response, that's a problem."

He points out that very often patients will experience a worsening of pain after the first few treatments before the pain steadily improves.

Dr. Lin also has found that, in general, the longer you have TN, the more sessions it takes to bring relief.

That may explain why the Chinese seem to get better results from acupuncture in TN – they turn to acupuncture at the first sign of pain. Americans tend to turn to it after conventional methods fail, many times years after the onset of pain.

"If you have TN only a year or two, it's easier to treat," says Dr. Lin.

U.S. doctors counter that that's true of conventional treatments for TN, too, most likely because the nerve injury hasn't yet become chronic and natural remissions are more common.

Acupuncture might not work for several reasons, says Dr. Lin. The acupuncturist might not be addressing the right spots on the body. The acupuncturist might not have enough experience or skill to use the right combination of sites. Or the patient might give up before the treatments have had a chance to begin taking effect.

How well does it work?

Although there have been several American scientific studies showing acupuncture's value in helping various types of pain, there's little in the medical literature about whether acupuncture is effective against TN. Much of the information is anecdotal from patients themselves… some say it helps; others say it didn't do anything for them.

The U.S. National Institutes of Health's National Center for Complementary and Alternative Medicine says research has shown acupuncture may be helpful in treating nausea, acute dental pain, headaches, temporomandibular joint dysfunctions, fibromyalgia and depression. TN and related face pains is not on NCCAM's list.

One institution where acupuncture has been used to treat TN is at the New York University College of Dentistry's Orofacial Pain Center.

"We've found acupuncture to be extremely useful in trigeminal neuralgia," says Dr. William Greenfield, the center's director. "We're getting a 70 percent success rate. What that means is 70 percent of the people are able to go about their day-to-day affairs in relative comfort. I think that's remarkable considering 100 percent of those people had failed in other previous treatments."

Like Dr. Lin, Dr. Greenfield says acupuncture seems to work best in patients who are in the early stages of TN and who have had no prior surgeries in the afflicted area.

Dr. Peter Teng, a dentist who has treated hundreds of TN patients with acupuncture over 30 years at NYU's Orofacial Pain Center, says acupuncture doesn't cure and doesn't help everybody. But he says it does provide many people with pain relief for weeks or months at a time.

Dr. Teng usually starts with twice-weekly treatments, usually using needles placed in the hand instead of directly into the painful or pain-triggering parts of the face.

Fairly typical is the experience of Jane Schwarzman, one of Dr. Teng's patients. After five treatments, "I was walking on air, I felt so terrific," she said in the Trigeminal Neuralgia Association's Fall 2001 TNAlert newsletter. "I could eat and talk."

About a month later, though, persistent coughing from a bout of bronchitis brought her TN pain back. Repeat acupuncture reduced the pain but hasn't stopped it altogether. She's been going back for monthly treatments to keep the pain at tolerable levels.

Several other recent acupuncture/TN studies have been done in the Orient.

In a 12-year study of 378 TN patients treated by acupuncture at the H.H. Yiu Acupuncture Clinic in Hong Kong, researchers reported "excellent improvement" in 88 percent of the cases. ("Excellent improvement" was defined by at least a 90 percent reduction in pain for at least six weeks after treatment.)

The acupuncturists in that study inserted needles in four locations around the face and stimulated them with light electricity. Patients got daily treatments for six days. Those who got relief got results within those six days in all but three cases. If acupuncture didn't help after two six-day sessions, treatment was stopped. About 10 percent of the cases had that outcome.

Heung-Hung Yiu and Dr. Kwong-Chuen Tam, the researchers in that study, said the success of acupuncture in TN "depends not only on the nature of the disease but also to a very great extent on the selection of acupuncture locations and the techniques of needle manipulation." They say more research is needed to ensure that acupuncturists who treat TN are using the best needle locations.

Another study – reported in a 1991 edition of the Journal of Traditional Chinese Medicine – claimed that 99 percent of 539 patients got initial relief from a 10-day regimen of acupuncture treatments. Over a period of one to six years, 44 percent had their pain come back.

Acupuncture treatments were repeated with similar results. On average, patients in this study needed an average of 26 acupuncture sessions to get their pain under control.

In one other 1987 Chinese study, 1,500 patients got acupuncture treatments every other day for a total of 20 treatments. At the end of the course, 54 percent had no pain, 28.3 percent were much improved, 16.6 percent were somewhat better, and only about 1 percent were no better at all.

However, a 1981 acupuncture study by Dr. William Sweet, the Boston neurosurgeon, turned out to be a lot less optimistic. He found that of 100 TN patients he surveyed who had undergone acupuncture treatment, 91 reported no benefit. Of the nine who reported initial relief, the pain came back in each case. None of those said they found relief upon a second round of acupuncture therapy, leading Dr. Sweet to conclude that the pain had coincidentally gone away on its own.

Others have questioned the quality of the Chinese studies, suggesting that the results are greatly exaggerated. A 1999 British Medical Journal review of nearly 3,000 Chinese acupuncture trials raised a variety of criticisms, such as reporting only short-term results, failing to report the level of help, failing to compare acupuncture treatments to no treatment and failing to report side effects.

Side effects and drawbacks

One of the attractive points about acupuncture is that it seems to be a low-impact therapy that presents little chance of any unwanted problems. For the most part, studies bear that out.

A pair of 2001 studies by members of the British Acupuncture Council found few complications and no serious problems in patients who underwent more than 66,000 acupuncture treatments.

A five-year study of more than 55,000 acupuncture treatments by 76 different Japanese acupuncturists turned up similar results – a few minor problems but no serious complications.

Both studies concluded that in competent hands, the risk of acupuncture is small.

That doesn't mean the procedure is risk-free.

A 1995 study published in the British medical journal Lancet surveyed 1,135 Norwegian doctors on experiences they had in treating patients who had undergone acupuncture. The survey turned up 66 cases of infections, 25 cases in which a needle had punctured a patient's lung, 31 cases in which patients' pain worsened after acupuncture treatment and 80 other assorted problems, including local bruising, hepatitis B, skin rash and nerve injury.

Acupuncturists also report that occasionally people faint during treatments, and a few experience temporary drops in blood pressure. All of these complications are treatable and usually temporary.

Infections can be virtually eliminated by the use of disposable or at least sterilized needles. Lung punctures also should happen rarely, if ever, in trained hands.

Therein lies part of the dilemma. Acupuncture training is not as standardized as Western medicine, and licensing rules vary widely from state to state. The bottom line is that practitioners may range from highly trained, highly experienced, state-licensed acupuncturists to ones who have very little training or oversight.

As Dr. Lin pointed out earlier, acupuncture is as much an art as a science, so finding an acupuncturist who is experienced in dealing with face pain can be as important as finding an experienced TN surgeon.

That alone can be a problem because many areas – especially rural ones – have few or no trained acupuncturists anywhere nearby.

Even among experienced acupuncturists, the treatments and diagnosis may vary widely. That means it's entirely possible that one acupuncturist will use one grouping of needle placements while another one will use a totally different set. The ensuing success of those therapies may vary accordingly.

A 2001 report in the Southern Medical Journal highlighted this disparity. In this study, a 40-year-old woman went to seven different acupuncturists over a two-week period and got five different diagnoses: "Qi stagnation," "blood stagnation," "kidney Qi deficiency," "yin deficiency" and "liver Qi deficiency."

The resulting treatment plans varied, too. The different acupuncturists said they would use anywhere from seven to 26 different needles in anywhere from four to 16 acupuncture points. These points varied from acupuncturist to acupuncturist, covering 28 different spots in all. Of these 28 different points, only four of them were prescribed by two or more acupuncturists.

That doesn't mean one plan is right and one plan is wrong or that there *is* only one plan that's going to work. They *all* may work – regardless of how many needles are used or where they're placed – if the source of help is endorphins, distraction and/or the power of suggestion. Or maybe there's more than one way and one place to unblock a Qi channel.

HELP FINDING AN ACUPUNCTURIST

Following are a few resources that may be able to help you locate an acupuncturist in your area:

- American Academy of Medical Acupuncture
  4929 Wilshire Blvd., Suite 428, Los Angeles, CA 90010
  1-800-521-2262 or 323-937-5514
  www.medicalacupuncture.org

- American Association of Acupuncture and Oriental Medicine
  433 Front St., Catasauqua, PA 18032
  610-266-1433
  www.aaom.org

- National Acupuncture and Oriental Medicine Alliance
  14637 Starr Road SE, Olalla, WA 98359
  253-851-6896
  www.acuall.org

- National Certification Commission for Acupuncture
  and Oriental Medicine
  Canal Center Plaza, Suite 300, Alexandria, VA 22314
  703-548-9004
  www.nccaom.org

Acupuncture's role in TN

So where does all of this leave acupuncture in the universe of face-pain treatment?

On the positive side, acupuncture does seem to help at least some, if not many, people – and with little chance of ill effects.

It's also a treatment that can be tried alongside other therapies, whether it's something conventional such as carbamazepine tablets or another CAM therapy such as hot-pepper cream, herbs or chiropractic adjustments.

You'll also know in a fairly short time whether acupuncture is going to help or not. Most people have an answer within a couple of weeks or after about 10 sessions.

Dr. Lin says he's also found that acupuncture is just as effective in so-called "atypical" TN (TN-2) as it is in classic cases. "It works about 85 percent of the time for atypical cases," he says.

On the down side, acupuncture is unlikely to be a long-term solution for face pain. Sometimes it lessens pain but doesn't quell it entirely. Even in cases where treatments knock out TN pain, it almost always comes back sooner or later. At the very least, most patients are advised to come back for regular maintenance sessions about four times a year even if the pain stays away.

If pain comes back, acupuncture can be repeated. Some studies report that ensuing rounds are just as effective as the first; others, like Dr. Sweet's, indicate that they aren't.

But unlike some of the conventional TN surgeries, there is no technical or physical limit to how many rounds of acupuncture a person can get over the years. As long as the treatments are giving relief, they can be repeated over and over again.

Another drawback is that acupuncture is rarely covered by insurance. That means most of the cost comes out of patients' pockets. First-time acupuncture visits typically cost more than $100, and follow-up treatments are usually in the $50-$100 range. So that 10-session trial can easily cost more than $500 out of pocket.

Says Dr. Teng: "I tell my patients, if you fail, you have lost a few hundred dollars, but that's all." Unlike surgery, he says, there are no permanent complications, and nothing will have precluded you from moving on to whatever other therapy you want to try.

CHAPTER 17

CHIROPRACTIC FOR FACE PAIN

"A typical head weighs 10 to 12 pounds, maybe 15 pounds, and it sits on a 2-ounce bone. It's like trying to balance a basketball on a ruler."
—Dr. Stephen Goodman, Lancaster, Pa., upper-cervical chiropractor

Ever since Iowa magnetic healer Daniel D. Palmer restored hearing to a deaf janitor in 1895 with an opportune slap on the back, chiropractors have been manipulating spines for all sorts of health problems.

At the heart of this profession is the premise that misaligned spines cause pressure on the spinal cord and/or spinal nerves. One of the results of that stress on the nerves can be pain.

The job of the chiropractor is to ferret out these misalignments and correct them, freeing the nervous system to work properly again.

About 80 percent of a typical chiropractor's practice involves treatment of low back pain, neck pain, headaches, whiplash and other skeletal maladies. Only a small percentage of cases involve facial pain, and TN is just one of the conditions that falls under that category.

"From a chiropractor's point of view, this is something you see very rarely," says Dr. Scott Haldeman, who is both a licensed chiropractor and neurologist in Irvine, Calif. For that reason, he says, TN is not a condition that's discussed in much detail, if at all, in chiropractic colleges.

Not surprisingly, standard chiropractic treatment isn't attempted that often in treating TN and related face pains, and when it is, success rates have been spotty at best.

However, the track record has been more promising with a specific type of chiropractic treatment that focuses on the very top of the spine (the cervix) where the spinal cord connects to the brain stem.

Although there have been no published studies to measure the success rate of this "upper cervical" treatment, practitioners and some TN patients who have tried it are reporting significant and sometimes complete pain relief.

The spine and face-pain connection

Upper-cervical chiropractors suspect that problems in the upper spine can cause pain in the face in two ways. One is by an injury, such as a fall or a car accident that traumatizes the upper spine. The other is a more gradual misalignment that develops as a result of aging, poor posture or neck-stressing repetitive actions.

Both of these focus on the top three vertebrae and particularly on the health and alignment of the top-most bone, the "atlas." The atlas is a doughnut-shaped bone that surrounds the spinal cord at its connection with the brain stem.

In an ideal posture, the atlas would be exactly horizontal, the spine would be gently curved in its normal fashion, and the head wouldn't tilt abnormally. But because so many of us have had our heads snapped back at one time or another or just have less-than-ideal posture, it seldom works out that way.

Chiropractors say it doesn't take much for misalignments to occur when you've got an anatomy that consists of a 10- to 12-pound ball (the head) held atop a narrow bone that houses the all-important spinal cord.

Minor tilting may not cause any noticeable symptoms. But when the tilting is severe enough or when a neck injury occurs, the spinal cord moves into an abnormal position within the spinal canal. This can create a chronic traction that can affect the nerve fibers that pass through the upper spine.

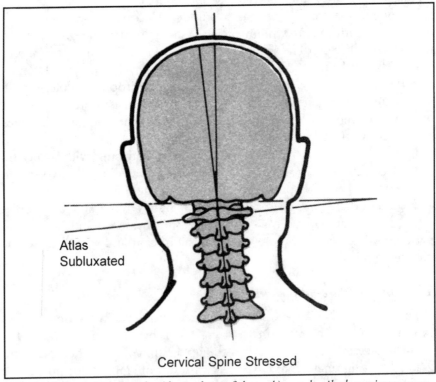

Atlas
Subluxated

Cervical Spine Stressed

This sketch shows how the atlas (the top bone of the neck) may be tilted, causing pressure on the nerves that run through it.

(Reprinted with permission of Vogel Enterprises, Inc.)

Chiropractors say this can translate into TN or related face pain because the very beginning of the trigeminal nerve – the *"trigeminal nucleus"* – reaches down into the first three vertebrae.

Some chiropractors suggest that TN pain is one logical result of injury to or traction on the trigeminal nucleus.

Dr. Roger Hinson, an Atlanta upper-cervical chiropractor who specializes in face pain, believes this might even be a common cause of TN – and one that goes hand-in-hand with the compressing blood vessel that neurosurgeons talk about.

Just as a compressing blood vessel at the nerve's root can make the whole trigeminal system "hyperexcited," Dr. Hinson suggests that traction damage to the trigeminal nucleus can have the same effect. He also suggests that it may take both of these offenses to cause TN in some people.

This, he says, might explain the cadaver studies that showed some people with nerve/vessel contacts near their brain but no TN. And it might explain why most people with misaligned upper spines don't have TN – they're lacking a compressing blood vessel in the skull as the final triggering factor.

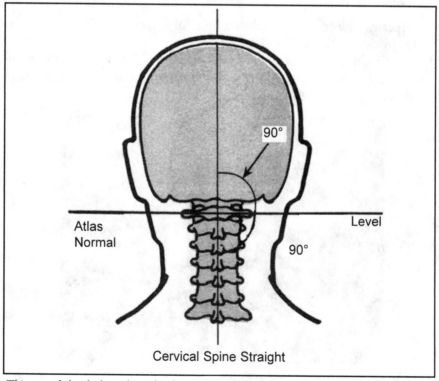

This second sketch shows how the the atlas should be orthogonal (aligned perpendicular) to the head and the axis of a straight cervical spine.

(Reprinted with permission of Vogel Enterprises, Inc.)

"If the tissues covering the spinal cord and brain have traction on them, unusual things happen," agrees Lancaster, Pa., upper-cervical chiropractor Dr. Stephen Goodman. "And one of them is trigeminal neuralgia."

Dr. Goodman also believes compressing blood vessels are a triggering problem that "add insult to injury. This is what brings (the pain) over the edge. At least that's the theory. We don't know for sure."

Boulder, Colo., upper-cervical chiropractor Dr. Erin Elster says she almost always finds signs of injury in patients whom she's treated for TN.

"It's very easy to cause injury in the upper spine and neck," she says. "There's a definite link between trauma to the head and neck and neurological problems. The trauma can be things like blows to the head, a car wreck or even a fall. Sometimes people aren't even aware they've injured themselves. They may fall, brush themselves off and walk away."

Dr. Elster says pain doesn't always occur immediately after a fall. "The time between an injury and the onset of face pain can be quick or it can be a long time," she says.

Searching for problems

Typically, chiropractors look for signs of injury and spinal misalignments by taking X-rays.

Dr. Hinson says he has taken X-rays of eight TN patients, and seven of them had grossly misaligned atlases. "We're seeing rotations in these people that are way outside the scale we'd normally see," he says.

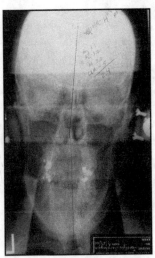 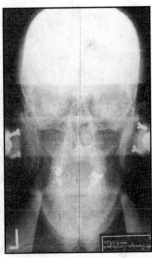

These X-rays of a trigeminal neuralgia patient's head show the alignment of the head both before (left) and after (right) chiropractic adjustments.

(Images courtesy of Dr. Roger Hinson, upper-cervical chiropractor, Atlanta, Ga.)

Chiropractors also may pick up signs of misalignments by looking for head-tilting, uneven shoulders, a tilted pelvis, restricted neck movement and one leg appearing shorter than the other because of increased muscle tension on the hip and pelvis on that side.

Dr. Elster also does thermal scans using a handheld device that measures minute temperature differences of the skin at various points. "When you pick up temperature differentials, that's usually indicative of a problem neurologically," she says.

Spinal misalignments or *"subluxations,"* as chiropractors call them, can occur for a variety of reasons.

Besides the injuries that Dr. Elster mentions, more gradual misalignments can occur because of poor posture, sleeping on one's stomach, improper lifting and stresses such as cradling a phone between the shoulder and neck or working overhead with the head tilted.

Dr. Hinson says aging is a contributing factor to TN because as we age, our spinal discs thin, the joint spaces get tighter, cartilage erodes and our necks shorten. The result is extra pressure on the spinal ligaments. He says that might help explain why TN is much more common in older people.

Fixing the misalignments

If pressure on the upper spinal cord is the root of the problem, then the way to fix it, according to upper-cervical chiropractors, is to move the upper spine back into place. The idea is to take pressure or traction off of the spinal nerves, or in effect, to "decompress" the nerves. In that regard, the aim is similar to what neurosurgeons are doing by moving a compressing blood vessel off of the trigeminal nerve root in a microvascular decompression surgery.

That's easier said than done, and there is a lot of disagreement on how – and even whether – to do it.

By some estimates, there are as many as 150 different chiropractic techniques. Upper-cervical is a specialized sub-field of chiropractic that's done by roughly only 1,000 chiropractors out of the estimated 60,000 chiropractors now practicing in the United States.

Even within this specialty are about 10 different sub-specialties that go by such names as Orthospinology, Atlas Orthogonality, NUCCA (those who are members of the National Upper Cervical Chiropractic Association), Palmer Specific, Blair Upper Cervical, Kale Brainstem, the Laney Technique and Upper Cervical Orthogonal (Cowin Technique).

Some use only the hands to manipulate the spine. Some use different types of machines. Some use supplemental therapies such as ultrasound, electrical stimulation and ice and heat treatment. Others don't. Methods of diagnosing vary. And the angle and degree of adjustment may differ from chiropractor to chiropractor, all of which prompts some to conclude that chiropractic is as much art as science.

Upper-cervical chiropractors say this field has become so specialized in part because of the precise adjustments that are needed when working in the upper spine.

"It's such a difficult area to treat that if you don't do it exclusively, it's hard to do it effectively," says Dr. Goodman.

Unlike the larger manipulations that are done for back pain, upper-cervical adjustments are generally less forceful. In some of the techniques, the adjustment amounts to little more than a slight tap or some mild vibrations.

Retired Alabama chiropractor Dr. Cecil Laney, himself a neuralgian, says it doesn't take much force to move the atlas. However, he says it does require a very precise movement by a skilled practitioner using accurate before-and-after X-rays.

"The cervical spine is a very complicated mechanical structure," Dr. Laney says, adding that more nerves go through it than any other part of the body. "Developing the measures to realign these structures has proven to be a very difficult task. It is very easy for the average chiropractor to twist or pull on the neck, move structure around and get some measure of results. This won't cut it on most difficult problems like TN."

Dr. Hinson agrees and says the larger, more forceful adjustments done in standard chiropractic treatments "are really hit or miss when it comes to TN. With an upper-cervical adjustment, it feels more like someone pushing you with a finger. It's a little tap."

Not all adjustments are that mild. Some techniques use more of a small, quick jerking movement. On average, the force used is only in the 2- to 3-pound range. In rare instances, though, movements have been sharp enough to cause potentially serious blood-vessel injury, which we'll discuss in more detail later in this chapter.

However the adjustment is done, the idea is to get the atlas to line up exactly perpendicular to the upper spine.

Sometimes it takes only one adjustment to do that. More often, though, the patient gets two or three adjustments each over two to four weeks to move the spine back into place.

One thing that all agree on... as Dr. Goodman says, "You can't put it back yourself."

Success rates

So how likely is it that upper-cervical treatments will help?

No one knows for sure since there haven't been any published clinical trials on TN and chiropractic.

Dr. Hinson conducted one pilot study in 2000 in which he treated eight TN patients between the ages of 47 and 79 who had their pain for an average of just over seven years. Each patient got between three and 12 spinal adjustments over an eight-week period.

Of the eight patients, two got complete relief after the first session and had no recurrence during the eight-week study. The remaining six all got significant relief over the first four weeks, averaging 69 to 78 percent pain reductions based on two different before-and-after pain questionnaires.

"All eight had significant decreases in pain scores during the eight-week intervention period," Dr. Hinson says. "Notably, not one continued to have lancinating pain at the end of the study, though several continued to have significant numbness and (abnormal) sensations from their previous surgeries."

Dr. Hinson adds that there was no difference in results between the five patients who had undergone previous TN surgery and the three with no history of surgery, suggesting that prior surgery might not affect chiropractic success rates.

Dr. Hinson also surveyed some of his upper-cervical colleagues who together had treated a total of 68 patients with TN. Those chiropractors reported that 73.5 percent of those patients got complete pain relief, 21 percent got at least some relief and only about 6 percent were not helped at all.

Dr. Elster says she's treated about a dozen TN patients and that "about 90 percent of them have been able to get back to tolerable levels. Some reversed all the way to no pain. The best results seem to be when we see people sooner rather than later and younger rather than older."

When chiropractic adjustments work, the results are usually quick and sometimes immediate.

That's what happened with Bob Moses, a neuralgian from New Jersey, at his first upper-cervical treatment.

"After the adjustment, which was almost unnoticeable, I was laid on my back to measure the length and evenness of my legs," Moses says. "The doctor then put out his arm to help me up off the table, and as I sat up, my pain was gone."

That's also been Dr. Goodman's experience with most patients.

"If the treatment is done right, the pain should be gone before you leave the office," he says. "The success rate is high immediately. Holding it is the difficult part."

Others say it's more likely to take at least a few treatments to notice the full effect, especially if you've had face pain for a long time.

"The prognosis should be clear really soon," says Dr. Hinson. "Maybe not after the first adjustment, but definitely within one to two weeks. If there's not any change in symptoms by then, we're probably barking up the wrong tree."

In the case of injuries, it may take a few weeks of adjustments for pain relief to happen, says Dr. Elster.

"The goal of care is to realign the spine so it's no longer interfering with nerve physiology," she says. "That time frame varies from person to person. As a rule of thumb, I tell people to give it 30 days."

Dr. Elster says that it may take some time for injuries to heal even if the spine is successfully realigned. She's also found that people who have had especially severe pain for a long time also take more time to see improvement.

Dr. Hinson says it's not unusual for patients to feel some temporary discomfort for a few days after an adjustment, particularly muscle stiffness related to the change in spinal position. That's the body readjusting to its new posture, he says. However, there should be no sharp pain, bad headaches or other adverse effects.

"When this is done by an experienced chiropractor, there are no complications," says Dr. Hinson.

He adds that patients should stay in close touch with their primary-care doctors before reducing or stopping their TN medications. "Patients are often eager to reduce dosages, but decreasing too quickly can cause significant, even dangerous, side effects," he says. "When patients do well initially but pain returns or becomes less responsive to (adjustments), it's usually because the patient has reduced medication too quickly."

Keeping the pain away

As Dr. Goodman mentioned, keeping the pain away seems to be a bigger challenge than relieving it in the first place.

"This is a difficult place to work," he says. "You think you have it and then it goes out again. These adjustments are harder to hold than for other pains like sciatica and back pain. The results aren't as long-lived as I'd like."

Dr. Elster says that when the ligaments around the spine are stretched, it takes some "retraining" to get them to tighten to the point where they can hold the spine in its new, corrected position. That's why a series of adjustments may be needed early.

"I try to taper down as people maintain alignment," she says.

Once patients are "stabilized," she still suggests they come back once every six months for a checkup. "If something has slipped out of place, we can adjust them even before the pain starts back up."

In addition to adjustments, chiropractors also usually attempt to figure out what might have caused the misalignment in the first place. If it's a posture problem, for example, the chiropractor may recommend different walking, sitting or sleeping habits. If it's a repetitive action like cradling the phone on the job, a headset may help.

If pain comes back, a new set of adjustments can be done. These can be repeated indefinitely.

Unfortunately, there is no data on whether ensuing treatments are as effective as first-time ones.

What patients say

Patient feedback doesn't shed much more light on chiropractic's overall effectiveness than the limited reports from chiropractors. Results run the gamut.

People like Dick Powell of Pennsylvania say it didn't help at all. "I tried upper-cervical treatments with two different chiropractors," he says. "Neither one gave effective treatments." He says he also was concerned about getting a "whiplash-type" neck injury from the way the adjustment instruments would suddenly let his neck drop.

Kate Borland of Virginia says her X-rays clearly showed a misaligned atlas, but her treatments only worked for the first two days – and even then didn't give complete relief.

Some have better results by combining chiropractic adjustments with other therapies. That's the route Tampa, Fla., TN support group co-leader Rohn Harmer took.

He got relief by getting a series of five lidocaine injections along with chiropractic adjustments. "After six weeks of both neural therapy and chiropractic adjustments, I had the first day without pain," he says. "My neck was severely misaligned due to a whiplash in June 1998. I didn't realize that this was the situation prior to seeing a chiropractor."

Nearly a year later, though, the pain came back suddenly and sharply. "I had 10 treatments over four weeks with a continuous reduction in the frequency and severity of the shocks beginning at four weeks and continuing for 12 weeks," Harmer says. When a more burning pain began at that point, he began getting shots of Vitamin B-12 and began a nutritional plan (both discussed in Chapter 18).

He's had a couple of 3- to 5-day flare-ups since then, both of which were stopped by additional spinal adjustments. "I visited the upper-cervical specialist and got a 'tune-up,'" Harmer says. "Both times, my neck had slipped out of position."

Some patients have had seemingly miraculous experiences from chiropractic alone.

One of the most striking accounts of upper-cervical treatment for TN involves James Tomasi, an Oklahoma man who suffered with on-and-off TN attacks for 10 years.

The pain finally flared so bad that Tomasi's wife, Rhonda, said Tomasi "wouldn't sleep four to five nights straight, crying, wishing he could die." One day Mrs. Tomasi heard a radio program about upper-cervical care and convinced her husband to try it.

"It was amazing," says Tomasi. "The doctor simply pressed on the side of my neck until the bone moved. I didn't feel a thing. In fact, as my wife led me to the car, I told her, 'What a rip-off!' Later that night, I had my first break in pain. By the next morning, I was having 20 minutes of no pain. Two days later and one more treatment, by that night the pain was gone."

Tomasi has been pain-free ever since and off medicine.

Elizabeth Markham of Texas had similar results after less than a month of adjustments. "During this time I was able to gradually decrease the amount of Tegretol I was using to control the pain," she says. "The pain decreased so much that I did not have to take any medication at all. Since that time I have not had any medication or any pain except for an occasional twinge in my face.

"I was only hoping to get some relief from my pain so I could have a life again," she adds. "I never dreamed we would get these kinds of results. I feel like I have a new lease on life."

Sherri Douglas of Ohio is another who got complete relief after two adjustments.

She turned to an Atlas Orthogonal chiropractor because of side effects from Tegretol. "I couldn't think clearly, my vision was blurry, and I was so drowsy I could hardly drive myself to and from work each day," says this 33-year-old mother of two.

Douglas was still having pain after her second adjustment, but the chiropractor told her her atlas was still in place and that the pain was most likely "healing pain."

"To make a long story short, that was the last time I had pain," she says. She got off Tegretol altogether and has been pain-free for six months (as of this writing) with just one other adjustment. "I was having a little tingling in my face, so I had him check my atlas, and it was out slightly," she says. "It is just amazing to me that a treatment that is so simple can change so much."

For Minnesota TN support group leader Mary Butcher, relief came more gradually, but once it did, she's been pain-free and off medicine for five years.

"At first, I had to go back every two or three months and then every three or four months because I couldn't hold the alignment," she says. "That time frame has gradually lengthened to five months, and now I haven't seen him for an alignment in eight months. I went for a check a few weeks ago, and I was still fine. When I'm out of alignment, it's obvious. I get the zings."

Then there are people who get at least some relief at first from chiropractic, but it doesn't last.

Moses, for instance, got dramatic improvement right away and was able to get off three of the four medications he was taking for his "atypical" TN (TN-2). Then the treatment seemed to stop working.

"We kept at it for just over a year with no good results," Moses says. "We tried going back to my original adjustment, adjusting out in the opposite direction of the adjustment that was working before my downfall. We even started from scratch with new X-rays. Nothing worked."

Since then, he's gone back on medication and begun looking into other treatments.

Maxine Payne of Tennessee is another neuralgian who got excellent upper-cervical results at first, only to have the pain return unabated after an auto accident.

Payne originally had TN on her left side and got rid of that with a microvascular decompression surgery. When she developed TN on her right side a few years later, she wasn't too crazy about another MVD.

The first MVD had left her with marked numbness.

So she turned to upper-cervical chiropractic treatment and got relief after five adjustments. "In a month, the pain was gone altogether and I was off medicine," Payne says. "The adjustments were so gentle. At first, I had the same reaction everybody has... it's so gentle it can't work. But when I started improving, I thought, 'Hey, there *is* something to this.'

"The chiropractic adjustments kept me pain-free and drug-free for a year and a half, then I had an auto accident with a bad whiplash," she says. "I haven't had a remission since."

Payne is now controlling her pain with a combination of medication and chiropractic adjustments.

Doris Ballew, who leads a TN support group in Knoxville, Tenn., also got relief for about a year after a three-month round of upper-cervical adjustments.

"I was never able to get off medication completely, but I was able to reduce the amount of Carbatrol I was taking," she says. "Then in November 2002, my pain came back fast and furious. Neither the chiropractic treatments nor acupuncture gave me any relief. I was unable to eat or talk on three separate occasions during 2003."

Ballew ended up trying a Gamma Knife radiosurgery, which also didn't help, and then got an MVD surgery, which knocked out the sharp pain. She is off medication but has some numbness and a bit of burning pain.

Sue Remmey, a TN support group leader from Philadelphia, got relief from a combination of phenytoin (Dilantin) and upper-cervical chiropractor for 10 years before ultimately getting an MVD surgery, which was successful.

"For me, I had reached the point where the adjustments were only successful half the time, and I was getting too many attacks to keep driving to Lancaster," she says. "Even though I eventually decided on the MVD, I know for sure the upper-cervical chiropractic treatment helped me to control the TN for many years... It takes perseverance to pursue chiropractic, but I think for those who have atypical pain or failed surgeries, it is worth trying for a month just to see."

Atlanta TN support group leader Patricia Sumerford, who has been treated successfully for four years by Dr. Hinson, agrees that there's little harm in at least trying this approach.

"I can tell whenever I'm getting out of line, and all he has to do is make the adjustment, and the edge of what might be oncoming pain goes away," Sumerford says. "There are some it doesn't work for, but for most it has been a blessing that they can get off the dreadful pain medicines and the side effects they cause."

What doctors say

Many, if not most, physicians have long discounted the whole underlying theory of "subluxations" and their connection to health. Many also doubt the long-term efficacy of adjustments, particularly in face pain. But medical doctors' biggest concern with upper-cervical treatments in particular is the possibility of serious blood-vessel injury.

At least some of the concern stems from a recent study sponsored by the American Heart Association and conducted by the Stanford (University) Stroke Center. The center asked 486 California neurologists about patients they might have seen during the previous two years who had suffered a stroke within 24 hours of neck manipulation by a chiropractor.

The survey turned up 55 such cases. One patient had died and 48 were left with permanent neurological deficits, including slurred speech, dizziness and inability to arrange words properly.

The neurologists attributed most of the cases to tears in the vertebral artery, an important vessel that's anchored to the base of the skull.

The Manitoba (Canada) College of Physicians and Surgeons also recently advised doctors to warn patients about the risks of spinal adjustments after six cases of manipulation-related brainstem injury were reported in that province within a three-year period.

And the May 2003 journal Neurology also wrote about the risks to the vertebral artery from adjustments and took the stance that the largely temporary and incomplete relief of these adjustments does not justify the risk.

"How common are strokes following neck manipulation? Nobody knows," says Dr. Stephen Barrett, who heads the QuackWatch web site. "No clinical research has addressed this problem, and chiropractic malpractice insurance companies have refused to make their data public. Most speculations run from one in 400,000 to one in 3 million. But when manipulations are done without valid reason – as they often are – no complication is excusable."

The May 27, 2002, issue of The Medical Letter, a newsletter for doctors, weighed in with this conclusion: "Spinal manipulation can cause life-threatening complications. Manipulation of the cervical spine, which has been associated with dissection of the vertebral artery, appears to be especially dangerous."

Dr. Hinson, the Georgia chiropractor, says such injuries are very rare and associated only with the more forceful adjustments that relatively few upper-cervical practitioners do.

"The mechanism of manipulation-induced stroke is usually forceful rotation of the upper cervical joints beyond their normal range of motion," he says.

He says this type of maneuver, called a *"rotary break"* in chiropractic, involves moving the joint in both directions. The adjustment also makes a cracking noise.

Most upper-cervical techniques involve much milder adjustments, he says, adding that "there is little potential for trauma to the vertebral artery with this type of adjustment."

Dr. William Jarvis, president of the Massachusetts-based National Council Against Health Fraud, warns that another potential chiropractic hazard is the repeated X-rays that some chiropractors do. That, he says, exposes patients to potentially cancer-causing radiation.

Again, there are differences from chiropractor to chiropractor. Some do more X-rays than others, and a few require none at all.

Chiropractic's role in face pain

Chiropractic's main appeal to face-pain patients is that it offers a possible way to get out of pain without the sedating side effects of medicine and the potential complications of surgery. These people hope that if all goes well, they won't face a lifetime of pills and won't have to make a decision that might leave them with a numb face – or worse.

Others turn to chiropractic only after they weren't helped by those more "mainstream" therapies. And still others use chiropractic as one cog in a multi-pronged approach that might include mainstream therapies and other CAM therapies.

The bright side is that some people report getting remarkably good results from just a few adjustments. Some are able to get off medication and at least get a temporary reprieve from pain.

Upper-cervical chiropractors say they're having equal success with those who have "atypical" TN and even anesthesia dolorosa – two conditions that don't respond as well to mainstream therapies.

And they point to the low (some would say no) risks and the fairly quick results.

The down side is that, at best, it's unknown how helpful spinal adjustments will be over the long haul. The long-term outlook from members of the Trigeminal Neuralgia Association so far isn't terribly promising. As with most other therapies, the pain often has a way of finding its way back, even despite a new round of therapy.

Repeat or regular adjustments can be done so long as it's helping, but that can get expensive. Some insurance plans cover chiropractic care and some don't. Initial visits with X-rays generally cost more than $100, and follow-up sessions typically cost between $25 and $45. Depending on how many treatments are needed, out-of-pocket expenses can easily run into the hundreds of dollars.

Beyond the expense, doctors warn about the blood-vessel risk (even if it's small).

Then there's the confusing issue of finding someone who offers the particular technique that's most likely to help you. As Dr. Jarvis puts it, "Chiropractic is a conglomeration of factions in conflict."

Given the relative few upper-cervical specialists, you may have trouble finding *any*, especially in rural areas. And if there's only one or two, you may not be able to choose whether you prefer, say, a hands-only Palmer practitioner over an orthospinologist using an instrument.

"There are tremendous differences in techniques," says Dr. Elster. "But there haven't been studies done that compare technique to technique."

That means the only way you're going to know if a particular chiropractor is going to help is to try it and see.

Dr. Elster advises patients interested in upper-cervical treatment to ask about chiropractors' training and experience and to ask what kind of success they've had in treating prior face-pain cases similar to yours. She also advises getting recommendations from other people.

"I encourage people that if they haven't had success with one upper-cervical chiropractor to try another one," Dr. Elster says. "You shouldn't give up on the whole concept because one technique didn't work."

HOW TO FIND AN
UPPER-CERVICAL CHIROPRACTOR

Besides checking in your local telephone book, different types of upper-cervical chiropractors have their own organizations that can help you locate members throughout the country.

Some of these organizations and other upper-cervical resources are:

- Academy of Upper Cervical Chiropractic Organization
  1637 Westbridge Drive, Unit H4, Fort Collins, CO 80526
  www.aucco.org

- American Chiropractic Association
  1701 Clarendon Blvd., Arlington, VA 22209
  1-800-986-4636
  www.amerchiro.org

- International Chiropractors Association
  1110 N. Glebe Road, Suite 1000, Arlington, VA 22201
  1-800-423-4690 or 703-528-5000
  www.chiropractic.org

- National Awareness Campaign for Upper Cervical Care
  5215 Colbert Road, Lakeland, FL 33813
  1-888-622-8221
  www.uppercervical.org

- National Upper Cervical Chiropractic Association
  2608 West Kenosha, Suite 224, Broken Arrow, OK 74012
  918-748-1900
  www.nucca.org

- Society of Chiropractic Orthospinology
  770-517-9921
  www.orthospinology.org

- Up C Spine
  an informational web site on all the techniques.
  Founded by patient Greg Buchanan, it also has lists
  of practitioners worldwide.
  www.uppercervicalspine.com

CHAPTER 18

NUTRITION THERAPY

"Eating a poor diet is like putting bad gas in a car. What does it do?
It sputters and spits. It's the same with our body when we don't eat right."
—Dr. Henry Gremillion, University of Florida College of Dentistry

Most of us – neuralgians or not – would concede that our diets are less than ideal. Americans are notorious for over-doing it with high-calorie snacks, fatty fast foods and sugar-laden soft drinks. As a country, we tend to over-eat and under-exercise.

That's not exactly a great prescription for good health in general. In fact, obesity and poor dietary choices have been linked to a variety of ailments, particularly heart disease, diabetes, high blood pressure and some cancers.

What's not known is the role diet and nutrition might play in trigeminal neuralgia and related face pain. Certainly, minimum amounts of a variety of nutrients are needed for the body and its nervous system to function properly. Deficiencies also can hinder the body from healing as it should and from fighting off disease.

But can a lack of a particular nutrient *cause* TN? Can it at least contribute to it? If so, which one or ones? How do we know how much is not enough? Are those levels the same for everyone or is an adequate level for one person a deficiency for another? Theories and suspicions abound.

That's not unusual for the field of nutrition, though, where all sorts of opposing theories still abound even when it comes to the big picture of what's a good diet and what's not. Some say we should be eating high-fiber, low-fat diets. Others say high-protein, low-carbohydrate diets are the way to go. One book claims we should eat more like the Japanese. The next one says we should eat more like the Italians.

It gets even more confusing when particular nutrients are linked to particular disorders. Just about the time one study tells us that coffee, for example, might raise our cholesterol level, another study comes along telling us it lowers the risk of colon cancer.

Every year seems to bring news of yet another food, vitamin or supplement that might cure or prevent an ailment. Vitamins A and C, oat bran, garlic, green tea, carrot juice from the juicer, coenzyme Q10, lycopene and fish oil capsules are just a few recent examples.

Sorting it all out gets very complicated. Most nutrition studies reach their conclusions by monitoring people's diets and comparing what happens health-wise. Isolating exactly what accounted for any differences is exceedingly complex, given the huge amount of variables involved.

Even when we think we have something figured out, does that mean we can pull out that particular nutrient and use it as a supplement to head off particular problems? Or do we have to eat the whole food to get the benefit?

It gets even more complicated if you believe some recent studies in cancer prevention. These studies suggest that nutrients may have a differing effect from person to person depending on our genetic, hormonal and enzyme makeup. If that's the case, doctors in the future might give prescriptions for certain diets that are tailored to each person's biological makeup and ailments.

In the meantime, we're stuck with a maze of often-conflicting studies, claims, counter-claims, changing recommendations and testimonials of all sorts.

Food links to face pain

In the world of TN, there have been no specific dietary studies – conflicting or otherwise. TN is just not a common enough disorder to justify the kind of large and costly studies that are done in more widespread problems such as heart disease and diabetes.

That pretty much leaves practitioners and individual patients to look for bits of information that seem to make sense. One approach is to focus on nutrients that have an effect on the nervous system in general. Another is to try nutrients or diets that seem to help other pains or somewhat related conditions such as multiple sclerosis.

One step that seems to make good sense is cutting back on anything that stimulates the central nervous system. The last thing you want to do is excite an already hyperexcited trigeminal nerve even more. Food-wise, the main culprit in that is caffeine.

Sylvia Escott-Stump recommends cutting out or cutting back on caffeine for TN patients in her book, *"Nutrition and Diagnosis-Related Care"* (Williams and Wilkins, 1998). Caffeine is most commonly found in regular coffee, tea, chocolate and many soft drinks.

One particularly striking caffeine case study was reported in 1991 by Dr. Stephen Glore, assistant professor of clinical dietetics at the University of Oklahoma.

Dr. Glore reported that a 45-year-old woman with TN got relief within three weeks by switching to decaffeinated coffee. The woman had been drinking three to four cups of regular instant coffee per day – more when her pain was worse.

On the low-caffeine diet, the woman remained pain-free for a year. When, as a test, she began drinking two cups of cocoa a day, the pain came back within a week. She also found that even one cup of regular coffee was enough to restart "moderately intense" pain.

At the time of Dr. Glore's report, the woman had been keeping her pain in check for two years with the low-caffeine diet.

Dr. Glore points out that one case doesn't offer much proof, but it at least might be something worth exploring for those with high caffeine intakes.

There's also been some evidence that nuts, chocolate and other foods high in arginine may contribute to post-herpetic neuralgia.

Dr. Richard Griffith, professor emeritus at the Indiana University School of Medicine, reports that he once had a patient who was a compulsive eater of nuts and chocolate who was about to have surgery for TN.

Dr. Griffith suspected the arginine in these foods might have been activating the herpes virus that can lead to post-herpetic neuralgia outbreaks. When the man cut back on those foods, the pain went away almost overnight.

Like Dr. Glore, Dr. Griffith points out that one case doesn't make a study. But as with caffeine, he says a small dietary change is worth trying before going ahead with a more invasive therapy.

Since then, one other neuralgian from California has alerted the Florida-based Trigeminal Neuralgia Association that she was able to get rid of her pain through a combination of L'lysine supplements and avoiding chocolate and nuts.

One other food ingredient that can heighten sensitivity to pain is aspartame, the artificial sweetener in NutraSweet and Equal. More than a few neuralgians have complained of seeming to have pain flare-ups soon after eating foods or drinking beverages with aspartame.

There may be a biochemical explanation for this one. Aspartame breaks down in the body into an agent that is chemically similar to a body chemical that's involved in the transmission of pain signals.

As with caffeine, anything that enhances our pain-signaling ability in an already hyperexcited trigeminal system is not a help. Small amounts of aspartame are unlikely to make a difference, but consuming larger amounts might.

Several other neuralgians have told TNA that they were able to reduce their pain by avoiding fatty foods and reducing overall fat in their diet to 20 percent or less of total calories.

"About two weeks later, I began to notice my TN was not as severe," wrote C.G. Hartland, a neuralgian from Wisconsin who used the American Heart Association's diet plan along with daily two-mile walks. "At first, I attributed this to a remission, even though I had never experienced one in the 12 years I suffered. Two weeks later, my TN disappeared. Several months later I splurged on a lasagna dinner, and the next morning the TN was back. I returned to my low-fat diet, and a few days later the TN went away again."

For what it's worth, a few other neuralgians say they've been helped by other diet-related measures, including adding yeast and acidophilus to their diets; avoiding gluten-rich foods; drinking daily fresh-vegetable juices made in a juicer; eating daily servings of alfalfa and mung beans, and switching to vegetarian or vegan diets.

Pain-triggering foods

Since the trigeminal nerve and its fibers are responsible for almost all sensations in the face, anything that creates a significant change in the mouth is a potential pain trigger. That especially includes foods that cause sensations of heat, cold, sweetness and sourness. The sharper the sensation, the more likely the food is to trigger signals that end up "crossing tracks" to set off the pain-signaling nerve fibers.

These foods can vary from person to person. Eating hot foods such as salsa, chili, hot sauce or even hot cinnamon candy may do it for some people. Other people might not mind that but have trouble with particular spices, such as cinnamon, ginger, nutmeg, salt or black pepper. Still others mind cool-sensation foods such as mint candy or mint-seasoned foods.

Even people whose primary trigger zone is the nose may get pain flare-ups when eating foods with strong odors, such as hot mustard, horseradish, garlic or onions. Vapors from these foods can sensitize the nerve endings in the nose and trigger a TN attack.

Dr. Neal Barnard, in his book, *"Foods That Fight Pain"* (Harmony Books, 1998), claims there are 12 foods that are common "headache triggers." These are: dairy products, chocolate, eggs, citrus fruits, meat, wheat, nuts, tomatoes, onions, corn, apples and bananas.

On the other hand, Dr. Barnard says there are some foods that are almost never implicated in pain by anyone. These so-called "pain-safe" foods include brown rice, cooked or dried fruits such as cherries, cranberries, pears and prunes, and cooked vegetables such as artichokes, asparagus, broccoli, chard, collards, lettuce, spinach, beans, squash and sweet potatoes.

It's unknown if some of these same foods might trigger TN pain as well as headaches. But if you suspect a dietary link to your TN pain, Dr. Barnard suggests sticking only with the "pain-safe" foods for about two weeks. If the pain eases, then gradually add other foods until pain starts to return. This, he says, may help you zero in on particular foods that might be a pain trigger for you. (That is, of course, unless TN's tricky maneuver of going into and out of spontaneous remissions fakes you out.)

Before tinkering around with *any* significant dietary changes, it's always a good idea to check first with your doctor.

Two main routes

Beyond looking for particular TN/food links, targeting face pain with a nutrition game plan can be done on two levels.

One is the big-picture approach of trying to take in the right amounts of the right nutrients to ensure there are no deficiencies that might be causing or contributing to the pain.

The other is a more focused approach that goes to the heart of the presumed cause of TN – a blood vessel compressing the trigeminal nerve. You'll recall that the reason this vessel is a problem is because it beats on and wears down the protective coating (myelin) of the trigeminal nerve fibers, thereby allowing the nerve to short-circuit much like an electrical cord without its insulation.

That got more than a few people thinking… what if we can come up with a way to heal that myelin or to prevent it from breaking down in the first place? Then it wouldn't matter if there's a blood vessel there or not. If the myelin is in place, the nerve won't short-circuit.

The big question is how to achieve that. Multiple sclerosis researchers have long been looking at gene therapy, diet, medicines and other means of restoring healthy myelin because that's also at the center of that disorder. Others have suggested megadoses of the nutritional building blocks the body uses to manufacture myelin.

Although some of these measures have been of some help to some people, so far the magic bullet of myelin reproduction (if there is one) hasn't been uncovered.

We'll take a look at some of these efforts later in this chapter, but first, let's look at Main Route 1: what a healthy nervous system needs to function.

The "healthy-nerve" diet

By eating a good diet (a definition that's hotly debated topic itself), you'll at least "help stack the deck in your favor," says Dr. Parker Mahon, professor emeritus at the University of Florida's Facial Pain Center.

A healthy, balanced diet will help ensure your body is getting the nutrients it needs to work right. That's all most people need to do, according to the American Dietetic Association, the nation's largest organization of food and nutrition professionals.

ADA's official position is that "most healthy people can get all the nutrients they need from food in a well planned diet... the best nutritional strategy for promoting optimal health and reducing the risk of chronic disease is to wisely choose a wide variety of foods."

People who eat poorly are likely to feel worse in general. And the less healthy you feel, the more you're likely to mind the pain you've got.

Good nutrition is a particular concern in TN because the simple acts of eating and drinking so often trigger pain attacks. As a result, some neuralgians curtail eating and drinking, which can lead to weight loss, poor nutrition and dehydration.

The first step, then, in "nutrition therapy" is to eat a healthy, balanced diet – one that the U.S. Department of Agriculture says is roughly 30 percent fat, 30 percent protein and 40 percent carbohydrates.

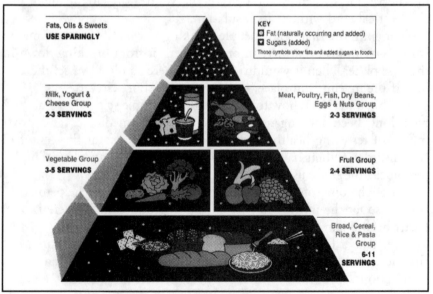

The Food Guide Pyramid is a graphic guide to what the U.S. government considers to be a healthy diet.

(Image by U.S. Department of Agriculture and U.S. Department of Health and Human Services)

USDA's Food Guide Pyramid is a graphic guide to achieving that. More U.S. nutrition guidelines are available online at USDA's Food and Nutrition Information Center (www.nal.usda.gov/fnic).

Some neuralgians are able to maintain a good diet by sticking with soft foods or by pureeing harder foods that are more difficult to eat. Some also say it's less painful to drink through a long straw than sipping directly from a glass or cup.

Another option for those who can't chew at all during particularly painful episodes is to use liquid supplements such as Ensure or to supplement their food with additional vitamins, minerals and other nutrients.

Dr. Mahon also says a good diet can help keep cholesterol and blood pressure under control for good circulatory health. "One major theory about the cause of TN blames it on blood vessels that pound on the trigeminal nerve," he says. "If an artery develops atherosclerotic plaque because of high cholesterol, it will pound even harder."

SEVEN GUIDELINES FOR A HEALTHY DIET

Following are seven main points that most nutritionists and the USDA recommend for a healthy diet:

- **Eat a variety of foods.** By varying choices from all five main food groups (breads and cereals; fruits; vegetables; dairy products, and meats), you'll be assured of getting a mix of the more than 40 different nutrients your body needs.

- **Maintain a healthy weight.** You'll have more energy, feel better and be less likely to suffer from obesity-related disorders. This also may help keep blood pressure down, which can be a factor affecting TN pain.

- **Use fat and cholesterol in moderation.** This can help you keep weight and blood pressure down.

- **Eat plenty of vegetables, fruits and grain products.** These are high in important vitamins and minerals and also supply fiber to help your body get rid of waste.

- **Use sugar in moderation.** Sugars are "empty" calories that contribute to weight gain and tooth decay without giving any nutrient value in return.

- **Use salt and sodium in moderation.** These cause your body to retain water and can help increase blood pressure.

- **If you drink alcohol at all, do so in moderation.** It also adds calories with little nutrient return and interacts with a variety of medications. Overdoing it can lead to a host of health problems, including liver and stomach disorders.

— Sources: USDA, American Dietetic Association

Nerve-related vitamins and minerals

Several vitamins and minerals are believed to be important to healthy functioning of the nervous system in general. Deficiencies of them could lead to nervous-system impairments, including nerve pain. Here's the list:

- **Vitamin B-1** (thiamine). It breaks down carbohydrates but also is needed for proper nerve function. Deficiency can cause depression, anxiety and beriberi, a potentially fatal condition that includes pain or tingling in the arms and legs.

  Found in cereals, peas, brewer's yeast, garbanzo beans, beef liver, egg yolks, soybeans, sunflower seeds, kidney beans, wheat germ, navy beans, pork, fish, rice bran, salmon steak, nuts, brown rice, whole grain products, rye and whole wheat flour. Recommended Daily Allowance (RDA): 0.8 to 1.3 mg for men, 0.8 mg for women.

- **Vitamin B-3** (niacin). Needed for proper nerve function. Deficiency can lead to degeneration of nerves.

  Found in liver, brewer's yeast, white chicken meat, halibut, peanuts, pork, salmon, sunflower seeds, swordfish, tuna, turkey, veal, breads, grains, flour, cereals, legumes and mushrooms. RDA: 16 to 23 mg for men, 14 to 16 mg for women.

- **Vitamin B-5** (pantothenic acid). Manufactures hormones and chemicals that regulate nerve function. Deficiency can cause nerve pain.

  Found in meat, poultry, fish, beans, peas and whole-grain cereals. RDA: 2.5 mg for men and women.

- **Vitamin B-6** (pyridoxine). Needed for proper brain and nerve function. Deficiency can cause lack of coordination, nervousness and convulsions.

  Overdose also can lead to nerve damage, so this is one you can overdo. For his patients, Dr. Mahon suggests supplements of 100 to 200 mg per day but only for three weeks at a time.

  Found in meat, poultry, avocados, bananas, broccoli, bran, brewer's yeast, carrots, cereals, dairy products, filberts, whole wheat flour, lentils, potatoes, sweet potatoes, rice, salmon, shrimp, soybeans, sunflower seeds, tuna and wheat germ. RDA: 1.8 mg for men, 1.5 mg for women.

- **Vitamin B-12** (cobalamin). Used by the body as a component in manufacturing blood cells and in the production of myelin, the protective coating around nerves. Gross deficiencies of Vitamin B-12 can lead to nerve damage (both pain and inflammation) and to anemia, depression and memory loss.

  Found primarily in animal products, such as liver, salmon, oysters, beef, lamb, veal, clams, flounder, herring, mackerel, sardines, eggs, milk and cheese. RDA: 6 micrograms.

- **Vitamin E.** Needed for proper function of nerves and muscles. Deficiency can cause nerve abnormalities.

  Found in vegetable oils, margarine, butter, wheat germ, cereals, green leafy vegetables, nuts and legumes.
  RDA: 9 to 10 mg for men, 6 to 7 mg for women.

- **Calcium.** Needed for nerve transmission. Found in dairy products, turnip greens, collards, kale, mustard greens, broccoli, oysters, shrimp, salmon, clams and sardines.
  RDA: 800 to 1,000 mg for men, 800 to 1,200 mg for women.

- **Potassium.** Regulates nerve sensitivity. Found in bananas, oranges, orange juice and other fruits, broccoli, legumes, mushrooms, nuts, sunflower seeds, meat, fish, poultry and whole grains. RDA: 40 to 80 mg for men and women.

- **Magnesium.** Regulates nerve sensitivity. Deficiency can cause tremors and twitching. Found in milk, cheese, broccoli, meats, seafood, spinach, tofu, popcorn, whole grains, legumes, nuts and wheat bran. RDA: 250 to 600 mg for men, 200 to 600 mg for women.

- **Copper.** Used in production of nerve fibers and myelin sheath around nerves. Deficiency occurs only in severe malnutrition. Found in liver, shellfish, meats, nuts, legumes and cereals. RDA: 2 to 3 mg for men and women.

- **Phosphorus.** Needed for proper nerve function. Found in chicken, milk, lentils, egg yolks, nuts and cheese.
  RDA: 1,000 mg for men, 850 mg for women.

The role of supplements

If you're not getting those government-recommended amounts in foods, another way is to take vitamin pills or supplements that contain the nutrients you're lacking. Some products contain just one particular nutrient; others combine many into a single multivitamin.

"Nutritional supplementation is indicated in many patients," says Dr. Mahon, "Particularly when you have a compromised trigeminal nerve, anything you can do to provide for a healthy environment for that nerve will tend to reduce the number of bouts you'll have with this excruciating pain."

The question is which nutrients and which amounts will make a difference? The research has been slim, and the effects may well vary from person to person.

Most of conventional medicine and nutrition look to the government-recommended amounts as the ideals for good health.

The ADA says that relatively few people need any supplements at all, and that evidence backs supplement use only in a few specific instances. Among them: extra iron for pregnant women; extra calcium for those at increased risk of osteoporosis and those allergic to dairy products; Vitamin B-12 supplements for strict vegans who have eliminated all animal products; Vitamin D supplements for those with limited milk intake and limited exposure to sunlight; and multivitamin and mineral supplements for those on weight-loss diets of under 1,200 calories a day.

Beyond those and a few others, any helpful effects are unproven — and possibly useless or even harmful, the ADA says.

Others, however, believe some of the government-set nutrition levels are woefully inadequate and that at the very least, some people may need much higher levels of selected nutrients than others.

Whole books have been written about the subject of megadoses of various nutrients. Studies back up some of the claims, but in other cases, the evidence amounts largely to case studies and patients reporting their own improvements following a switch to a diet- or supplement-related plan.

Either way, doctors offer a few cautions when it comes to taking megadoses.

"Many people began to take B-complex vitamins in megadoses after they were reported to be good for the nervous system," says Dr. Mahan. "Unfortunately, high doses of vitamin B-6 can actually damage nerves within just three months, interfering with 'proprioception' – your sense of orientation of your body in space. Individuals who took 500 mg per day for a year began to stumble frequently and lose their balance."

A few studies have reported an increase in kidney stones in people who were taking more than 1,000 mg of Vitamin C supplements a day, and high levels of Vitamin A also have been linked to headaches and other neurological disturbances.

"When vitamins are consumed in excess of the body's physiological needs, they function as drugs rather than vitamins," says Dr. Stephen Barrett, who runs the QuackWatch web site. "A few situations exist in which high doses of vitamins are known to be beneficial, but they must still be used with caution because of potential toxicity."

Of particular concern are Vitamins A, D, E and K, which can be stored in the fat. If excess amounts of these are taken in day after day, levels can build up and become harmful.

The ADA says that when supplements stay within the government-recommended levels, there's little risk of adverse effects. It's when amounts start to greatly exceed those levels that push risks into uncharted territory.

Even when the body simply excretes nutrients it doesn't need, that's at the very least a waste of money, says Dr. Barrett.

Those who believe in the merits of supplements, on the other hand, say this might be the best money you've ever spent if it gets rid of the awful pain. As Pennsylvania health counselor Emily Jane Lemole points out, the number of people harmed by diet supplements is minuscule compared to the numbers harmed by prescription drugs.

A doctor or nutritionist may be able to help you figure out what nutrients you might be lacking, what products might best help and what levels are safe and helpful.

Most of the nutritional plans neuralgians use are tailored around the above list of vitamins and minerals that play a role in nerve function. And that brings us to Main Route 2: ways that might specifically address TN and related face pains.

Vitamin B-12 and myelin

If damaged myelin is at the heart of the trigeminal nerve's short-circuiting pain, then fixing it would seem to be a logical goal. Neurosurgeons address this problem by seeking to move a blood vessel away from the area where the vessel is beating on the nerve and wearing down the myelin.

The nutritional approach is to figure out ways to encourage the body to heal injured myelin and to prevent it from wearing down. Because Vitamin B-12 is thought to play a role in myelin production, it's been one of the most common nutrients used in combating TN.

Researchers were exploring Vitamin B-12 injections and pills as a TN treatment as early as the 1940s and 1950s. In three different studies between 1952 and 1954, more than three-quarters of the 49 patients studied got complete or marked relief from Vitamin B-12 shots given daily for 10 days. The daily doses ranged from 100 to 1,000 micrograms.

The studies did not, however, follow up to see how lasting the pain relief was. Then when the prescription medications Dilantin and Tegretol came along, B-12 research was largely abandoned.

The only recent study has been one from Japan that linked the methylcobalamin form of B-12 to the prevention and treatment of

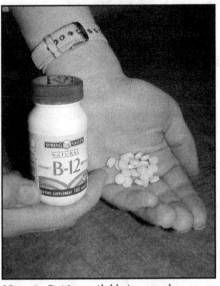

Vitamin B-12, available in over-the-counter tablets in a variety of doses, is thought to play a role in nerve myelin production.

(Photo by George Weigel)

such disorders as chronic fatigue syndrome, Parkinson's disease, neuropathies, Alzheimer's disease and muscular dystrophies. The researchers suggest that high doses of methylcobalamin might help regenerate myelin and nerve cells.

U.S. doctors occasionally suggest B-12 injections or supplements, and it's a cornerstone of almost all nutrition-related TN plans. But since there have been no detailed, double-blind studies into its effectiveness and dose rates, there is no protocol for its use in TN.

Some neuralgians report that B-12 helped them tremendously.

One Kentucky woman who wrote to the *"Dear Dr. SerVaas"* column in the Saturday Evening Post claims she got rid of TN in 1960 with B-12 shots and again during another flare-up in 1980. She says she takes B-12 tablets every day and has had no major flare-ups since.

Another San Diego woman wrote in the San Diego TN support group's newsletter about getting relief from several days' worth of 3,000-microgram sublingual Vitamin B-12 tablets. (These are placed under the tongue to dissolve.)

But others have tried the exact same kind of program only to find no help. Philadelphia TN support group leader Sue Remmey, for instance, tried B-12 injections for several weeks and saw no measurable improvement. Other support group leaders report similar findings – occasional help but a lot of "no-improvements."

B-12 tablets are easy to find in the vitamin section of pharmacies and supermarkets. Typically they come in sizes ranging from 25-microgram to 1,000-microgram tablets. Most contain the cyanocobalamin form of B-12. The methylcobalamin type is often a bit harder to find.

In her 1987 book, *"The Right Dose: How to Take Vitamins and Minerals Safely"* (Ballantine Books), nutritionist Patricia Hausman reports that there is little risk of taking too much B-12. She says Swedish doctors found no problems in patients who took single doses as high as 100,000 micrograms or in patients who took 500 to 1,000 micrograms daily for three to five years.

In rare cases, some people have had allergic reactions after B-12 injections. These are usually limited to skin problems such as acne, eczema or a swelling and crusting of the skin around the lips, although one person reported in the medical literature had a severe enough allergic reaction to B-12 injections that death resulted.

Concludes Hausman: "I have little reason to suspect that those who take B-12 supplements orally will be harmed, even at very high doses. As vitamins go, B-12 simply is one of the safest."

Nevertheless, it's always a good idea to discuss any therapy with a trusted health practitioner first.

Nutrition-based plans

More often, B-12 is just one arm of a multi-faceted approach that includes dietary changes, other supplements and changes in lifestyles.

One of the few published plans is one suggested by Dr. Abram Hoffer and Dr. Morton Walker in their book, *"Putting It All Together: The New Orthomolecular Nutrition"* (McGraw-Hill, 1998).

Their plan suggests B-12 injections of 1 mg (1,000 micrograms) "several times each week and tapering off depending on progress," or sublingual B-12 tablets of 1 to 2 mg (1,000 to 2,000 micrograms) each day. In addition to that, they recommend ascorbic acid (Vitamin C) in doses of "at least 6 grams daily," L'lysine up to 3 to 6 grams daily and B-complex vitamins. (Note that the level they suggest of Vitamin C is well above the level that some studies have found to increase the risk of kidney stones.)

Using that as a starting point, Lemole (the Pennsylvania health counselor) and her husband Dr. Gerald M. Lemole, a cardiac surgeon and author of *"The Healing Diet"* (William Morrow, 2000), tailored a comprehensive plan for their sister-in-law, Gwen Asplundh, who was still having TN pain despite a Gamma Knife surgery, acupuncture and numerous medications.

The program started with B-12 injections, L'lysine and Vitamins B and C, but it added Vitamin E, folic acid, niacin, cod liver oil capsules and multi-mineral tablets with calcium, magnesium, zinc, selenium and manganese.

The plan also included avoiding dairy products, sugar and caffeine; drinking a daily blended mix of fresh fruit, flax seed oil and lecithin, and switching to a high-fiber diet rich in so-called "good fats" (i.e. flax seed oil, olive oil and avocados), fruits, vegetables, whole grains, garlic, onion, beans and soy products and cold-water fatty fish such as salmon, cod, herring, sardines and mackerel. (See the accompanying box for the exact plan.)

Dr. Lemole says that the entire plan is geared toward supplying the body with all of the "building blocks" it needs to maximize the production of myelin, which is composed mostly of cholesterol and essential fatty acids.

"The (myelin) sheath degenerates in many instances because you don't have the sufficient building blocks and enzymes to make it come back and regenerate," he says.

He adds that as people age, they no longer absorb B-12 as well as they once did.

What's not yet proven is whether megadoses of B-12 can stimulate the regeneration of injured myelin, including in people who aren't deficient in B-12. Experiments involving B-12 in treating multiple sclerosis (also a disorder related to damaged myelin) haven't turned out to be very promising.

The explanation is that myelin apparently is produced only when enzymes are available in a proper ratio. Adding mass quantities of one ingredient won't do the trick, the thinking goes, and the body will just excrete the B-12 it can't use.

In any event, the Lemoles' plan worked wonders for Asplundh.

"After two to three weeks of this program, I felt like a miracle had happened," she says. "I was able to go off Neurontin, we could discontinue the B-12 injections and I was pain-free!"

She has had a few flare-ups in the years since but each time knocked the pain back down with a new one- to two-week round of B-12 injections and hot-pepper (capsaicin) cream. (B-12 injections must be prescribed by a doctor although the sublingual tablets are available over-the-counter.)

THE LEMOLES' TN PROGRAM

Following is the program Dr. Gerald and Emily Jane Lemole recommend for neuralgians and those with related face pain:

Vitamins:
• Vitamin B-12. Daily injections of 1 mg for the first week, tapering off to three times a week until pain is relieved. Then either 1 mg weekly injections or 3,000 microgram (3 mg) daily sublingual tablets of B-12, preferably the methylcobalamin type.
• High-potency multivitamin with minerals, with at least 50 mg of B vitamins included. One daily.
• Vitamin E. 400 I.U. daily. (Begin with 100 I.U. daily and increase gradually in those with hypertension or diabetes.)
• Vitamin C. 1,000 mg capsules, two at a time three times daily. (Note: Some studies have shown that taking more than 1,000 mg of Vitamin C per day can increase the risk of kidney stones. Also, high doses of Vitamin C and E may alter the effect of blood-thinning medications such as Coumadin.)
• Niacin. 640 mg capsules, three times a day until pain is gone, then reduce to one daily.
• B-50 complex. One capsule daily.
• Folic acid. 800 microgram capsules. Take two at a time twice daily.

Minerals:
• Multi-Mineral tablets that contain calcium, magnesium, zinc, selenium and manganese. Take two in the morning and two in the evening.

Amino Acids:
• L'lysine. 500 mg capsules, take two at a time three times a day until pain is gone, then reduce to 500 mg daily.

Essential Fatty Acids:
• Max EPA fish oil. Three gel caps daily.
• Ultra GLA (Gama-linolenic acid). One daily.

"Magic Drink:"
• In a blender, combine 8 ounces of fruit juice, one fresh fruit (banana, peach, pear or kiwi), 2 tablespoons lecithin and 1 tablespoon flax seed oil. Drink one or two daily. Optional additives: nutritional yeast, psyllium powder, wheat germ, green magma, soy protein powder.

Diet:
• Eat liberally: high-fiber foods, "good" fats (flax seed oil, olive oil, borage oil, evening primrose oil, avocados), fruits, vegetables, whole grains, nuts, beans, soy products, garlic, onions, cold-water fish such as salmon, cod, herring, tuna, sardines and mackerel. (Note: Garlic and onions can be pain-triggering foods for some neuralgians.)
• Avoid: Animal fats, homogenized milk, fried foods, most processed foods, hydrogenated fats (cakes, cookies, etc.), caffeine, sugar.

"I know it's hard to believe that something this easy can be effective," Asplundh says. "I also know that what works for one person may not work for another. But doesn't the reward of being without pain and off drugs make it worth giving the natural path a try?"

Several members of the Philadelphia TN support group tried the plan but didn't have as good a result as Asplundh, Remmey reports. It's unknown how many others might have tried this program and what their results have been.

Emily Jane Lemole stresses that it's important that the program be done as a whole as opposed to attempting to split out just parts of it. "It's all related to myelin reproduction and nerve generation," she says.

She also advises giving the program at least six weeks – "although you'll probably see improvement sooner." Even if the program doesn't stop the pain, she says, at least the diet changes will be good for overall health.

"The worst thing about this is that it won't get rid of your pain," Lemole says. "But at least you haven't compromised any of your body's systems."

"It seems sensible to me that the risk you take doing this for six weeks is far outweighed by the benefits you get," says Dr. Lemole.

If it doesn't work, he adds, "you've screened out the people who need further, more invasive and more risky medical therapy."

As with any program involving significant nutrition changes, the Lemoles stress that this program should be tried *only* under the guidance of your own doctor. They say this is especially important for those who are pregnant and those who are taking prescription drugs.

Other nutrition and lifestyle efforts

Other people have tried programs similar to the Lemoles' plan, and still others have combined nutrition-based plans with other therapies. A few examples...

Rohn Harmer, co-leader of the TN support group in Tampa, Fla., has been getting relief from a combination of upper-cervical chiropractic treatments, dietary changes and "a nutritional plan that includes about 90 percent of the Lemole plan."

He originally got B-12 injections for six weeks but now takes a daily sublingual B-12 tablet (3,000 micrograms of the methylcobalamin type) in addition to the daily "Magic Drink" and other supplements in the Lemole plan (except for a different dose of lecithin).

Harmer also follows a dietary regimen recommended for multiple sclerosis patients (the "Dr. Swank Diet," available online at www.swankmsdiet.com). It involves very limited red meat; skinless turkey or chicken in moderation; fish three times a week; three to five eggs a week, and liberal amounts of raw vegetables, almonds, seeds and freshly blended fruit and vegetable juice. He avoids packaged snacks and any foods with trans fats or hydrogenated oil.

"During the three years on this diet, my pain has been manageable, my cholesterol has dropped from 221 to 176, my triglycerides have returned to a normal range... and my blood pressure is now 90 over 60," Harmer says.

Vicki Lord, a neuralgian from Georgia, has kept her pain to "occasional zingers" by combining a nutrition plan with low doses of the anticonvulsant topiramate (Topamax).

She uses the Hoffer/Walker supplement plan, including B-complex, Vitamin C and a multivitamin along with L'lysine. "They advocate B-12 shots," says Lord, "but I've been successful with sublingual tablets – two 1,000-microgram tablets daily, unless I'm feeling pain, then I use 5,000-microgram pills. I always try increasing my B-12 before increasing my Topamax... I know most doctors think its hogwash, but all I can say is that three-and-a-half years ago, I was barely functioning on high doses of anticonvulsants, and now I have my life back."

Another neuralgian from San Diego reports that a combination of acupuncture and 1,000-microgram sublingual B-12 tablets daily have worked for her, along with supplements of B-complex, a high-potency multivitamin, lecithin and flax oil capsules.

Several members of the Dallas TN support group say they have been helped by taking daily capsules or tablets of B-50, which is a blend of all the B vitamins in one 50mg dose.

FOR MORE INFORMATION ON NUTRITION AND HEALTH...

Four good online resources that offer more detailed information on nutrition, health, supplements and the role of individual nutrients are:

- The U.S. Department of Agriculture's Food and Nutrition Information Center at www.nal.usda.gov/fnic

- The American Dietetic Association at www.eatright.org

- The National Institutes of Health Office of Dietary Supplements at http://ods.od.nih.gov

- The American Society for Nutritional Science at www.nutrition.org/nutinfo

And Kathie Mitchell of Arizona said her answer was a wholesale lifestyle change, including a major dietary revamping based on Dr. Norman W. Walker's book, *"Fresh Vegetable and Fruit Juices"* (Longman Trade/Caroline House, 1995). The heart of it is avoiding meat, bread, cereals, pasta and other starchy foods and eating raw fruit and vegetables and drinking three quarts of fresh, raw fruit and vegetable juice daily.

Mitchell says it "is not a diet that got me well, it is a lifestyle change... The other aspects of this lifestyle change are: exercise, purified water, plenty of fresh air and sunlight, temperance (especially no MSG and aspartame), proper rest, trust in God, an attitude of gratitude and benevolence."

She adds that these changes have kept her pain-free without medication for more than five years.

Success, precautions and limits

Surgeons and TN support-group leaders will tell you that for every success story like the above, there are plenty of others who say, "Been there, done that and it didn't help." Others find that the changes are so sweeping that they can't stick with them or that the results aren't as quick and comprehensive as they had hoped.

So long as the programs are not potentially harmful, most doctors don't discourage their patients from trying nutrition therapy. Even if it doesn't knock out the pain entirely, sometimes a well designed nutrition plan can improve other aspects of health or allow patients to get by on lower doses of medication.

The concern arises when plans suggest supplements that go well beyond the conventionally accepted levels or when diet plans focus too narrowly on certain food groups to the exclusion of others.

The ADA, for instance, says science still only has a limited understanding of all the nutrients in various foods and how they work together for our overall health. "Because there are so many constituents in foods, it is difficult to specifically identify those responsible for positive health effects," it says in a 2001 Journal of the American Dietetic Association report. "There may be more than one active substance, and the matrix in which they appear may also be important."

In other words, breaking out what we think might help into a supplement doesn't guarantee it'll have the intended effect. And more of even a good thing isn't necessarily better.

Sometimes taking too much can lead to unexpected risks, as researchers found in recent studies involving beta carotene. Three studies set out to investigate whether this nutrient (found in carrots, pumpkins, sweet potatoes and other red/orange fruits and vegetables) could reduce the risk of cancer. All three trials found no beneficial results, but two of the three unexpectedly showed *increased* lung cancer rates in smokers and asbestos-exposed workers. Researchers believe that at the tested supplemental doses of 20-30 mg, beta-carotene interferes with other cancer-preventing compounds, such as canthaxanthin, lutein and lycopene.

The ADA says we only scarcely understand effects like that. It warns that when we take in a megadose of one apparently beneficial nutrient, we may be interfering with the important workings of something else.

Studies have shown, for example, that high doses of Vitamin E interfere with Vitamin K and increase the effect of blood-thinning drugs. Others have shown that high levels of calcium inhibit the body's absorption of iron, that folic acid can mask symptoms of Vitamin B-12 deficiencies, and that high doses of zinc can lower copper levels.

For that reason, the ADA says it's best not to tinker with megadoses before we know what we're doing and before we know what levels are safe and effective. It's only been since the 1990s that the U.S. government has begun assessing safe upper levels of various nutrients, the ADA reports, and even then five of the first 17 nutrients couldn't adequately be assessed because of the lack of data.

"Supplements are neither regulated nor tested by the government for safety or effectiveness, so their use is largely a world of the unknown," ADA says. It adds that "only food can provide the ideal mixture of vitamins, minerals and other substances for health... Vitamin and mineral supplementation for curative purposes should only be done under the supervision of a physician."

A FEW TIPS ON SUPPLEMENT SHOPPING...

• Is there good reason to invest in a particular supplement? Do you have a particular need for it that you can't get in your diet? Or are you taking supplements on a "just-in-case" basis?

• Is there good evidence to support the intended benefit of the supplement?

• How reliable is the source of your information? Is it from a trusted, knowledgeable, unbiased source or is it from the same person who has a stake in selling the supplements?

• Don't be swayed by medical-sounding lingo. If you don't understand something or if it doesn't make good sense, ask more questions or do more research. It's always a good idea to research more than one source.

• How much will you need to take and for how long? Are these levels within safe ranges?

• Will the supplement conflict with any medications or other supplements you're taking? It's always best to check with your doctor first, but it's especially important for those who are pregnant, nursing or being treated for a chronic condition.

• Look on the product labels for the "USP" symbol. This indicates the product has met the strength, purity and dissolution standards of U.S. Pharmacopeia, a national testing organization.

• Check the expiration dates to make sure the product is fresh. At home, store supplements in a cool, dry place and out of the reach of children.

— Sources: Mayo Clinic, FDA Center for Food Safety
and Applied Nutrition, QuackWatch

CHAPTER 19

TIPS FROM THE "VETERANS"

"We know what it's like to hurt."
—Cindy Ezell, TNA's Patient Information Coordinator
and a veteran neuralgian

"Veteran" TN sufferers have come up with all kinds of strategies and practices to deal with their pain attacks.

Some of these ideas make pretty good sense and even have some scientific basis behind them, while others are somewhat more off-beat. Either way, most people figure that if something helps even a little bit and isn't harmful, why not give it a try?

None of the following tips are likely to stop your pain dead in its tracks, but some of them may help "take the edge off" your pain or give you some self-help coping ideas until you reach a more permanent solution.

Following are some of the day-to-day tips TN sufferers say they've employed to strike back.

• *Cold compresses.* You wouldn't think these would help since cold weather so often makes TN pain worse. But cold packs held against the painful and/or trigger areas numb the nerve endings and deaden the pain for at least some people.

If you don't have commercial ice packs, try using bags of frozen peas. They work great and mold to the face. Plus they can be refrozen and used again and again. (Just don't eat them after repeated freezes and thaws because they'll be soggy.) Another option is mixing one part alcohol to three parts water and freezing the mixture in a sealable plastic bag.

Most people prefer the above cold packs to ice in a bag because ice is hard and uncomfortable.

Apply cold packs for 20 to 30 minutes at a time. Use a pillow case or other thin cloth between the cold pack and your skin to absorb moisture. Don't use towels or thick cloth because they'll absorb too much of the cold.

Repeat the ice treatment each hour if the pain returns.

• *Heat treatments.* Here's a paradox. While cold helps some people, others find that hot towels or heating pads work better for them.

A few people who have experimented with both heat and cold say they get best results by alternating cold packs and hot towels. This likely helps by depleting the nerve endings and slowing the nerve-firing rate to lessen the perception of pain.

• *Hot creams.* Over-the-counter heat rubs such as Ben-Gay and Icy Hot apparently do not work the same way or with the same anti-TN effectiveness of the hot-pepper or capsaicin cream discussed in Chapter 15. But some people say they've nevertheless had some relief from these other over-the-counter heat creams, most likely because their burning sensations temporarily take precedence over other stimuli.

If nothing else, they're a little less expensive than capsaicin cream.

• *Menthol creams.* Others have found relief from creams that contain menthol or from straight peppermint oil.

"Heaven on Earth I call this one," says Sheila Vives of Florida, who swears by the over-the-counter Bio-Freeze Pain Relieving Gel she uses. "I apply this over the nerve areas being affected. Be sure to hit the temple area since so many nerves and pains come from that region."

Bio-Freeze (www.biofreeze.com, 1-800-246-3733) contains 3.5 percent menthol and 0.2 percent camphor and is sold in health food stores and some medical supply stores and chiropractic offices. Menthol acts by changing the way the nerves fire in painful situations. It uses the same receptors as some narcotics.

Vives says it temporarily numbs the area and can give hours of relief. "Just don't get it too close to the eyes," she says. "And give it time to take effect before driving as the vapors can make the eyes water and squint at first and the nose run."

She buys the sample pack size so she can carry them in her purse and glovebox for "emergency" relief.

A 76-year-old Australian woman also reports getting relief from her post-herpetic neuralgia by using two or three drops of peppermint oil on the painful area. She reapplies the oil three or four times a day and gets up to six hours of relief at a time.

• *Avoid burning eyes.* For those using capsaicin, heat or menthol creams, Australia TN support group leader Irene Wood offers a tip on keeping these creams out of the eyes.

She says some of her group members realized that it was usually when taking a shower that the creams washed off and got in their eyes. To prevent that, Wood suggests washing the face separately *before* taking a shower – "with a face cloth and lots of soap and warm water, repeated a couple of times."

• *Gum-numbing rubs.* "About the only thing that gave me relief was by using Anbesol on my lower jaw," says Fred Lehman, a Pennsylvania neuralgian. "I would put it on cotton balls and let them lay between my cheek and jaw, and when the numbness wore off, I would soak the cotton again."

Like the local anesthetics dentists inject, this approach may work by temporarily desensitizing TN trigger points. The active ingredient that's absorbed into the nerves is very much like the anesthetic lidocaine. Keep in mind that gum-numbing rubs can be overdone, so don't exceed the label directions.

• *Give the nerve the "cold shoulder."* Along the same line is using cold foods to desensitize any trigger zones you might have in the mouth.

One California neuralgian says she eats "a lot of Popsicles to keep the nerve half-frozen." Another neuralgian from California says he got relief in his pre-Tegretol days by keeping ice chips in his mouth at all times.

And a neuralgian from Canada says she prefers slushy cold foods like Slurpies and Freezies. "Ice cubes are too hard and ice chips are too jagged," she says. What *really* worked best, she adds, is eating a cold Slurpie or Freezie while taking a really hot bath. "It looks ridiculous and sounds ridiculous, but for some reason the combination worked for me. And there are locks on most bathroom doors, so no one has to see you."

• *Eating tips.* When eating, it may help to choose easy-to-chew foods or to liquefy foods in the blender during peak pain periods. Even eating foods of varying consistency may allow nerve fibers that pick up varying pressures on the teeth to rest.

If drinking triggers the pain, you might try using an extra-long straw to "bypass" most of the mouth. (This worked for the Trigeminal Neuralgia Association's patient information coordinator Cindy Ezell.)

When chewing, take small bites so you don't have to open the mouth wide or chew more vigorously than necessary. Also chew slowly and on the opposite side of the pain.

If it's cold drinks that seem to make the pain worse, switch to warm beverages. Often, room-temperature or body-temperature drinks work best since that's less of a change in either direction, making the nerve fibers that detect temperature change less likely to fire.

• *A nerve-calming tea.* Texas TN support group leader Shelly Wilson had a member who always seemed to have fewer TN attacks after drinking decaffeinated chai tea.

When they mentioned it to a doctor, they learned that chai tea has small amounts of bromine, which was an agent that 19th-century doctors used as one of the first anticonvulsant medications because of its nerve-quelling properties.

• *Teeth tips.* If brushing teeth triggers pain, try using a soft cloth or an anti-bacteria, anti-plaque mouthwash. Some neuralgians say they clean their teeth with a Water Pik set on low. And avoid teeth whiteners, which can erode the teeth's dentin and make them more sensitive, which in turn can increase the chance of pain being triggered.

• *Chew gum.* If researchers are right about how neurochemical levels limit the duration of TN attacks (see Chapter 3), it would seem possible to continuously stimulate the nerve so it can't "reload" and keep firing off pain attacks every few minutes.

Some people say that by constantly chewing gum, they find the nerve is unable to "save up enough power" to fire off a major attack at the first new touch to the face or gums. While that wording isn't quite scientifically correct, the idea behind it has some medical merit. The nerve can be desensitized by repeated firing with this activity, making it less able to fire a pain pattern.

Again, there's no harm in trying it, other than the increased chance of tooth cavities if you chew sugared gum.

• *Facial massage.* You'd think this would trigger TN attacks, but it's generally light touches – not deeper pressure – that ignite those painful nerve firings.

The medical explanation is that the deeper rubbing is triggering the nerve fibers that sense deeper pressure, pre-empting the firings of the light-touch fibers in the same area that are the ones that normally set off TN attacks.

Massage also may loosen tight muscles and cause the release of endorphins, the body's natural pain-killing chemicals.

Rather than massaging the face, some people have found it helps to simply press the painful area with their hand and hold it there. It may even be possible to short-circuit an attack by trying pressure as soon as a pain spasm comes on.

• *Massage the ears.* This tip comes from Florida acupuncturist Larry Han, who says the ears have many points that respond well to acupuncture needles.

He says manually massaging the ears for 10 minutes at a time three times a day also often helps alleviate face pain.

In China, massaging the ears is an ancient practice thought to promote longevity and general good health. It's also free.

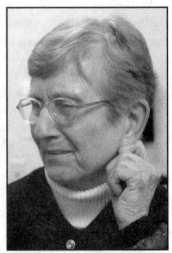

Acupuncturists say massaging the ears daily stimulates acupuncture points that ease face pain.

(Photo by George Weigel)

• **Chin adjustment.** Here's one that comes via the San Diego TN support group.

"Open your mouth as wide as you can. Then place your hand on your chin, push your jaw back gently toward the painful side of your face. Repeat this several times at a sitting about four times a day. It has helped many."

Other than possibly reducing muscle tension in the jaw, it's unknown why this might work. But it's also free, easy and unlikely to harm anything – unless, of course, jaw movements are one of your pain triggers. In that case, never mind.

• **Flex the neck (or not).** Some say they are able to prevent or stop TN attacks by flexing their neck or otherwise changing their head position.

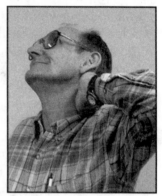

One theory behind that is that the change in position might be enough to temporarily move a compressing blood vessel off the trigeminal nerve. But considering the vessel and nerve are deep within the skull and sometimes wrapped around or embedded in one another, simple changes in posture aren't likely to make much of a lasting difference, if at all.

Some neuralgians say they get relief by flexing their neck.
(Photo by George Weigel)

Pittsburgh neurosurgeon Dr. Peter Jannetta says between one-third and one-half of his patients say certain postures seem to aggravate TN attacks. Another 2000 study reported that flexing the head forward seems to be a fairly common pain-triggering action for many neuralgians.

By identifying and avoiding those postures or actions, it's possible to head off at least some attacks. However, there's been no evidence of certain postures being capable of curing TN altogether.

If you embrace the chiropractic theory that at least some TN cases are caused by a misaligned upper vertebrae, neck-flexing may have a similar effect to a chiropractic adjustment – if you're able to move the vertebrae in the right way and keep it there.

Whatever the theory, if it works, keep doing it. Just be gentle.

• **Clever sleeping strategies.** Sliding the face against the pillow or bed may be enough to trigger an attack, so it makes sense to keep the affected side up whenever lying down.

Other people come up with all sorts of creative sleeping positions to keep the face from contacting anything. One described on the Facial Neuralgia Resources web site (www.facial-neuralgia.org) is folding up a pillow and placing it under the chest to raise the face and shoulders off the bed. That way only the forehead touches the bed. (Forget that one if your trigger point or pain is in the forehead region.)

• *Get proper rest.* When you're tired and worn out from lack of sleep, any pain feels worse. Try to maintain regular sleep habits and don't short-change yourself by trying "burn the candle at both ends."

One of the few non-cruel traits of TN is that once you're asleep, the pain lets you alone. Usually. It's seldom that a pain attack will wake you in the middle of the night.

• *Set the alarm for a nighttime dose of medicine.* This is definitely one to discuss with your doctor first. Many people say their worst pain is first thing in the morning. That makes sense because it may have been eight hours or more since the last dose of medication.

One way to prevent that wakeup agony is to get up in the middle of the night to take a pill and thereby keep the medication more constant in the bloodstream. On the other hand, once you're awake, you may open yourself to nighttime attacks that might make it difficult to get back to sleep.

Another option is to discuss with your doctor the possibility of switching to one of the newer extended-release versions of carba-mazepine, such as Tegretol XR or Carbatrol. These have longer-acting effects that can spread pain relief out for more than eight hours.

• *Stay away from face-touching activities as much as possible.* Duh. You've probably already figured that out, but the question is how to do it. You can't stop eating or brushing your teeth or washing your face.

But you can grow a beard instead of shaving (if you're a man... or don't mind being a hairy woman). You can forgo using cosmetics. You can use a wash cloth vigorously to clean the face since it's usually light touch instead of firm pressure that triggers attacks. Or you can try a mild astringent on cotton to wash the face, if you find that works better.

• *Cover the face outside.* A light breeze across the face is one of the most common pain triggers. Some people use a Neoprene mask when-ever they go outside, especially in cold weather. (Cold itself also can be a pain trigger.) Others use a scarf. The best facial covers for TN are those that are either tight-fitting or those that protect but don't touch the face. What you *don't* want is a loose-fitting cover that can suddenly rub up against the face, creating a light touch that can trigger the pain itself.

• *Loosen those glasses.* Ontario neuralgian Keith Ennis one day noticed that his glasses fit so tight that they were leaving an impression on the skin of his face.

"I wondered if there was enough pressure to impact the trigeminal nerve, so I added a small piece of sponge to the inside of the temple," he says. "That moved the frames outward enough to clear my face. There is now no indentation, and my facial pain has been substantially reduced."

Like loose-fitting clothing that can brush against the face, it's possible Ennis's glasses were acting as a light-pressure trigger that was aggravating his TN.

• *Cut out nicotine.* There's evidence that this substance, found in tobacco, also can increase our sensitivity to pain. It may help to cut down on or quit smoking. Your lungs will thank you even if it doesn't help your TN.

• *Try to limit other "stressors" in your life.* Stress, lack of sleep, poor diet and other tensions in your day-to-day life might not cause a TN attack, but they can make the attacks seem to hurt worse. Take care of yourself and your body, and you at least won't be contributing to the problem.

"If you don't take care of the ship that carries you, you'll sink," says Dr. Michael Langan, associate professor at the University of Florida School of Dentistry.

Stress-management techniques range from relaxation tapes to self-hypnosis to yoga. See Chapter 20 for more on this.

• *Prayer.* Don't overlook the power of praying. Many patients say it's their single biggest ally in coping with TN.

"I've never appreciated the Lord as much as when I was going through this," says Pennsylvania neuralgian Ray Land.

Singer Norma Zimmer, a long-time neuralgian, says words from Psalm 42 have helped her get through many painful periods. It reads: "But, oh, my soul, don't be discouraged. Don't be upset. Expect God to act, for I know that I shall again have plenty of reason to praise Him for all that He will do. He is my help. He is my God."

"Folks who have faith have more hope," says Pennsylvania counselor Dorina Saul, adding that hope is a key to maintaining a good attitude that helps one cope with chronic pain.

For more on the role of faith in face pain, see Chapter 20.

• *Strenuous exercise.* "I've noticed that when I'm outside gardening for a few hours, I never get an attack," says Marian Shartle, a neuralgian from Pennsylvania.

Land also says he never got attacks when riding a bike, playing basketball or doing any sustained exercise.

The dilating of blood vessels or the release of endorphins may offer physiological reasons for why exercise may prevent attacks. Exercise also refocuses your attention away from pain and builds a stronger, healthier body that's better able to cope with pain.

• *Fresh air?* Tennessee neuralgian Barry Schlatter says his TN improved drastically soon after he installed a filterless air purifier system in his house.

He thought it was coincidental at first until his dentist mentioned that he seemed to have larger-than-average passageways in the canals above his teeth roots (where nerve branches traverse.)

Schlatter says his dentist asked if he had been outside hunting or fishing a lot. "I told him no but explained the air purifier," Schlatter says. "He likened it to being about the same."

The theory is that the fresh air (albeit filtered indoor air) encouraged the opening of these nerve pathways, which could mean less pressure on the nerves. There's no scientific proof of any link between TN and filtered air, but Schlatter's not planning on tinkering with his filtration system anytime soon.

• *Keep a "pain diary."* The idea of this isn't to remind yourself how bad it hurts but to keep track of medicine dosages and pain peaks and valleys. If you've gone a few weeks without pain, you may be able to cut back on your medicine for awhile.

This is also a way to determine if the peaks are getting worse and the remissions less, which is helpful in making a decision about surgery or other treatment. If nothing else, a diary might help you put together any possible pattern to the pain, which might help you eliminate situations or factors that seem to make the pain worse.

• *Play detective.* Whether you keep a diary or not, look for possible links to what makes your pain ebb and flo.

If your pain gets worse after certain activities, cut them back or cut them out. Look for dietary links or posture links and some of the other factors mentioned above.

• *Prioritize your activities.* If the pain is worse at certain times of day or if you tire by midday, plan your daily activities around those factors.

You may want, for example, to tackle your highest-priority jobs in the morning so at least those things are done in case you're too tired to get everything done. Or you may plan on doing certain activities only if you feel up to it that day.

It may help to schedule breaks or naps, if you can. And if you've found coping techniques that help (i.e. meditation, self-hypnosis, yoga, ice packs, etc.), be sure to schedule those into your day.

•*Avoid vibrations.* Bumpy roads, humming and even sitting next to speakers at church or at a concert have brought on attacks for many TN patients.

It may be impossible to avoid all vibrations – especially unexpected ones – but you may be able to pick seats as far away from the speakers as possible.

•*Avoid bright light.* For other people, light is a particular pain trigger. Members of the Pacific Northwest TN support group have found that wearing good quality sunglasses with the proper ultraviolet (UV) protection help avoid light-sensitivity problems.

Particularly helpful, they add, are the wrap-around sunglasses that are often sold at sporting goods stores. Besides keeping light out, they help keep wind and dust particles from sneaking in the eyes.

In the car, attachments can be bought to extend windshield visors farther down.

•*Dry-eye help.* For those who have dry eyes as a side effect of medication or as a complication from surgery (or for those who just have naturally dry eyes), the Northwest Pacific group recommends artificial tears, which are available over-the-counter at drugstores.

The members say they've had good results with such brand names as Genteal, Celluvise and Refresh. They advise using the drops early in the day before the eyes start feeling "scratchy."

Keep in mind that artificial tears or tear-replacement drops are different from eye drops that remove redness. The latter constricts blood vessels.

•*Attitude boosters.* The Northwest Pacific TN support group's May/June 2002 newsletter offered a few more "gems of knowledge from fellow TN'ers," such as:

"Find what makes you happy, and do what you can to keep your spirits up. Give yourself permission to take your breakthrough medications when needed; never torture yourself. Say no when you don't feel like doing something, and don't feel guilty about it. Take some time off to play. Do breathing exercises and learn to relax."

CHAPTER 20

COPING WITH FACE PAIN

"If you have pain all the time, it doesn't take a heck of a lot
of it to wipe you out."
—Dr. Peter Jannetta, Pittsburgh neurosurgeon

Holly Berenschot of California called it her "nightmare." She could tell you the exact date she felt her first jolt of TN pain (Aug. 29, 1982), and she never forgot what triggered that first awful attack (biting into a cookie.)

"I went to the dentist the next day, thinking there was a tooth problem," she said. "He assured me there was not." Eventually an ear, nose and throat specialist suggested that the pain was "tic douloureux," not a tooth problem.

"This doctor, who was a complete stranger to me, looked at me with so much sympathy and said, 'Oh, I hope not ... that is one of the most painful things you could have,'" Berenschot recalled. "I had never heard of tic douloureux, and his comment certainly did not help, but at last and at least I had a name for my condition."

Berenschot got temporary relief from a series of glycerol injections before undergoing a successful microvascular decompression surgery in 1988. She was pain-free until she passed away from unrelated bone cancer in May 1995. But she never forgot those electric attacks.

"It is difficult to list all the things that change in one's life with this kind of pain," she once said of her TN ordeal. "I could no longer promise to be anywhere at a particular time and feel confident I could make it. Every time my husband started to kiss me, I turned my cheek so he would not touch the right (painful) side of my face.

"Putting a blouse on over my head triggered pain when the cloth barely touched my nose. There were days when I drove the freeway to work being careful not to touch my tongue to my gums in fear of triggering pain. There were days when I would not risk driving at all and my husband took me to work, then I sat at my desk dreading when the phone would ring because just talking often triggered an attack.

"In one three-week period when I could not eat or drink without triggering pain, I lost 18 pounds. I believe I ate less than an 8-ounce cup of yogurt in that time but forced myself to drink water. Brushing my teeth was an impossibility at times and washing my hair or face was terrible agony.

"The last seven weeks before my surgery, I was flat on my back. Everything triggered the attacks: sitting up, lying down, in fact any motion, just shifting my eyes toward the ringing telephone. My daughter-in-law got in the habit of calling each night to see how I was doing. I loved her for caring but dreaded having to move and talk. When my family came to visit, I could not speak. All they could do was look down on me."

Not everyone ends up on her back like Berenschot. But her experience is not that unusual when it comes to describing what TN patients go through.

Lots of exams, no answers

Terah Biszantz of California bounced around among 11 different doctors and dentists over a three-year period before she was even diagnosed with TN. At first she had a root canal done by a dentist who thought her problem was an infected upper molar. When that didn't work, an endodontist redid the root canal.

"When he put the post into the tooth, my face exploded into pain," remembers Biszantz. "Nothing seemed to help the pain. Novocaine did not help, nor did massive amounts of codeine, to which I became addicted... I had two extensive sinus surgeries and even had the root-canal tooth pulled. Nothing helped.

"One doctor shrugged his shoulders and said to me, 'What do you think I have, a magic pill?' This was a devastating experience as my pain was constant and increasing. I did not think I could survive with this much pain every day for the rest of my life."

Fortunately, Biszantz was able to locate two fellow TN patients through the then fledgling Trigeminal Neuralgia Association and from them found out about Dr. Steven Graff-Radford at Cedars-Sinai Medical Center in Los Angeles. He quickly diagnosed TN and started her on Tegretol and later Dilantin and baclofen.

Like Berenschot, Biszantz also eventually underwent a microvascular decompression surgery to get relief. But also like Berenschot, she says this is a pain you never forget. "Each morning, as I wash my face, I say a little prayer of thanks for the relief of my pain," Biszantz says.

TN affects more than just the face

The dread... the constant vigilance over those sensitive trigger points... the tiring pain that seems to get ever worse, even after you've told yourself it *had* to be at its peak. This is all a part of what it's like coping with TN day after day.

Living with the sharp and chronic pain of TN is tiring, it's a strain on emotions, and it's a strain on families and relationships.

Trigeminal neuralgians often experience anxiety or even panic attacks while worrying when the next major TN attack will hit. They may take on a pessimistic attitude. They may feel like they're "losing control." They may experience guilt or even grief at not feeling up to doing the things they used to do.

What used to bring joy and laughter may become a bother. Smiles may disappear, not only because the joy is gone but because the mere action of smiling may be enough to trigger an attack.

Frustration levels often soar, first at the all-too-often difficulty in getting an accurate diagnosis and then at the ongoing treatment if the pain keeps breaking through.

"Emotionally, it's so destructive," says Chuck Lewis, a neuralgian from Pennsylvania. "You're always tensed, waiting for the next episode."

It can be just as vexing for doctors, and that can lead to conflicts between patient and doctor. "It's such a frustrating condition," says Dr. Jack Carey, a retired neurosurgeon from Maryland. "You think you have it under control, and all of a sudden it flares up."

Some TN sufferers end up withdrawing into a shell and stick as close to home as possible. Others find their tempers flare much quicker than before. Sluggishness and sleepiness from the medications add to this emotional brew. It all boils down to a problem that's as much mental and emotional as physical.

It's not unusual for neuralgians, at some point, to wonder if the whole thing really is in their head – which is easy to imagine since all of the tests typically come back "normal."

"'Is this real or am I crazy?' That's what so many of my patients ask," says Dr. Graff-Radford.

Even when patients themselves have no doubt the pain is quite real, they often feel like others think it must be all in their mind, says Dr. Steven Hickman, a psychologist and instructor at the University of California at San Diego.

He says that's understandable because "pain in general is hard to measure. You can't see it on a blood test or MRI. You don't have a little meter on your head."

Reacting to the pain

Not everyone reacts to TN the same way, of course. Some seem to adapt to and cope with the pain better than others.

One obvious reason is that not all pains are of equal intensity. Some cases flare worse than others, and even in any single case, the pain fluctuates over time. But we all also have learned to perceive and cope with pain in differing ways. Things like our upbringing, our past experiences, our current psychological state and our general outlook on life are just a few of the factors that influence how we tolerate pain.

Ever notice how some people seem able to tolerate high doses of pain while others appear to be in mortal agony with the exact same injury or condition? While the actual injury may be the same, the way we react is both situationally and culturally variable. Our tolerance to pain also can change day to day, and we can affect that process. Research has shown that how individuals react mentally and emotionally to pain has a lot to do with the degree of pain experienced.

"Ever hear anybody say your pain is all in your head?" asks Pennsylvania psychologist John Weigel. "Well, they're right. Pain centers *are* in your brain. That's where you experience pain."

Some of the way we experience pain is learned.

For instance, a child who hears a parent talk about how painful a dental visit was may grow up with an exaggerated fear of dentists. On the other hand, a child who grows up in a family or culture that teaches "no pain, no gain" is likely to be conditioned to accept higher levels of pain.

Athletes often tolerate pain better than others because they're accustomed to pushing themselves beyond comfort levels to achieve goals.

One pain study even compared two groups of men undergoing the same surgery – wounded war veterans vs. non-veterans. The combat veterans required less pain medication after surgery, most likely because they considered the surgery to be a relatively minor matter compared to what they had been through in the war.

To a degree, pain perceptions can be "relearned" to our advantage. While finding a war to fight in isn't exactly an ideal way to go about doing that, we do have some control over how we let pain affect us.

"There is a connection between the brain and the body, and that connection can be your best friend or your worst enemy," says Weigel.

He points out that there's a difference between pain and suffering. "The sensation of pain is one thing, but how you experience it is entirely different," says Weigel. "I can be in pain without suffering."

Pain becomes suffering when it controls our lives and makes everything seem bad.

Dr. Beree Darby, a University of Florida psychologist, immunologist and biochemist, says research verifies that our mental and emotional states have a direct effect on our physical state.

In one study, for example, cancer patients healed faster in pleasant surroundings with a view of trees and gardens outside.

In a 1975 study of mice bred to be cancer-prone, 92 percent of those placed in a high-stress environment got cancer while only 7 percent of those in a low-stress environment developed the disease.

Dr. Darby says that even expectations make a difference. "People tend to get better when they *expect* they're going to get better or believe they're *supposed* to get better."

Time and again, research backs up a connection behind mind and body. People who are under stress or who are suffering from depression consistently report feeling painful stimuli much more sharply than non-stressed, non-depressed individuals.

Worrying can lead to an upset stomach or a headache. And who hasn't gotten sweaty palms or "butterflies" in a nervous situation?

Those who constantly bemoan how bad the TN pain hurts, worry about the next attack and let the condition interfere with their lives are the ones most likely to suffer the worst. On the other hand, those who manage to keep a positive attitude and who don't dwell on the pain may not be able to stop attacks, but at least they are better equipped to cope with the situation.

It's not easy, of course, to be your usual optimistic, cheery self when it feels as if there's a lightning bolt erupting in your face. But there are techniques that can be learned to "close the gate" to pain, which we'll discuss later in this chapter.

Fighting the mental battles

Those who don't learn to cope well can spiral into a host of secondary woes, including denial, anger, substance abuse, workaholism, anxiety and/or depression. "Pain is a stressor," says Dr. Hickman. "And that causes a reaction in our body."

Some of these reactions are very similar to what people go through following the death of a loved one. Florida psychologist Rennie Manning, who came down with TN on her 50th birthday, says many people need to go through a sort of grieving stage over the loss of their health.

She says some even go through the whole five-stage loss process that Elizabeth Kubler-Ross wrote about in those who learn they're going to die. These stages are: 1.) denial and isolation; 2.) anger and resentment; 3.) bargaining with God; 4.) depression, and 5.) acceptance.

Dr. Cynthia Belar, also a Florida psychologist, says reaching the point of acceptance is a key step in keeping face pain from overwhelming your entire life.

"We have learned that an important part of dealing with pain is acceptance and ownership of it," Dr. Belar says. "That doesn't mean liking it, giving up and being resigned to it, or blaming yourself for it. It does mean you accept the fact that the pain may not go away and take responsibility to manage it as best as you can. An important part of taking responsibility is to set goals in three areas of your life – life, work and recreation. That will help you to maintain a positive identity so that your life isn't just about pain."

"Accepting" pain, though, is often the last thing people are inclined to do. "Most people want to get away from pain," says Dr. Hickman. "But it's like a Chinese finger puzzle... the more you pull away, the tighter its grip."

Coping with the reality of pain instead of going into an emotionally draining "fight or flight" mode often requires the help of a caring spouse, a trusted friend or relative, and maybe even a health-care professional.

"When you hear someone say you ought to go to a psychologist, that doesn't mean they think you're cuckoo," says Dr. Graff-Radford. "The reason is that they want you to enhance your brain's ability to deal with your affliction."

So-called "cognitive behavioral therapy" – which focuses on how you assess and react to the current environment as opposed to the "tell-me-about-your-mother" approach of Freudian psychotherapy – has been particularly helpful in gaining pain-coping skills.

Dr. Graff-Radford says he believes all chronic pain patients should have some sort of behavioral therapy, whether it's counseling or learning relaxation and stress-management techniques.

The depression connection

If left unchecked, it's easy for all of these swirling, changing feelings to cause TN sufferers to slip into chronic anxiety and depression. Anxiety and depression in turn can lead to a variety of secondary ills, including a rise in blood pressure, sleeplessness, loss of appetite, weight loss and ulcers.

EIGHT MYTHS OF PAIN

1.) **"If you look good, you can't be in THAT much pain."** Looks aren't everything. Even X-rays and MRIs appear normal in TN, but try telling anyone who's ever felt TN pain that they're exaggerating.

2.) **"If psychological methods work, that proves it must be 'all in your head.'"** Counseling and mental techniques may help people cope with pain better, but that doesn't mean the pain isn't "real." Also, our mental and emotional health has a direct bearing on our physical health. Healing one can help heal the other.

3.) **"Pain is always a warning signal."** That's what it's designed to do. But when illness or injury damages the pain-transmission system, chronic pain such as TN results. In other words, the warning system overreacts.

4.) **"Pain is punishment."** Being a "bad" or "mean" person doesn't make you any more likely to get pain than being "good" insulates you from it. TN is an equal-opportunity employer. Otherwise, why don't more criminals have it? Why do priests and pastors and philanthropists sometimes get it?

5.) **"Someone is to blame for this."** Pain happens. Just because we can't figure out why doesn't mean someone or something improper "caused" it. Misguided blame is a waste of energy that can drag us down instead of helping. Besides, maybe some good will come of this problem someday. Or maybe you'll end up being a better, stronger person in the long run.

6.) **"If you ignore the pain, it'll go away."** Don't we wish. Sometimes that's true. But many other times, if you do nothing to address underlying problems, pain may get worse.

7.) **"It's possible to control pain or 'will' it away."** That can be true to some degree sometimes. Mental techniques such as hypnosis and biofeedback may help. But most times you're also going to need to take steps to fix or treat the underlying problem.

8.) **"Medical science can cure everything."** We're getting better, but we're not *that* good. Some pains we can fix. Some we can make somewhat better sometimes. But other times there are pains that even the best doctors can't do much to help.

— *Source: Dr. Cynthia Belar, Florida psychologist and author*

Anxiety over the pain can be almost as troubling as the pain itself. Researchers have even documented that the anxiety level of TN patients is higher than the normal population even when the pain is in remission or controlled by surgery.

Doctors at the Medical College of Virginia stumbled across that finding in 1990 when testing TN patients for numbness six months to three years after surgery. The patients took a 40-question anxiety test to measure possible anxiety over the sensory testing, but the results turned up significant levels of anxiety in general.

"This altered stress level might be expected under conditions of continual, intermittent attacks of pain," the researchers reported in the Journal of Oral Maxillofacial Surgery. "However, because these patients reported a 90 percent pain relief from their pain, it is conceivable the neuralgia had a permanent psychological effect on these people."

If TN leads to depression, it's important to seek professional help because depression is a separate and distinct condition. It's also one that's readily treatable – if it's recognized.

Some of the key signs of depression are loss of energy, a decrease in usual interests, sudden changes in sleeping or eating, mood change, irritability, withdrawal from people, trouble making decisions, and thoughts of hopelessness or suicide. All aren't required to be considered "depressed," but the more symptoms a person has from that list, the more likely that he or she needs professional help. Psychological tests can be given to confirm depression.

Dr. Karen Stennie, a University of Florida psychiatrist and anesthesiologist, says several studies have found that depression occurs in between 40 to 80 of people with chronic face pain. It's especially prevalent in those with so-called "atypical" TN (TN-2).

"Yet depression remains seriously under-treated, probably 50 percent of the time," she says. "If it's unrecognized, it goes untreated."

One reason depression goes untreated is because people often are "reluctant to portray themselves as 'weak,'" says Dr. Stennie. "They may rebel if you suggest it's 'in their head.'"

The truth is, depression is not a "weakness." It's a physical condition that can be traced to changes in brain chemistry. In this case, it's a secondary illness spun off TN.

Interestingly enough, the same brain chemical found to be lacking in people with depression – serotonin – is also involved in the transmission of pain. That's why antidepressant drugs that increase the body's supply of serotonin are sometimes helpful in treating pain as well as depression.

Antidepressants are sometimes even found to be more helpful in treating "atypical" cases (TN-2) than anticonvulsants.

Depression treatment usually involves counseling and one of the approximately 30 antidepressant medications now on the market. Anxiety also can be treated with counseling and anti-anxiety medication.

"When you have pain, that affects your life," says Dr. Graff-Radford. "And when it affects your life, you can become depressed, you can become anxious, you can become a grouch. You can become so absorbed with your pain because it's so overly consuming that that's all you can think about in life."

"Willing" the pain away?

All of this is a normal and maybe even expected reaction, says Philadelphia psychiatrist Dr. Richard Saul. He knows all too well. He suffered with TN pain for eight years and went through the mental and emotional battles along with the physical pain.

"I was 52 and strong and healthy," he says. "I never had any diseases, never had any conditions. Suddenly I came down with left-sided facial pain that was excruciating. The first thing I did was deny it, feeling that the next day it would go away.

"Then I became very angry. I thought that if I had to suffer this much pain, I might as well have cancer and die. I may as well have a 'real' disease that's going to finish me off."

Dr. Saul put up with cycles of pain for years, always worrying about when the next attack would strike. "The anticipatory agony that you suffer in terms of doing something that might precipitate an attack is terrible," he says.

He even tried "outsmarting" the pain by trying to will it away but quickly found he had no control whatsoever over the attacks. "You just suffer with it until it's good and ready to be over. There's very little you can do to stop it," he says.

Dr. Saul eventually grew tired, angry and frustrated and slipped into a depression. "It was making me a crazy person," he says. "It was changing my personality."

Dr. Saul eventually went to Pittsburgh and underwent a microvascular decompression surgery by Dr. Peter Jannetta in January 1994. Although the surgery stopped the pain, he was left with partial numbness in his left lower face, which he considers more than a fair tradeoff for ending the pain.

"I would do it again in a minute," he says. "The suffering you do is so tremendous that the complications are nothing compared to the pain I had."

You don't have to "learn to live with it"

Contrary to what you might be told, it's not necessary to "learn to live with the pain." Accepting the reality of the pain you have today doesn't mean you're resigning yourself to having it tomorrow. After all, TN is not a fatal disease, and there are many treatment options.

Each option offers potential relief, and people have a great deal of control over which option to try and when. But seeking physical relief is just one way to deal with the pain.

The other is to learn what psychologists call "coping strategies" – techniques that help individuals better tolerate the pain they have.

Among these strategies:

• *Don't let helplessness take over.* One of the biggest mental threats is to feel as if you have no control over the pain and there's nothing you can do. When that happens, you lose motivation, slip into depression and stop trying to find new ways to cope.

Experiments using animals put into helpless situations have found that when helplessness sets in, animals won't even try to escape when they're allowed to go free.

This same kind of situation can happen to humans suffering from TN pain. While you may not be able to stop attacks, neither do you have to feel defeated by them. The truth is that there are more treatment options than ever and nearly all TN sufferers ultimately find relief. So keep plugging away.

• *Use distraction to your advantage.* The more we focus on pain, the more it bothers us. Conversely, the more we're able to focus on other things, the less it seems to hurt.

Example: It's not uncommon for people to be so absorbed in a thought or a job that they didn't notice they had just cut themselves.

"One of the tricks those fire-walkers use when walking barefoot over hot coals is to not think that they're walking on hot coals," says Weigel. "Their minds are somewhere else disassociated from their bodies."

When pain strikes, think about something pleasant, pray, meditate or get your mind on anything other than the attack.

• *Don't turn it into a 24-hour pain.* TN pain normally isn't constant, yet many TN sufferers find themselves fretting about the pain even between attacks and during remission periods. That only turns a part-time pain into a full-time one.

"Many sufferers of TN develop a habit of checking or monitoring themselves for signs of the next flare-up," says Dr. Toby Newton-John, a clinical psychologist at Royal North Shore Hospital's Pain Management and Research Centre in Sydney, Australia. "You need to be aware of pain flare-ups so that you can take appropriate action, but anxious monitoring will only increase your distress and your body's hypersensitivity. Try to shift your awareness onto how well you are coping or how nice it is to be in less discomfort rather than focus on when you are next likely to be in pain."

Take advantage of those breaks to get on with your life as much as possible.

• *Stay busy.* One of the worst things you can do is to quit your job, quit your hobbies and stop taking vacations.

"Don't sit at home in a chair waiting for the next pain to occur," says Florida psychiatrist Dr. Alberto de la Torre. "Make your life constructive… don't become obsessed with the pain."

Keeping busy not only prevents TN from defeating you, but it also is a great way to keep the mind distracted from pain.

• *Stay positive.* Focus on as many positive emotions as possible. Don't dwell on TN at the expense of other good things that probably are going on in your life if you take the time to notice them.

• *Try not to become too still and rigid.* One common trait of a neuralgian is a tendency to avoid moving the face and head so as to avoid triggering a pain attack. This can work against you when carried to the extreme.

"There is evidence that chronic pain sufferers who stop or drastically reduce using the body part in pain become increasingly sensitive to any movement of that body part," says Dr. Newton-John. "It seems that the brain 'turns up the volume' on nerve inputs from a region when it has stopped routinely receiving them."

When new movement finally does occur, it can send an exaggerated barrage of stimulation signals to the brain.

Dr. Newton-John suggests trying to stay as flexible and mobile. "You may have to be gentle and slow in your movement of the affected areas, but that is preferable to avoiding movement, which can lead to that area becoming hypersensitive and more painful. Gentle stretching of the entire body, but especially the neck, shoulders, jaw and upper body on a regular basis can help to keep the brain receiving normal signals from all body areas and not turn up the volume any more than it already has."

• *Focus on the present.* Don't worry about all the attacks you haven't had yet or what you're going to do if the pain gets worse. Cross that bridge when and if you come to it.

Concern yourself only with the nature and amount of pain you've got today. If the pain is tolerable, get on with your life. If it's not tolerable, it's time to consider another treatment option.

This doesn't mean you shouldn't take the time to educate yourself on the options available if the pain gets worse. Just don't dwell on it.

• *Treat yourself to the things that bring you joy and pleasure.* Get out and do what you like to do. Don't give up your passions. When TN is active, the attacks will come on whether you're in bed or out dancing anyway.

Just realize that sometimes you might need to be more flexible than before. You may need to reschedule at the last minute or leave early if the pain is just too bad. And the people you're with will need to learn to adjust as well. That's better than giving up activities altogether.

COPING WITH SUDDEN PAIN FLARE-UPS

Clinical psychologist Dr. Toby Newton-John says that coping with a TN flare-up "is a bit like riding a wave... you can't stop it, but you can stay on your feet and flow along with it until it eventually subsides."

He advises neuralgians to view flare-ups not as a "disaster" but as a "challenge." "How are you going to respond," he asks, "with an increase in anxiety and frustration and distress, which will inevitably worsen the pain, or with as much calmness and rational thought as you can muster?"

Here are some tips he offers on dealing with flare-ups of face pain:

• **Try not to panic.** The aim is to retain a sense of control despite being in severe pain. Try different ways of coping with the pain until you find something that helps.

• **Prioritize.** Recognize that you might not get everything done that you planned. Decide what you can put off and what you can cancel altogether until the pain is under control.

• **Communicate with others.** Let others know what's going on so they don't worry if you become suddenly quiet or need time alone.

• **Do relaxation exercises.** Breathe deeply. Learn and use such techniques such as progressive muscle relaxation, meditation, self-hypnosis and others discussed in this chapter.

• **Try some light activity.** Even if the pain isn't completely gone, try a few non-vigorous activities such as watering the plants, ironing, polishing shoes, etc. for no more than 15 minutes. It may help distract the pain.

> ...*Coping with Sudden Pain Flare-ups Continued*
>
> • **Rest.** Take a time-out for 15-20 minutes to lie down or sit in a comfortable chair to regain some energy. It may help to listen to music or watch TV. Avoid doing nothing for too long because the distraction of activity can help.
>
> • **Gentle stretching.** So long as it doesn't trigger pain attacks, try stretching or going for a slow walk for 10-15 minutes. Exercise and relaxing muscle tension often help relieve pain.
>
> • **Distraction.** Try an even more distracting activity, such as a hobby or a conversation (if possible) or a light job that takes some concentration.
>
> • **Reflect.** Once the flare-up has passed, ask yourself what helped the most. This is also a good time to learn about other techniques that might help next time.
>
> • **Reevaluate.** If the pain is becoming worse or breaking through your current treatment, contact your doctor and/or consider other treatments. (For very severe attacks in which you need immediate medical help, see the tips under "What to do about surprise attacks" in Chapter 8.)

Relaxation

One of the best approaches you can take is to learn relaxation techniques, which have been called the "aspirin of behavioral techniques."

Most Americans are notoriously unskilled at this, as our high blood-pressure levels and near-frantic lifestyles attest. Relaxing can be learned, however.

Dr. Hickman says a good place to start is with deep breathing exercises several times a day. He suggests taking deep, slow breaths from the abdomen, especially whenever you're in pain.

You'll know you're doing it right if you lie down and put a book on your stomach and the book goes up and down as you breathe. This is the same technique that women are taught to use during childbirth.

This kind of breathing not only brings in adequate oxygen but relaxes tensed muscles.

A second exercise is "progressive muscle relaxation." This is where you slowly tense and then release various muscles, starting with your feet and working your way up. (See the sidebars on the following pages for more details on both of these techniques.)

Mental imagery

Another good way to get your mind on "your team" is to focus on peaceful, pleasant and relaxing thoughts. It's a way of bumping anxiety and pain thoughts out of the way.

"The brain responds to the biggest, brightest, loudest stimuli first," says Pennsylvania language therapist Dorina Saul. "You can use that to your advantage by giving yourself something bigger, brighter and louder than the pain."

One of the oldest techniques is imagining yourself in a favorite spot, whether it's the beach, a relaxing mountain retreat or a favorite resort. The more you can focus on that, the less attention is left for the pain and its aftershocks.

Saul suggests recruiting as many of your senses as possible – picture three things you see at your favorite spot, then three things you hear, three things you feel, three things you smell and so on.

DEEP BREATHING EXERCISES

1.) Loosen tight clothing and sit in a comfortable position with your back supported. Some people prefer sitting in a cross-legged position and others prefer lying down with their head on a small pillow. Close your eyes.
2.) Place one hand on your upper chest and the other on your abdomen just below the breastbone. Try to breathe so that the hand on your abdomen is the one moving.
3.) Now place both hands on your abdomen below the ribs. Breathe in slowly through your nose, allowing your abdomen to rise as your diaphragm moves down.
4.) Pause for a few seconds between breaths, then breathe out slowly through your nose, feeling your abdomen fall as your diaphragm relaxes. Let as much air out of your lungs as possible.
5.) Repeat three or four times. Try to relax your muscles and concentrate on your breathing during the process.
— *Source: The Encyclopedia of Healing Therapies (Dorling Kindersley, 1997)*

She says this exercise stimulates the creative part of your brain and "transports you from a place of pain to a place of no pain."

Another "imagery" technique is to think of a peaceful color in one hand and a brash color in other hand that represents your pain. In your mind's eye, move both closer together until the peaceful color moves in front of the pain color. Or move the peaceful color to the foreground and send the pain color farther away.

Weigel says it sometimes help to repeatedly visualize the pain going away. Instead of picturing colors or beaches, picture being able to touch your face without triggering an attack or being able to brush teeth or chew food without pain.

It might sound like hocus-pocus, but research has found this kind of visualizing sometimes work.

"There have been studies in cancer patients where tumors have shrunk when patients visualized them shrinking," Weigel says. "These things are possible because the body and mind and emotions are all connected."

Audiotapes are also available to help people recruit their minds as a pain-fighting aid. The tapes usually combine soothing background music or sounds with a narration that guides the listener into a relaxed state and then into an imaginary place of peace.

Guided Imagery Inc., an Ohio company that produces one of the most popular tapes, says they're often used to help people with pre-surgery anxiety and post-surgery recovery. But they're also commonly used for any kind of anxiety. (More details on those tapes are available by writing: Guided Imagery, 2937 Lamplight Lane, Willoughby, OH 44094, calling 440-944-9292 or visiting online at www.guidedimagery-inc.com.)

Numerous books on mental imagery also are available, and most psychologists can offer tips on this centuries-old idea. As Dr. Saul, the psychiatrist with TN

PROGRESSIVE MUSCLE RELAXATION

1.) Lie on your back, close your eyes and try to breathe slowly and deeply, emphasizing the out-breath. Pause before you breathe in again.

2.) Tense the muscles in your right foot, hold for a few seconds, then release. Tense and release the calf, then the thigh muscles. Repeat the process with the left foot and leg.

3.) Tense and relax each buttock in turn, then your stomach muscles. Clench and release your right fist, then all the muscles in your arm. Repeat the process with the left arm.

4.) Lift your shoulders up to your ears. Hold for a few seconds, then lower again. Repeat two or three times. To relax your neck, rock your head gently from side to side.

5.) Yawn, then relax. Twist your mouth into a pout and release. Frown, scrunch up your nose, then let go. Raise your eyebrows, then relax all the muscles in your face. (This is assuming none of these actions are pain-triggering ones for you.)

6.) Focus on your breathing again. Imagine yourself feeling warm and peaceful. Then wriggle your toes and fingers and ease your back muscles. Gently bend your knees and roll onto one side for a while, then slowly get up.

— *Source: The Encyclopedia of Healing Therapies (Dorling Kindersley, 1997)*

---

pointed out above, you're not likely to be able to "will away" the pain, but you may at least be able to reduce anxiety, stress and pain intensity.

Hypnosis and self-hypnosis

Ever drive down the road, deep in thought, and suddenly realize you have no recollection of what you passed for the last 10 miles? That's a form of hypnosis.

There are a lot of misconceptions about hypnosis because it's sometimes been presented as entertainment – usually in exaggerated form with the seemingly robotic subject willing to do anything that's suggested.

Dr. Darby says hypnosis is really nothing more than a state of mind in which a person hyper-focuses on a thought, setting or object.

She says subjects don't turn into zombie-like creatures; they're just in a temporary, altered state of consciousness that they can go into and out of when they choose. "If someone doesn't want to go into hypnosis, they won't," she says. "And you can come out of hypnosis in a split second whenever you want to. You do *not* 'get stuck' in hypnosis."

Most people are familiar with the mystical figure dangling a watch to put people into a "hypnotic trance." In hypnosis therapy, it's not necessary to use a watch – or anything else, for that matter. In fact, individuals can be taught how to hypnotize themselves.

When used as therapy, the idea of hypnosis is to deeply relax and then focus on a pleasant setting. While surrounded by these positive images, the patient then focuses on a suggestion.

In the case of TN, the suggestion might be a soothing warmth on the face while lying on a beach. Or it might be eating a favorite sandwich (without pain) in a wooded cabin. It's very much like combining the relaxation, distraction and visualizing techniques mentioned earlier.

One neuralgian from New Jersey says he was able to greatly diminish his TN pain by daily self-hypnosis sessions in which he imagined blood vessels moving off of his trigeminal nerve.

Like imagery, hypnosis also may sound like so much hocus-pocus. But it has helped people get rid of chronic pain, shrink tumors, reverse AIDS and even have surgery without anesthesia, says Dr. Darby. "It's amazing what our unconscious mind can do when you give it permission," she says, adding that this part of the mind is what controls all of the hundreds of millions of biochemical reactions in the body.

According to the National Institutes of Health, studies show that 15 to 20 percent of "hypnotizable" patients with moderate to severe pain can get total relief with hypnosis. Even if hypnosis doesn't help with the pain itself, it may help reduce related anxiety and stress.

Most people can learn self-hypnosis in three or four sessions with a trained hypnotherapist, Dr. Darby says. Audiotapes can be used to help. Insurance sometimes covers hypnosis therapy done by trained and licensed professionals.

About 95 percent of people are able to go into light hypnotic states, Dr. Darby adds. About 55 percent can reach a medium level, and 20 percent can go into deep levels.

Meditation

This ancient technique is somewhat similar to hypnosis. The idea is to become deeply relaxed while hyper-focusing the mind on a particular object, activity or sound. Only in this case, the goal is to drain the brain of all thoughts. No suggestions are introduced.

Meditation developed in the East and Far East, and has almost always been used in a spiritual context. In the West, though, it's been primarily a non-religious stress-reduction technique.

Meditation sessions usually last about 15 to 20 minutes and involve deep breathing, relaxing and focusing on nothing but a selected object, activity or sound. Some use flowers, a burning candle, a picture or rosary beads. Others repeat a relaxing sound over and over again. Whenever the mind wanders or is distracted, the meditator returns to the object or sound.

What this does is counteract the body's "fight-or-flight" response. Whenever the body is threatened (either for real or just perceived), the brain tells the adrenal glands to produce hormones that get the body ready to fight or flee. Blood pressure, heart rate and muscle tension goes

---

HOW TO HYPNOTIZE YOURSELF

1.) Lie or sit in a quiet, comfortable place where you're likely not to be disturbed for 20-30 minutes. Relax, breathe deeply and release any tension in your body.
2.) To induce a relaxed, focused state of mind, imagine yourself walking down a long path or descending a staircase, counting down from 10 to zero.
3.) Repeat to yourself key statements that you'd like to accomplish. In the case of TN, it could be something like, "My face is warm and relaxed," or "I feel calm." Keep the statements positive (i.e. *not*, "I don't feel pain" or "My face doesn't hurt.") You could also play a tape that has your statement recorded.
4.) When you're ready to come out of self-hypnosis, do step one in reverse, for example, climbing back up the stairs and counting up from zero to 10.

— Source: The Encyclopedia of Healing Therapies (Dorling Kindersley, 1997)

up, and breathing becomes faster and more shallow. All of that is a good thing when an acute threat is taking place, but in chronic cases, it's draining and potentially harmful.

Brain-wave tests during meditation sessions have found that a deep state of meditation is somewhere between sleep and full consciousness. Other tests have found that meditating reduces stress hormones and improves blood flow to the brain.

As with hypnosis and imagery, meditation is unlikely to cure pain, but it can reduce anxiety, stress and some of the negative effects those pain side effects have on blood pressure, heart health and the like.

Meditation can be learned from books, tapes, videos, meditation classes or one-on-one from a teacher.

Biofeedback

In the 1920s, German neurologist Dr. Johannes Schultz began to develop a series of six mental exercises aimed at "teaching" the mind to consciously control body functions that are normally subconsciously controlled, such as heart rate, body temperature and blood pressure. The aim is to counteract the otherwise harmful effects of stress and anxiety.

This so-called "autogenic training" employs many of the same

HOW TO MEDITATE

1.) Find a warm, quiet place where you're not likely to be disturbed for 15-20 minutes.

2.) Sit in an upright chair with your back straight and your feet on the floor. Or sit on the floor in a cross-legged position. Rest your hands on your lap or knees and imagine a straight line connecting your navel with the tip of your nose. Close your eyes and relax.

3.) Breathe slowly and rhythmically. Inhale through your nose, and feel the breath move down to your abdomen. Notice which parts of your body are most tense, and as you exhale, imagine the muscles loosening.

4.) Focus on the object of your meditation. This can be an object such as rosary beads, a candle, a picture, flowers or whatever relaxes you. Or it can be a word, phrase or sound that's repeated over and over again.

5.) Allow your attention to become passive. If your mind wanders, return to the object of meditation.

6.) Try to stay as still as possible. You may feel sleepy at first, but this usually passes and you'll become more alert.

7.) When you're ready, after about 15 minutes or so, open your eyes. Take a minute or so to become fully aware of your surroundings. Then stretch and stand up slowly.

— *Source: The Encyclopedia of Healing Therapies (Dorling Kindersley, 1997)*

techniques as the above therapies – deep breathing, muscle relaxation and imagery.

The original method involved focused concentration and repeated phrases, such as "My forehead is cool" or "My arms are heavy" – kind of a blend of self-hypnosis and meditation.

In the 1960s, advances in technology made it possible to add immediate electronic feedback to the training so people could tell if their mental exercises were having the desired effect. This offshoot of autogenic training became known as "biofeedback."

In biofeedback, electrodes are attached to the skin that monitor minute changes in skin temperature, electrical conductivity, muscle tension and/or heart rate. Feedback from these measurements are converted into a form that the person can readily recognize – usually beeps, flashes or moving needles on a dial.

If the relaxation techniques are working, the person should hear the beeps slowing, indicating that heart rate is slowing, muscle tension is easing and the skin is warming.

Usually after about six half-hour sessions, most people have learned what works well enough that the monitoring is no longer needed. In effect, it's a way to teach the mind how to reduce stress's effect on the body.

There's now even a variation of biofeedback called *"neurofeedback"* that uses electroencephalographic electrodes attached to the scalp to monitor brain waves. By projecting the waves on a video screen, people can learn to self-regulate their brain activity.

Biofeedback has been most effective in treating stress- and anxiety-related disorders, including depression, insomnia, ulcers and high blood pressure. But it's also proven effective in helping epilepsy, migraines and other types of chronic pain.

One case study reported by the First Step Wellness Center in Lincoln, Neb., tells of a 46-year-old woman with TN who gradually reduced her pain and got off medicine by using a combination of biofeedback, neurofeedback, deep breathing, cognitive behavioral therapy and stress management. In all, the woman underwent 29 neurofeedback sessions over 37 weeks.

As with the other relaxation techniques, biofeedback is more likely to help with the anxiety and stress involving TN as opposed to causing any drastic reductions in the pain intensity. But used as part of a multi-pronged effort, every little bit helps.

Insurance sometimes covers biofeedback. If it doesn't, out-of-pocket expenses may run $50 to $125 per session.

Prayer

People of faith will tell you that prayer isn't just another "coping strategy" – it's their front-line therapy, and all other treatments and decisions flow from regular visits with the "Great Physician."

The most common benefit of prayer is that it's a source of hope, strength and guidance to those in pain. Regular talks with God can be calming, they can motivate people to keep going when they feel like giving up, and they can help in the treatment decision-making.

"I think anybody who has this disorder knows what being out of control feels like," says Sue Remmey, a TN support group leader in Philadelphia who found her strength in God during 10 years of off-and-on pain.

She says it was her faith and the prayers of people in her church that gave her the courage to ultimately pick up the phone and schedule a microvascular decompression surgery.

Instead of being a nervous wreck before having her skull opened, she was surprisingly calm and peaceful. "The morning of my surgery at 7:30, a group of women had gathered to pray for me," Remmey says. "It really touched me when I found out they were planning to do that. I think that is one reason I was so peaceful the morning of the surgery... I know it was not of myself since I get anxious when I make a wrong turn driving. God was merciful to me and gave me the peace to go through it. Even my family noticed."

What really took her aback was when her surgeon, Dr. Benjamin S. Carson Sr., himself a man of faith, asked if a lot of people had been praying for her. "He said he could tell because he can sense when patients are being prayed for," Remmey said. "For me, it was an amazing affirmation in the power of prayer and the power of our Lord to intervene directly into our lives."

"We need to remember that people are physical, mental and spiritual beings," says Dr. Carson. "The spiritual aspect is what distinguishes us from other animals and provides us with an actual connection to God. I have found that even though it sounds very strange, I can tell when a lot of people are praying for a patient upon whom I am operating. It seems that things go much more smoothly, and I feel as though I am in a 'zone.' There is absolutely no way to prove this, and many people would say that it is foolishness, but then again if one could prove it, there would be no need for faith."

Dr. Carson also believes prayer has positive physical effects on patients.

"It has been well documented that stress exacerbates any medical condition, and I strongly suspect trigeminal neuralgia is one of them," he says. "A strong faith in God dampens the level of anxiety and stress and can have an ameliorating effect on a host of diseases. So even though some people say that prayer and faith are just coping mechanisms, it is quite possible they actually have a physical effect on the electrochemical systems that control our bodies."

Other doctors have noticed the effects of prayer. Dr. Harold Koenig at Duke University Medical Center in Durham, N.C., realized once in his hospital rounds that people who prayed or read Scripture seemed to be coping better with their medical problems.

So he and a team of researchers at Duke recruited 4,000 senior citizens from the Durham area to take part in a six-year study. The senior citizens were surveyed about their health condition and asked if they prayed, meditated or read the Bible.

At the end of six years, the researchers found that those who rarely or never prayed died at a nearly 50 percent higher rate than those who prayed at least once a month. The difference held even when the cases were controlled for risk factors such as smoking, drinking and social isolation, according to a report on the study published in the Journal of Gerontology.

Other studies have found that intercessory prayer (praying for others) can affect healing even when the patient doesn't know he or she is being prayed for.

One of the best known studies is one done by Dr. William Harris at St. Luke's Hospital in Kansas City, Mo. Dr. Harris studied the outcomes of 1,000 heart patients admitted to the hospital.

Half of the patients had five volunteers pray for them daily over four weeks. Those doing the praying only knew the patients' first names and did not visit the hospital. They were instructed to pray for a "speedy recovery with no complications." The patients did not know they were being prayed for. The other half of the patients got the same care but no prayers.

At the end of four weeks, Dr. Harris measured results using such indicators as chest pain, pneumonia, infection and death. He concluded in a 1999 report in the Archives of Internal Medicine that the patients being prayed for fared 11 percent better.

A similar study in 1988 at San Francisco General Hospital found that heart patients being prayed for had lower rates of congestive heart failure and could go home from the hospital sooner.

And another study reported in the American Heart Journal found that patients about to undergo angioplasty (a procedure to unclog heart arteries) had fewer complications when they were prayed for.

Critics, however, point to a few other studies in which prayer seemed to make no difference, including a 2001 Mayo Clinic study of 800 heart patients that found no difference in results after 26 weeks.

Critics also argue that linking prayer to health makes those who don't get better feel guilty for "not praying hard enough" or not being a good enough person. And they question the ethics of using any therapy on people without their knowledge.

Dr. Blair Justice, a University of Texas psychobiologist and long-time prayer/healing researcher, says, however, that enough studies have been done over the years to provide solid evidence that "this isn't some product of a good imagination."

Neuralgian Jennifer Devlin of Alabama will tell you that she's not imagining the sudden end of pain in her left cheek immediately after an unusual prayer experience.

She says one night in November 2002 she "woke straight up in my bed around 3 a.m. with the worst TN strike yet – on top of Tegretol and Keppra. I felt like all my teeth on the left side of my face had cracked out of my head. I had a terrible feeling of discouragement for what my path would be from now on."

After getting her son on the school bus the next morning, Devlin went to her bedroom, got down on her knees with Bible in hand and prayed. "I can't even describe what happened that morning, except for the fact that the Holy Spirit was with me and in me in such a way that I have

AMERICANS' THOUGHTS ON THE HEALING POWER OF PRAYER

ICR Research Group surveyed 1,000 adult Americans in 1996 about their opinions on prayer and healing. Some of what the poll found:

- 80 percent believe that prayer and similar spiritual faith can help people recover from illness or injury.

- 56 percent believe their faith has helped them to recover from a health problem in their own lives.

- 64 percent say they pray for their own health.

- 82 percent say they pray for the health of others.

- 63 percent believe it's good for doctors to talk to patients about spiritual matters, but only 10 percent had ever had a spiritual discussion with a doctor.

never experienced before," she says. "I started praying for healing in my face, and I *know* that exactly at that moment, I was healed."

That morning was the last attack of pain she's had. "I know not everyone will have a healing experience like I did, nor will most people understand what a miraculous thing this is," she says, "but God allowed this in me to bring glory to Him... My husband stands by me in amazement and sweetly has said, 'Welcome back,' because I am finally the person I used to be."

Whether cases such as these are coincidental remissions, examples of the mind's healing power or true miracles, they do happen.

Even if the results aren't as striking as in Devlin's case, prayer is free. And as Dr. Harris points out, there are no side effects.

Humor as therapy

Groucho Marx once said, "A clown is like an aspirin, only he works twice as fast."

Research in the last 20 years is backing up that idea and the age-old folk wisdom that "Laughter is the best medicine."

Study after study highlights the benefits of humor and laughter, not only in relieving stress and anxiety but also in warding off colds and flu, reducing pain and even extending life.

"Finding something to laugh at when you're in pain can help reduce the pain at the same time that it substitutes a more positive mood for a negative mood and lifts your spirits," writes Dr. Paul McGhee, author of *"Health, Healing and the Amuse System"* (Kendall/Hunt, 1999).

Humor's role in healing got a huge boost in the late 1970s from Norman Cousins' book *"Anatomy of An Illness as Perceived by the Patient"* (Bantam, 1991) in which he told about his miraculous recovery from an often fatal and very painful spinal disease.

Aware of research that negative emotions were harmful to health, Cousins figured the opposite also must true. So despite being given 1 in 500 odds of surviving, he checked out of the hospital and spent most of his time with friends watching "Candid Camera" shows, Marx Brothers films and other comedy programs. He beat the odds and survived.

While there's no direct evidence that laughter cured the disease, Cousins' experience encouraged a variety of studies about humor, hope, optimism and maintaining a positive attitude. Some of the findings:

- Pain levels in patients at a long-term-care facility went down after watching funny movies.

• Senior citizens who are optimistic about their health have lower death rates than those with pessimistic outlooks.
• Cancer patients who express greater hope at the time of diagnosis survive longer than those who express less hope.
• The death rate of older people increases sharply following the death of a spouse. The greater the level of depression, the greater the increase.
• Heart patients with a pessimistic outlook were more than twice as likely as optimists to die within one year.
• Heart patients who scored high on tests for sadness and depression were eight times more likely to die within 18 months.

The link between positive attitude and health is so strong that doctors consider it one of a patient's best allies. When Cousins, for example, later surveyed 649 oncologists on the importance of various psychological and social factors in combating cancer, more than 90 percent of the doctors attached the highest value to attitudes of hope and optimism.

There are some physical explanations about why humor and laughing can help across such a wide spectrum of ailments.

One is that the mere action of a belly-laugh tenses and relaxes muscles – a known stress reducer. It's essentially a form of "self-massage."

Laughing also results in deep breathing, particularly exhales that get rid of oxygen-depleted residual air in the lungs. When we're stressed, we tend to breath shallow and rapidly. That discourages us from emptying our lungs and replacing the oxygen-depleted air with fresh, oxygen-rich air.

Perhaps most importantly, research has found that laughter reduces levels of at least four hormones that build up when we're under regular stress. This effect is similar to that seen in such other therapies as progressive relaxation, exercise, biofeedback, guided imagery and meditation.

Researchers also have found that watching as little as 30 minutes of a comedy video can increase the body's level of an antibody (immunoglobulin A) that fights off upper-respiratory illnesses such as colds and flu. Laughter has been linked to increases of two other antibodies.

Other researchers have speculated that laughing reduces endorphins, the body's natural pain-killing chemicals. However, research hasn't verified that suspicion.

What's more certain is humor's effect as a distraction tool.

"Many patients say that their pain is worsened when they feel depressed or when things seem hopeless," says Dr. McGhee, who also is president of The Laughter Remedy, a Delaware company that teaches the benefits of humor in the workplace. "It is reduced, on the other hand, when they're distracted or doing something enjoyable."

Humor, at least temporarily, draws attention away from the source of discomfort. Actor Robin Williams demonstrated the idea well in the film "Patch Adams," in which he clowned, told jokes and did magic tricks for hospital patients.

But taking time to laugh and choosing to view the glass as half full instead of half empty also has an impact on our overall mood and attitude, which, in turn, affects our perception of pain as well as our overall health.

"Part of the health-promoting power of your sense of humor lies in the fact that it helps keep the negative events that occur in your life from disturbing your mood," says Dr. McGhee. "It helps you keep an upbeat, optimistic outlook, even in the face of stress... Your sense of humor is one of the most powerful tools you have to make certain that your daily mood and emotional state support good health."

HOW TO LAUGH YOUR PAIN AWAY

Dr. Paul McGhee, one of the world's foremost experts on humor and health, offers eight ways to bring more humor into your life.

- **Discover the nature of your own unique sense of humor.** Humor is in the eyes of the beholder. We don't all find the same things funny. Take stock of what makes you laugh... Dry humor? TV sitcoms? Jokes? If you're not sure, sample different types and see.

- **Cultivate a playful attitude and a sense of fun.** Adults too often lose these common childhood traits. Overcome "terminal seriousness" by letting out the playful child in you. Spend more time with fun people or take time to play with children. Make a list of fun things and try to do at least one of them every day.

- **Laugh more often and more heartily.** Laughing is a skill that most of us don't practice enough. You may need to force laughs at first or post "laugh reminders" around the house. Try watching or listening to things you find funny or spend more time around laughers. It'll become more natural.

- **Practice telling jokes and stories.** Start with one or a few and get really good at it. Also ask others if they've heard "any good ones" lately.

Continued on next page...

Dr. Justice, the Texas psychobiologist, goes a step farther in his book, "*Who Gets Sick: How Beliefs, Moods and Thoughts Affect Health*" (Peak Press, 2000). He says that "those who get sick the most seem to view the world and their lives as unmanageable."

That's not to say that lack of laughing can bring on TN. But as with the other coping methods already mentioned, laughing can't hurt – unless you laugh a little *too* hard. Dr. McGhee offers some tips on how to introduce humor into otherwise humorless situations in the accompanying sidebar and through numerous articles at his www.laughterremedy.com web site.

...How to Laugh Your Pain Away Continued

- **Create your own verbal humor.** Think up puns. Try to solve riddles. Watch for unintended or double meanings in what you read (i.e. a church bulletin that read, "At this evening's service, the sermon topic will be, 'What Is Hell?' Come early and listen to the choir practice.")

- **Find humor in everyday life.** Funny things happen all the time if you take time to notice. Kids are especially good sources. Share stories about the funny things you see, write them down so you can remember them later when you need a laugh, and ask family and friends what funny things they've seen lately.

- **Learn to laugh at yourself.** This is a hard one, but there's a liberating quality about laughing at yourself. It helps to remember that no one's perfect before sharing one of your past blunders.

- **Find humor in the midst of stress.** Make a conscious effort to have a lighter attitude about whatever stresses you. Recruit family and friends to help you with whatever is most likely to cheer you up when you're down. Keep funny props around.

— *Source: Dr. Paul McGhee in a "Humor and Health" Internet course at* www.corexcel.com/html/body.humor.htm.

CHAPTER 21

HELPING PEOPLE WITH FACE PAIN

"They are not seeking your pity or sympathy, they simply want your compassion. Some will need your help. Just listen, they will tell you how."
—Sherri L. Connell, author of *"But You LOOK Good!"*
(Invisible Disabilities Advocate)

The emotional battle over pain isn't limited just to the TN patient.

"Pain is a family problem, not an individual problem," says Florida psychologist and author Dr. Cynthia D. Belar. "Family members often feel guilty or feel responsible for a person's problem."

"Even with the most love and caring in the world, no partner has the ability to turn off the pain when it flares up," says Dr. Toby Newton-John, a clinical psychologist at Royal North Shore Hospital's Pain Management and Research Centre in Sydney, Australia. "Partners need to understand that it is not a shortcoming of theirs, nor should it be an expectation of the sufferers."

In other words, TN is not anyone's fault. So step one is avoiding blame and guilt and focusing instead on addressing the problem at hand.

Even with that issue out of the way, though, there's no getting around the fact that chronic pain impacts everyone's living habits.

"It changes the whole system at home," says Dr. Steven Hickman, a psychologist and instructor at the University of California at San Diego. "It's like a new member of the family that moves in and affects everybody."

The effects of chronic pain can spill over into all sorts of family dynamics, including family outings, dealings with the kids, who does what jobs around the house and so on. It also affects relationships with friends, co-workers and potentially all interactions.

When the National Chronic Pain Outreach Association in 1994 asked 204 chronic-pain sufferers about how their pain was affecting their lives, 87 percent said the pain "interferes significantly." Seventy-one percent said it was affecting their personal relationships.

Surveys of caregivers have found that two-thirds of them believe the illness has put a strain on their marriage, one quarter of them say they've felt despair, and a large majority say they have experienced fatigue, frustration and stress as a result of caregiving.

"Chronic pain affects family relationships because family members distance themselves for fear of causing pain," says Dorothy McConaghy, a psychiatric nurse and former TN sufferer from Florida. "My children grew up knowing which side of my face could be touched and when I was having a 'jaw ache' and could not speak."

Supporters help with coping

Friends, spouses and other family members can play a big role in helping a TN sufferer cope with the pain. It's often not an easy job because you may get conflicting signals from the neuralgian. Sometimes neuralgians want company, sometimes not. Sometimes they want to talk about the problem, other times not.

Those who learn to maneuver these new boundaries can make a huge difference in how a person copes with pain.

Researchers at Vanderbilt University Medical Center in Nashville, Tenn., recently studied 181 people one year after they had completed a pain-management program. The researchers found that those who said they had no family support needed more medications, reported more pain and scored higher on emotional stress tests than those who had supportive families.

There's no mistake about it – support helps people cope.

Norma Zimmer, the singer who appeared for years on Lawrence Welk's TV program, said her husband, Randy, was a tremendous aid in helping her to cope with TN.

"It became difficult to look to my left without getting a shock, so Randy always made sure I sat where I could look at people to my right," she says. "Quite an accomplishment!

"Randy was marvelous. He cared for me with such love and protection and he was always so thoughtful and tender. He always accompanied me on my appearances, guarding my every move.

"Walking became difficult, as each time my heels hit the floor, it would cause pain. Randy even devised some rubber cushions to place in my shoes that eased the problem."

When the pain got so bad she couldn't even chew, Zimmer says her husband began pureeing her food.

What's not always easy for a spouse, relative or friend is figuring out exactly what helps and what doesn't. Go too far in helping or comforting and it might come off as "babying" the person or making them feel useless or helpless.

Or, a TN patient might get upset when a spouse continually asks about the pain but then get equally upset when the spouse stops asking.

Said one exasperated husband of a long-time TN sufferer: "My wife doesn't want me to kiss her because it might set off an attack, but then she criticizes me for not showing love and support."

Clearly, there's a fine line here that isn't always easy for family and friends to walk.

How others react

Dealing with the effects of your pain is just as new of an experience to your family and friends as it is to you. Most people have no idea how to react.

The most detrimental move is bailing out altogether. "My husband has threatened to leave me because, in his words, he 'can't take it anymore,'" lamented one Tennessee woman with atypical TN in an online message group. "How nice. I am in unbelievable pain, and *he* can't take it anymore!!!"

Others don't know what to say or do, and so they react by either avoiding contact or at least avoiding the subject of pain. That's not much more helpful than total abandonment, writes Sherri L. Connell in her booklet, *"But You LOOK Good!"* (Invisible Disabilities Advocate, 2003).

"If you are there by their side to hear their concerns," she advises friends and family, "they will gain the strength to continue to fight. But if you refuse to be there for them to listen, it will only make their losses seem greater because now they have lost you as well."

Dr. Newton-John says the best approach is for everyone to be open and honest about what they're thinking and feeling, about what they need and what they don't need. Trying to "mind-read" usually leads to misunderstanding.

"These are the keys to keeping the relationship healthy despite the pain," Dr. Newton-John says. "The pain is stressful enough without the added component of relationship stress, and the best way to prevent that is to practice talking together. Talking about pain in this sense is not complaining. It is a discussion where the sufferer and partner sit down together as a team and chat about how well the team is performing."

A good team, he adds, will encourage one another, give each other credit for their efforts and try to come up with ideas on how to improve the situation.

Maintaining good communication can be tough because sometimes neuralgians tend to "crawl into a shell" and want to be left alone. While that's understandable, it can alienate would-be help.

"I didn't understand this condition and couldn't explain it," wrote one Canadian neuralgian in an online account of her battle with TN. "Besides, there was nothing anyone could do anyway... I also clung to the hope that I would be one of the lucky ones, and this would disappear forever. So I said nothing. I now can readily see how that may easily be interpreted as a lack of trust. I am not saying that you have to advertise this (pain) to everyone, but those you care about and who care about you have a right to know something *is* going on. By not telling them, how can they possibly understand what is happening with you? You have taken away *their* choice to try and understand."

"As pain increases and treatment does not give relief, communication becomes more important but also more difficult," says McConaghy. "The care-giver will do well to remember that warmth and the ability to convey a sense of understanding of what the person in pain is experiencing are as therapeutic as any medicine and surgery."

Most of the time, friends and family truly want to help. They're just not sure what they *can* do.

"My wife would go to give me a kiss and I'd move away," says Dr. Richard Saul, a psychiatrist and neuralgian from Philadelphia.

"Well-meaning friends and family would come over to cheer my spirits," says Sue Remmey, a neuralgian and TN support group leader from Philadelphia, "but they would often leave quickly when they realized that even laughter and smiling would trigger the frightening attacks."

Flo McTaggart of California didn't know what to do as she watched her husband, John, suffer increasingly intense attacks despite medication.

"He would just sit on the end of the bed and wail," she told her local newspaper. "I was helpless. I just didn't know what to do. At a couple of points, he would say if he had a gun, he would use it. You never knew if he'd get through a supper without almost dropping to his knees in pain. All of a sudden, wham, it would hit, and the whole next hour or two would change."

McTaggart eventually got rid of his pain via a microvascular decompression surgery in San Diego.

Hard to understand

It's often hard for others to understand the intensity of TN pain. After all, you may look perfectly fine, and all the tests came back "normal."

"Often the most difficult part of having a chronic, debilitating illness is the lack of understanding sufferers encounter," writes Connell, who's battled both multiple sclerosis and TN. "People are accustomed to thinking that they have to see someone is bleeding before they can believe they are hurting... Most people cannot comprehend what it is like to be sick and/or in pain day after day because they are accustomed to going to the doctor, taking some medication and soon feeling better."

A 26-year-old Kentucky neuralgian says she's been distressed at how "non-trigeminal people just don't understand. How do you explain to a potential date that you can't go out with him because you're afraid 'it' will happen? You can't. So you stay home, alone."

Sometimes others end up making things worse when they try to be empathetic. They'll say things like, "I know how it must hurt," or "Just ignore it like I do when I get a headache and it will go away," or "I know just what you're going through… I sprained my wrist last summer and for weeks I could barely move it."

"It took me awhile to get past the frustration when someone said something like that," the Canadian neuralgian says. "In reality, however, so few have even heard of this they have nothing to relate it to, just as I had nothing to relate it to when it first started for me. Sure, I can describe it as being like being hit by a bolt of lightning over and over in your face, but how many people know what that feels like?"

The lack of reference or understanding about TN often causes others to wonder why you keep having pain. They may say things like, "Why don't you snap out of it?" or "Why can't you just tough it out until it passes?" Even when nothing is said, people in pain can often sense when others have a "buck-up-and-live-with-it attitude," as Connell calls it.

"Most people do not 'give in' to illness," Connell writes. "In fact, it is ingrained in our nature to fight to survive as hard and as long as humanly possible… Creating limitations for oneself is one of the hardest things a person can do. It goes against everything we are and everything we hoped to be. No one *wants* to be sick, and no one *chooses* to give up those things in life which bring such joy."

The sooner friends and family accept that, the better they'll be able to help, she says. Connell's advice is to trust the person's pain description, don't try to write it off as "no big deal" and don't make the person feel as if they are "weak" or somehow at fault. That will only make them feel more alone and isolated.

"I DON'T GET IT!"

The following is a poem the spouse of a neuralgian wrote about dealing with TN:

I don't get it! I don't understand! I know you're in pain. I have been in pain myself. But it has never incapacitated me as your pain immobilizes you. What is this pain that takes you away from me…that steals our time that we could enjoy together?

It's been so long since I last kissed you or caressed your lovely face. I hesitate to even hug you for fear that I might just graze your face and start the pain that can bring you to your knees.

I want to help you but don't know what to do. I want to ease your pain but don't have that power.

Help me to understand. I really need to know and understand just what you are going through.

"People tend to minimize it," says one neuralgian from Pennsylvania. "They don't think anything is wrong with me."

Things that <u>don't</u> help

Connell's booklet lists several specific approaches that are likely to discourage people in pain. These are some excerpts:

- **Do not treat them like they have chosen to have pain.**
  Avoid saying things like, "Why didn't you…" and "You could get better if you wanted to." No one chooses to have pain, and "trying harder," "having a better attitude" and "using mind over matter" won't get rid of it.
- **Do not expect them to be happy.**
  Do not demand them to see the "bright side" or to "cheer up." Sometimes they need to stop and mourn what they have lost and work through their changes. Telling them to "be positive" will only cause heartbreak and frustration.
- **Do not assume or put words in their mouths.**
  Avoid saying, "You must be having a good day!" or "You're doing better, aren't you?" This shows you do not really want to ask how they are doing because you do not really want to know. Instead ask how they're doing and be prepared to accept the answer.
- **Do not disagree with them because you can't see anything wrong.**
  When you say things like, "But you don't look sick," you are really saying, "But I don't care what you are telling me; because I can't see it, I don't believe it."
- **Do not disregard their new limitations.**
  If they have to say no to you, it's not because they want to. It is because they *need* to. Respect their limitations without inducing a guilt trip. Pain is exhausting. Odds are they're already pushing themselves beyond their limits.
- **Do not point out what they "at least" have.**
  Most people in pain are already thankful for little things they can achieve each day, and they don't need to be reminded that "at least they have" this or "at least they have" that. Instead try to see their will to keep going despite their pain.

• **Do not minimize their situation.**
Unless you're in their shoes, you have no right to tell someone, "It's not that bad" or "It could be worse." It can always be worse for anyone in any situation, but how does that help make their pain or losses any less?

• **Do not act like you can relate.**
Unless you have a chronic illness, you do not know what it's like. You don't have to empathize in order to show compassion. Most people in pain resent comments like, "Join the club," because the well person does not have the right to think they are in the same boat.

• **Do not act like fixing the problem is simple.**
Avoid comments like "Why don't you just..." or "Why can't they just..." Chances are the person has already thought of or tried that and already spent lots of money and seen lots of doctors. If there were an easy fix, it probably already would have worked.

Things that <u>do</u> help

On the other hand, Connell has found several other approaches that people in pain usually find encouraging. Excerpted from her booklet, these include:

• **Acknowledge their situation.**
Let your loved one know you understand and accept their situation and that you're there to help them in whatever way you can. This will let them know you believe them, love them as they are and respect them for their perseverance.

• **Acknowledge their losses.**
It helps to say things like, "I'm so sorry you can't work anymore!" and "I can't imagine what you've been through." This shows you have compassion for what they can no longer do or enjoy. It also lets them know you understand that this isn't something they chose to have.

• **Show them you are listening.**
Try asking, "How are you doing?" instead of, "How are you feeling?" This is more likely to spark an answer that tells how they are dealing with their challenges and struggles. You don't have to come up with solutions to the struggles... just taking the time to listen and care is often enough.

- **Show them you are aware of their circumstances.**
When someone in severe pain shows up to a gathering, let them know you appreciate the effort it took them. Say something like, "I am so glad you made it. I know it can be difficult for you."
- **Show them you are willing to help.**
Little things like picking up something at the grocery store or washing the dishes can be huge and much appreciated helps. Offering to help doesn't have to be a big commitment. People might need help, but neither do they want to become a burden on anyone.
- **Let them know you enjoy their company.**
Everyone wants to be appreciated. People in pain often feel like others don't want to be around them. Little comments like, "I'm so glad to see you," and "I enjoyed visiting with you yesterday" can be big morale boosters.
- **Show them your admiration.**
It takes a lot of strength, perseverance and determination to carry on in the midst of chronic pain or illness. Think of how you feel when you're sick for only a day or two. Imagine that every day. A simple comment such as, "You amaze me," can counteract a lot of negative feelings the person might otherwise have.
- **Let them know you appreciate your health.**
Nothing is worse than a healthy person complaining to an ill person about all of the things they had to do. These are usually things the ill person only wishes he or she could do. Instead, say something like, "You really make me appreciate being able to do things I never even thought about before."
- **Give them a compliment.**
Notice positive things about your loved one and let him or her know you noticed. Everyone likes compliments, but they're especially appreciated in tough times. Examples: "You look very nice today," "You have good ideas," and "Wow, you know a lot about…"

(Connell's "But You LOOK Good!" booklet is available through the Invisible Disabilities Advocate web site at www.InvisibleDisabilities.org or by sending a self-addressed, stamped envelope to: IDA, 41553 Madrid Drive, Parker, CO 80138.)

Walking that fine line

Probably the trickiest issue for a friend or family member is learning how to be helpful, supportive, understanding and compassionate without crossing over into making the person in pain feel like a pitied, useless burden.

That line varies from person to person and even from time to time, depending on how the pain is "acting" that day.

Most people appreciate offers of specific help but usually resent it if you just start doing everything for them – especially things they normally do.

"Sometimes one of the best things a spouse can do for a person in pain is let that person take care of himself or herself," says Dr. Hickman.

"You can actually undermine a patient's self-confidence about how to manage pain," adds Dr. Belar. "When that happens, they start to lose their identify and feel *more* helpless."

An understanding, supportive friend or relative will stay positive and upbeat. They'll show an interest in the person's condition without constantly bringing it up, especially during remissions. They'll learn about the medications and the treatments and other things the TN patient can do to get well and remind him or her about those options if helplessness starts to set in.

As Dr. Albert L. Rhoton Jr., the Florida neurosurgeon, puts it: "A physician's best ally in the treatment of any neurosurgical illness is a well-informed patient. And that means a well-informed family as well."

Friends and family also can help by encouraging the patient to remain active and involved and to continue doing things he or she enjoys, whether it's painting, boating, going to museums or going to movies (to the degree the person is able, that is). These activities can bring both enjoyment and distraction – two of those factors that help "close the gate" to pain.

If the person just isn't up to an activity, though, don't push. Being flexible and being willing to make allowances will help everybody.

"Families may have to learn to be more spontaneous," says Nancy McMahon, a registered nurse who works with Cincinnati neurosurgeon Dr. John M. Tew's TN patients. "For instance, grab the chance to do something when the patient is having a good day. It's OK to be angry when a family member's TN upsets your plans, but you need to explain that you're angry at the disorder, not the individual who has it."

Likewise, the patient needs to understand that TN is frustrating for the family as well. It helps when the neuralgian can spell out exactly what's helpful and what's not and realize that the situation is stressful for others as well.

Above all, don't just give up and avoid a person in pain. There may be days when the person really wants to be alone and will say so. That's fine. There may be other days when the person is hurting and just wants someone to sit with them. Then there may be days when the pain is gone, and the person suddenly seems like his or her "old self."

"Spending time with friends and family who care gives incredible strength and will to keep fighting the battle," says Connell.

The Canadian neuralgian tells of one friend who got it exactly right…

"It brings a smile to my heart when I think of one particular friend I talk to almost every day," she writes. "I don't know how he puts up with me some days. But he is there to listen if I want to talk about it, or to talk about other things if I don't. He never questions. He never 'advises.' He is just there. And always, always he can make me laugh, which is a great medicine. He's a very cherished friend."

The effect on children

Dealing with pain in the family can be particularly perplexing for kids. They may not understand the problem at all or they may feel somehow responsible, maybe even afraid.

The solution is to be frank with children and grandchildren. Try to explain to them as clearly and simply as you can what's wrong.

Explain to them why you sometimes jerk your head in agony for seemingly no reason. Explain to them that you're not mad when you're not speaking. Explain to them that it's not that you don't care about them when you can't play or go places.

When the pain subsides, take advantage of the break to spend time and go places with your children or grandchildren. Even when the pain is active, you may be able to share "quiet-time" activities such as coloring, putting together a puzzle or watching a favorite video together.

Encourage children to share their feelings about your pain. Don't let unanswered questions or worries silently fester.

Keep in mind that children may assume that this is a permanent problem or that it may get worse or that it may even be fatal. Try to be optimistic and convey to them that you are taking steps to solve the problem.

Remember, if TN is confusing to adults, think how much more confusing it must be to children.

An effective doctor

The final link in the TN "coping team" is a supportive doctor. Whether it's a neurologist, neurosurgeon, family doctor or a complementary/alternative practitioner, the patient's primary TN doctor plays a key role in how well the condition is managed.

Some are obviously better at this than others, depending on such factors as time demands, interpersonal skills and the clinician's knowledge and understanding of TN.

Chronic pains such as TN are often among the most difficult for doctors to treat, and finding a good solution may just as frustrating for them as it is for patients.

When treatments aren't working, there's sometimes a tendency for doctors to assume the pain must be psychological and to shuffle these patients off to the psychologist. Although that attitude is changing, it's still around.

Lack of time is usually the biggest hindrance to good patient/doctor communication.

Rare is this neurologist described by the online Canadian neuralgian: "He devoted two full hours explaining the diagnosis. He went through diagrams of the brain and showed me the course of the nerve. He outlined a course of treatment, being very sure to reassure me that at any time this could disappear and never return but that it could just as easily return with a vengeance. He began to explain the surgical options and choices I *might* have to make if drugs didn't work anymore. But there was no way I was ready or willing to listen to that. I was still pain free and didn't want to believe there would ever come a day when I would have to choose this option – and yet just weeks before he could have done whatever he wanted."

On the other hand, a neuralgian from Pennsylvania tells that her neurologist had her in and out in minutes with a medication prescription and little else. "My doctor didn't even explain what it was that he was diagnosing me with," she says. "He simply made the diagnosis and prescribed Tegretol. Everything that I have learned about TN has been from the web."

In general, TN patients give high marks to doctors who explain the problem in plain English, who clearly lay out the options and who simply take the time to listen, understand and respond to their patients' feelings and preferences.

Dr. Joanna Zakrzewska, in her medical textbook *"Trigeminal Neuralgia,"* (W.B. Saunders Co. Ltd., 1995), lays out an excellent game plan for physicians on how to manage TN cases. She advises TN doctors to:

1.) Allow plenty of time to explain the initial diagnosis and to answer patients' questions.

2.) Determine how much the patient already knows about TN, and just as importantly, how much the patient *wants* to know.

"Some patients want to know everything," Dr. Zakrzewska says. "Others only want some information." Either way, she adds, the doctor should make sure the patient knows the "lines of communication remain open" whenever they do have a question or need.

3.) Give information in small chunks and in plain English. The basic options should be clearly outlined, and any murky understandings should be clarified. Charts, diagrams and written hand-outs help.

"This kind of hope and knowledge at the beginning of treatment is very important," says South Carolina neurosurgeon Dr. Stephen Haines. "That way if you find one treatment isn't working for you, you can ask to move on to the next level."

4.) Listen to and respond to the patient's feedback. "Reactions to the diagnosis can include disbelief, shock, fear and anxiety," Dr. Zakrzewska says. "Many patients feel anger, which can be directed toward clinicians."

At this stage, the doctor should be prepared to function more as a counselor.

5.) Be prepared to suggest a treatment plan that takes into account the prior discussion with the patient. Whether the plan involves a specific treatment and follow-up visit or a referral to another specialist, the patient should leave with the feeling that the doctor stands ready to help if the patient further needs it.

Dr. Zakrzewska also believes doctors can do a great service to patients by offering them pain-coping strategies and details on support groups and other sources for more information.

"Patients have become experienced consumers who understand that they have rights," she says. "They have become less inclined to leave all the medical decisions to the doctors."

HOW TO HELP YOUR TN DOCTOR HELP YOU

Good medical care is a team effort between your doctor and you. Following are a few tips on how to get the best care possible:

• *Educate yourself.* This book is a good start. Information also is available through hospital libraries, public libraries (if your hospital library is not open to the public) and the Trigeminal Neuralgia Association, 925 Northwest 56th Terrace, Suite C, Gainesville, FL 32605 (phone: 352-376-9955).

The Internet also is loaded with TN information, including TNA's web site at www.tna-support.org. See Chapter 24 for other helpful web sites as well as tips on how to make sure you're finding accurate and reliable information.

• *Do some homework before choosing.* Ask friends, neighbors, co-workers, relatives and your family doctor for names of specialists they would recommend. (With TN, the specialist is usually a neurologist or neurosurgeon.)

Members of a TN support group are ideal for advice on how well particular doctors handle TN cases specifically – if your area has such a group. Choosing a highly regarded doctor in the first place is one of the best things you can do.

• *Be ready to give specific, detailed information.* Since there is no lab test to diagnose TN, the doctor depends on you to give an accurate description of your pain so he can tell if it's TN or some other problem. Even if it is TN, the exact nature of your pain may play a role in determining the best course of treatment.

Prepare for the visit by writing down such details as exactly where it hurts, when it hurts, what kind of pain it is, what makes it better or worse and whether it's constant or episodic. Don't depend on memory.

Some people keep a "pain diary" to help them accurately remember what the pain has been like or to help them link factors that seem to make the pain better or worse.

• *Give a thorough medical history.* Doctors usually ask pretty detailed questions to get at any possible adverse reactions to treatments they have in mind. If not, make sure the doctor knows about any allergies you have, any other illnesses, any other drugs you're taking and any other conditions, such as being or planning to be pregnant.

• *Don't be afraid to ask questions.* There is no such thing as a stupid question when it comes to your health. If you don't understand something, ask. The doctor may have drawings, charts, brochures or a better way to explain the point you don't understand.

If the doctor seems rushed or unwilling to take the time, consider asking for a longer appointment next time or seek out a new doctor who is willing and able to take the time.

Also ask about your doctor's feeling on the use of email questions. Some find this to be an effective and time-efficient way to keep in touch with patients. And patients often are willing to pay for this service, figuring it's worth the benefit of getting quick answers to a question or two without having to drive to visits, wait for appointments and pay for full-blown office visits.

Continued on next page ...

... Continued from previous page

• **Write down questions.** Questions and issues inevitably pop up between visits, but it's easy to forget them when you're finally in the doctor's chair. By writing down the questions, you'll have answers the next time the situation arises.

Take your list of questions along to your appointment. And jot down notes on the information and recommendations you receive so you don't forget later. Remember, your memory may not be working at peak levels if you're on medication.

• **Take someone along to doctor visits.** A spouse, other relative or close friend can help you remember what was said and make sure your questions are all asked and answered.

"Sometimes people with TN simply can't cope with doctors because they're in too much pain or are groggy from medication," says Trigeminal Neuralgia Association board member Brian Cronin, whose wife has TN. "At such times, the well spouse may have to become the logical, thinking partner and, if necessary, the 'attack dog' to make sure treatment is swift and appropriate."

• **Come away with a game plan.** Each doctor visit should end with a clear understanding of what the next step will be, whether it's sticking with the current treatment, trying a new dose or new drug or being referred to a surgeon or different specialist.

Make sure you understand how and when to take any new medications and what side effects may occur, especially ones that should be reported to the doctor.

Also, be sure to find out what's to be done if the pain suddenly flares between visits. Is the doctor or someone else in his practice always on call? If not, who can you call? Or does the doctor have an alternate dosage schedule you can use in case the pain breaks through the current dose? Whatever the case, be ready to deal with flare-ups.

• **Call the office if the game plan isn't working.** A doctor isn't going to know if a treatment isn't working unless you tell him or her.

Sometimes minor adjustments can be made that can make a major difference even without the need for an office visit. Other times a new option can be tried or a sooner appointment can be scheduled. In any event, don't suffer in silence figuring there's nothing that can be done until your next scheduled appointment.

• **Work as partners.** A good relationship is one in which the doctor and patient can discuss the options and come up with a treatment plan satisfactory to both.

Don't view the doctor as the ultimate authority who has the one and only right answer every time. On the other hand, doctors generally do not appreciate semi- or ill-informed patients who come in demanding a particular treatment.

The truths are: doctors aren't always right; what works for one patient may not work for the next one; not all patients feel the same way about the various treatment options, and the best solution often comes after some trial and error.

Good communication, patience and understanding from both parties make sure everyone is on the same wavelength. If it just isn't working, consider seeing a different doctor.

The "burden" on caregivers

Caring for a loved one in chronic pain can be difficult, taxing and stressful. It can even lead to physical and mental problems that psychologists have begun calling *"caregiver burden"* and *"caregiver burnout."*

Caregiver burden is the strain or load borne by a person who cares for an elderly, ill or disabled loved one. Caregiver burnout is when the burden progresses to the point where the situation threatens the health of the caregiver.

Helping someone in a chronic situation often requires a lot of extra emotional energy as well as physical energy. Besides taking on extra jobs that the person in pain is unable to do, the worry, frustration and feelings of helplessness alone can be draining.

In the short term, many people are able to cope well with these changes. But as time goes along, it's common for feelings of being burdened to grow, regardless of the emotional attachment to the person. This, in turn, often brings on feelings of guilt.

If these feelings aren't addressed in the early stages, psychologists say the burden can swell into burnout.

Caregiver burnout can take on many forms. Physical symptoms can include indigestion, changes in appetite, headaches, fatigue, weight loss or weight gain and insomnia. Mental and social symptoms can include social withdrawal, difficulty concentrating, irritability, increased use of sarcasm, increased anxiety and increased feelings of helplessness.

If burnout isn't addressed, depression can result.

Psychologists have come up with several questionnaires to help assess the burden on caregivers, which is a problem most agree is greatly under-reported and under-treated. One of the most used indexes is the Zarit Burden Interview, a set of 22 questions developed by Dr. Steven Zarit, head of the Penn State University Department of Human Development and Family Studies. (See Chapter 23 for the questions.)

If the burden is becoming a problem, some of the measures that might help are:

- *Take regular breaks from caregiving.* If the person in pain has remissions, those can be refreshing periods. If not, even getting away for a few hours every now and then can help.
- *Recruit some help.* Are there other family members, friends or neighbors who can check in or visit while you get away for a little while?
- *Seek professional counseling.* Counselors can help you sort out and "validate" conflicting feelings, offer some fresh insights or alternatives, and give a safe place to vent.

• *Do more research.* By learning all you can about the condition your loved one has, you'll feel better prepared and equipped to offer help. It's also a productive use of time that may lead to a resolution of the pain.

• *Take time for yourself.* It's not healthy to spend 100 percent of your waking hours caring for others. Don't give up your hobbies, your friends or your social life. Make at least some time to do things you find enjoyable.

• *Seek out support.* Support groups can be a huge help in sharing some of the burden. It's the one group where everyone understands what you and the person in pain are going through.

A support group for neuralgians

One morning in 1978, Claire Patterson of Barnegat Light, N.J., was putting on her makeup as she did every day. But on this day, something happened that would change her life – and the lives of thousands of TN sufferers – forever.

When she touched her face that day, Patterson felt a sudden pain like she had never felt before. "It was like an electric shock on the tip of my nose," she recalls. "You never forget that pain. I've had five children, have had broken bones and other problems, but there is no other pain like this one."

Patterson went to an ear, nose and throat specialist, who anesthetized the nerves in her nose. That helped briefly, but then the shooting pains came back. So she went back to the doctor and had the procedure repeated.

Same story. The pain came back.

The third time, she went to an internist, who quickly diagnosed the pain as trigeminal neuralgia. "My first question was, 'Will I die from it?'" she recalls. "And he said, 'No, but you may wish that you would if it gets bad enough.'"

Like most people, Patterson had never heard of TN. It was only after the sharp, electric-like pains came that she realized that the intermittent jaw aches she had had previously for two years were actually precursors to a full-blown case of TN.

Patterson started on medication and put up with the pain for nearly nine years. "During my first regimen of anticonvulsant drugs, I went into remission for a couple of months," she says. "But every time it came back, the pain was more severe. It started with just the tip of my nose, but nine years later the whole upper and lower side of my face was affected and eventually the back of my throat. Everything was irritating – a breeze, putting on makeup, eating and eventually even swallowing."

As the pain increased, so did her prescribed dose of medicine – to the point where she finally landed in a hospital. Doctors there told her her only option was to have the nerve severed to stop the pain.

Patterson balked at that. Cutting the nerve meant permanent numbness on that whole side of the face. She was convinced there had to be a better way.

There was.

With the help of her internist, Patterson located an article in the New England Journal of Medicine about a procedure called *"microvascular decompression."* In 1987, Patterson flew to Pittsburgh to have that operation performed by the neurosurgeon who had developed it 20 years earlier – Dr. Peter Jannetta.

Dr. Jannetta found an artery was compressing Patterson's trigeminal nerve and was able to lift it off and insulate it with a Teflon felt pad. Patterson woke up pain-free and hasn't had any of those terrible jolts since.

The beginnings of TNA

Something else happened after the surgery. Patterson happened to hear a woman in a nearby room crying and sobbing.

"I asked the nurse what was wrong with that woman, and she said, 'She has the same thing you do,'" says Patterson. "Later that night I went back and talked to her, and she broke down in tears and said, 'I had this disease 13 years, and I've never talked to anyone else who had it.' Well, I'd had it almost 10 years and I never talked to anybody else who had it either."

When Dr. Jannetta came by to see her, Patterson mentioned that it was a shame no one had ever started some kind of organization or support group for TN sufferers. Dr. Jannetta shot back: "Why don't you start one?"

That was the beginning of the Trigeminal Neuralgia Association.

By March 1991, Patterson, a former director of senior citizen groups from a remote New Jersey barrier island, had incorporated TNA as a national tax-exempt organization and shepherded the formation of the first few local trigeminal neuralgia support groups.

With Dr. Jannetta's help, a TNA Medical Advisory Board made up of some of the nation's top TN experts was appointed.

"I have to give Dr. Jannetta credit," says Patterson. "If he hadn't slipped that (challenge) right back at me, I don't know if I would have done it. It's pretty hard to say no when you've been cured of the worst pain in the world."

TNA's office started in the dining room of Patterson's home. It has since moved to Gainesville, Fla., and grown into a national organization that has helped spawn more than 200 regional support groups and telephone contacts in 40 states. It also has helped begin support groups in Canada, the United Kingdom, Israel and Australia with telephone contacts in Finland, Hong-Kong, India, Italy, the Netherlands, New Zealand and Singapore.

TNA also:

- Offers a periodic TNAlert newsletter and other educational materials, including this book.
- Has a web site (www.tna-support.org) that includes face-pain information, medical papers, links to other sites for treatment help, answers to common questions, tips for researching medical information online and more.
- Has a patient representative who's available to consult first-hand with neuralgians and their families.
- Has a board of directors, officers and staff who encourage research, attend physician conferences and spread the word about TN and its treatments.
- Sponsors a biannual national conference in which patients and many of the nation's leading TN doctors and experts get together for four days of seminars and meetings.

"Claire has shown that one person can make a difference," says Dr. Jannetta.

Patterson says she'll never forget what it was like to suffer for so long with very little information and without knowing anyone else going through the same thing.

"If I'd have known I had other surgical options those last five years I dealt with this," says Patterson, "I would have had surgery much sooner. When I was in dire straits, all I was told was, 'All we can do is sever the nerve.'"

A main part of her vision for TNA has always been to make sure future TN patients get thorough information so they can make informed decisions. "I want there to be informed patients, not helpless victims," she says.

Support makes a difference

Having such a resource and support group in place can be a tremendous help to people – especially in a case like TN in which there has been precious little written about it in the popular press.

Most people never heard of it before they got it, and before TNA came along, it was difficult to find any understandable information or even other people suffering from the same affliction.

That only makes the problem worse.

Without knowing there are other options, people may lose hope. Without knowing there are others, people feel isolated and wonder, "Why me?" And when there is no one else around who truly understands the pain and how bad it hurts, people tend to withdraw and isolate themselves even more.

"'You are not alone.' That's probably the best first thing to tell people," says Dr. Molly Nemann Patterson, a Cincinnati neuropsychologist.

Here's what *"The Prevention Pain-Relief System"* (Bantam Books, 1992) says about support groups for chronic pain: "You may withdraw emotionally and perhaps even physically from the people who are closest to you. You may avoid social events because they're just not fun anymore. Your pain may make it difficult to dance, bowl, sit for very long or even focus on a conversa-

---

TNA'S PURPOSE

The Gainesville, Florida-based Trigeminal Neuralgia Association's mission is to serve as an advocate for patients suffering from TN and related face pains by providing information, encouraging research and offering support. It's a patient-centered organization that provides programs that give patients access to credible information about face pain.

TNA's five specific goals are:

1.) To provide information and to support and encourage those who are afflicted with TN/facial pain and their families, by assisting in the development of support groups and personal contacts.

2.) To encourage sound research on the causes of TN and related facial pain conditions and the results of current treatments; and to disseminate this information among the medical and dental clinicians and the general public.

3.) To urge the continuing search for new medications and treatments.

4.) To advocate the development of effective pain management techniques amongst professional health-care providers for those with ongoing discomfort from TN and related facial pain conditions.

5.) To advocate for public policy which is supportive of the needs of those with rare disorders.

tion. Being with people who don't seem to understand your pain can put a knife-edge on those feelings of loneliness and depression ... That's why some people consider it something of a miracle when they finally meet others who mean it when they say, 'I know how you feel' or 'I understand.' That's what support groups are about."

"It is reassuring to meet other people with TN," says Audrey Parker-Dryden, a TN support group leader in Alaska. "When they look at us and say, 'I understand what you are going through,' they truly do! This helps to reduce our feelings of isolation that come from having such a painful disorder... and mitigates our feelings of 'Why me?'"

Support groups can help in many ways. Obviously, those in a group can help each other by lending a sympathetic ear and sharing a few words of hope and encouragement.

Members also can share coping skills and trade practical advice on what works to limit attacks.

HOW TO CONTRACT THE TRIGEMINAL NEURALGIA ASSOCIATION

The Trigeminal Neuralgia Association is a non-profit organization dedicated to helping trigeminal neuralgians and their families. It is supported almost entirely by donations from individuals. To contact TNA, write:

**Trigeminal Neuralgia Association
925 Northwest 56th Terrace, Suite C
Gainesville, FL 32605**

TNA's web site is:
www.tna-support.org

The TNA office also can be reached in these ways:

Office telephone: 352-376-9955

Office fax: 352-376-8688

e-mail: tnanational@tna-support.org

**Patient representative:
352-376-3608**

Patient representative e-mail:
patientrep@tna-support.org

They can take some of the burden off of family members by becoming a kind of "second family" that shares a common bond.

And group members can share helpful information on treatments – things that worked for them and things that didn't, doctors who helped and doctors who didn't.

That kind of information can help ensure that patients don't miss a potentially helpful option as well as help others avoid options that just about always turn out to be a waste of time and money.

Some groups even have doctor referral services to help direct new members to the doctors that the "veterans" in the group have found to be most helpful.

Support can add years?

There's even research that shows that support and support groups can help people live longer. According to the Mayo Clinic Health Letter, researchers at Stanford University and the University of California at Berkeley found that breast-cancer patients in professionally led support groups outlived those not in groups by an average of nearly 18 months.

A Yale University study of heart-attack patients found that those with at least two sources of emotional support were twice as likely to survive as those who didn't have such support.

And other studies have found that those in support groups are less reliant on their doctors and tend to comply better with suggested treatments.

FINDING A TN SUPPORT GROUP

New TN groups continue to crop up around the country. As of this writing, there are more than 200 groups and phone contacts in 40 states.

To find out if there's a group or contact person near you, call TNA at 352-376-9955 or write to: Trigeminal Neuralgia Association 925 Northwest 56th Terrace, Suite C Gainesville, FL 32605

Support-group information also is on the TNA web site at www.tna-support.org.

If there are no groups in your area, TNA urges individuals to take the "Jannetta challenge" and start a new one. The TNA office has materials to help new leaders get started.

Some TN groups meet monthly, some meet a few times a year. Some meetings include guest speakers such as neurologists, neurosurgeons, pharmacists, pain-management experts, dentists, oral surgeons, acupuncturists or chiropractors. At other meetings, members talk with one another and discuss questions, new findings and/or how they're coping with TN.

Between meetings, other members are always just a phone call away. A lot of a group's activity occurs by phone, mail or email, group leaders say.

The goal of the groups is for people to help each other. Leaders therefore are careful not to let meetings turn into a "pity party" in which everyone takes turns complaining about how bad the pain hurts. For a group to help, members have to *want* to take control of the situation and learn ways to cope with the pain or to get the problem corrected.

"We've had people come to support groups who sit back and the attitude is, 'OK, save me now. Do something for me,' " says Dr. Laura Hitchcock, executive director of the National Chronic Pain Outreach Association in Bethesda, Md., in *"The Prevention Pain-Relief System"* book. "Those people will never get any help from support groups because they want someone else to take care of them."

Groups also may not be terribly helpful for very shy people or for those who are easily upset by others' woes. But for the majority of people, support groups are an important source of strength and hope.

"Although support groups are not substitutes for appropriate medical or psychological care," says the Chronic Pain Letter, a New York-based publication for chronic pain sufferers, "by pooling medical information and coping strategies, group members report that they derive significant benefits.

"So important are support groups for those with chronic pain that pain-management programs routinely graduate patients into such groups as insurance that they will hold on to their gains. Increasingly, physicians and other professionals who treat or counsel people in pain are instrumental in getting their patients to join or start a group."

As a result, the number of support and self-help groups has ballooned in recent years. As of 1986, the American Self-Help Group Clearinghouse had 332 associations in its roster. By 2003, it had more than 1,100 – and counting.

Dr. John C. Norcross, a professor of psychology at the University of Scranton, says research indicates that at least 18 percent of Americans will visit at least one support group in their lifetime. The main reason: they want to connect with others who are going through the same problems.

Irene Wood, a TN support-group leader in Australia, once asked her members what they thought after attending their first meeting.

She got such answers as, "I was relieved to know that I was not the only sufferer," "It was a great comfort to me and made me feel that I am not a freak with a strange pain," and "I realized I needed to be part of the group on a long-term basis for my own good but also to be able to help others, if possible."

Dr. Norcross cites three large, federally funded studies that have shown that support-group meetings are as effective or nearly as effective in treating substance abusers as professional counseling.

These and other studies also have shown that people who go to medical self-help groups tend to feel better, comply more with treatments, improve in health, and their families tend to be more involved and more knowledgeable about their condition.

"There's nothing like people taking an active role in their care," says Dr. Hickman, the San Diego psychologist. "I think that's the most important thing for all of us."

Support group by Internet

One other current phenomenon that Dr. Norcross points out – there's been a sharp increase in people using the Internet for health information. He says about 80 percent of people with access to the Internet already have used it to look up health information.

Not only are people reading about their health conditions online, some are taking part in chat rooms, mailing lists and online forums. These are essentially functioning as "virtual" support groups.

One of the oldest and most developed of these is the TN-L Internet Support Group, a patient-based email list that links TN and related face-pain patients from around the world with one another 24 hours a day.

Members can opt either to get emails directly from other members or go to a password-protected web address and read past messages.

This free online service was started by a group of patients in 1992 and is hosted by the University of Arkansas with Polly Potter and Jet Duddridge as moderators.

TN-L says it picks up where "medical science leaves off – the human side... Here you can speak with people who understand what you are feeling. Our doctors may provide us with medical treatment possibilities and pain medications. They may understand us from a neurobiological point of view. They cannot feel what we feel. They cannot know what we know about this rare disorder."

What TN-L offers is a "deep understanding from fellow sufferers... the ones who understand why we might find ourselves screaming in the darkest moments... the ones who have been there and are there, too. Here we can find feedback to our most serious questions that the doctors cannot answer."

• To join the TN-L list, send an email message to listserv@listserv.uark.edu with the following in the body of the text: sub TN-L *Your Name*. (For example, Jane Doe would type: sub TN-L Jane Doe. The "sub" is short for "subscribe.") You'll then receive an email from TN-L that details how to join.
• The Facial Neuralgia Resources web site also has details and direct links to TN-L at http://facial-neuralgia.org/support/tnl_info.html.

Facial Neuralgia Resources itself is a goldmine of patient contact. Its home page at http://facial-neuralgia.org has both "Guest Book" and "Personal Stories" sections that offer hundreds of personal stories, comments and questions from neuralgians around the world. If you'd like to share your story with others, there's also a "Share Your Story" section that lets you do that – either anonymously or with your first name and email address listed so others can contact or respond to you.

The site also has links to TNA and other support resources, links to drug-company patient-assistance sites and a wide array of information on TN, atypical TN, atypical facial pain and anesthesia dolorosa.

• Massachusetts General Hospital is another resource that offers web forums on all sorts of neurological disorders, including TN and related face pains. Rather than using direct, person-to-person emails, this free site allows members to post messages for all to view. Then others who read the message can post responses.

This service is at Massachusetts General's BrainTalk Communities pages at http://neuro-mancer.mgh.harvard.edu/cgi-bin/Ultimate.cgi. Once there, click the "specific neurological conditions M-Z" button and navigate to the trigeminal neuralgia pages.

Massachusetts General also has another "Trigeminal Neuralgia Chatroom" site where people can message back and forth immediately. The down side here is that other people have to be logged in at the same time you are. The address for this site is: http://neuro-mancer.mgh.harvard.edu/echat42/Trigeminal_Neuralgia.

• If you want to talk with British neuralgians about their experiences, the United Kingdom Trigeminal Neuralgia Association has both a live chat room and a forum where past messages are listed, topic by topic. You can also send emailed questions to British TN experts through an "email support" button. The address for this web site is: www.tna.org.uk.

• The Trigeminal Neuralgia Association of Canada and the Trigeminal Neuralgia Association of Australia also have web sites where you can read past newsletters. Neither has chat rooms or forums as of this writing.

TNA Canada is at www.tnac.org and TNA Australia is at http://tnasydney.freeservers.com.

18 WAYS TO HELP A NEURALGIAN IN THE FAMILY

1.) Be patient. At times he or she might not want to talk about the pain. It's healthy anyway to talk about other things.

2.) Be informed. Learn about TN and the various treatments so you're ready to help with a new option if the current treatment isn't working. Also be familiar with your relative's particular case – his or her painful areas, how long he or she has had the pain, what treatments have been tried, what makes the pain better or worse, etc.

3.) Know how your relative is doing lately. You may need to communicate that information to doctors if your relative is having trouble talking. Examples: What's the frequency of pain attacks? Is the severity increasing? Any side effects from medicines? Where are the trigger points?

4.) Accompany your relative to the doctor. People in pain and on sedating medication may not always be able to comprehend everything the doctor says. Besides, you may be able to give the doctor important observations you've noticed.

5.) Help your relative contact others with TN. Not only might these people be able to offer valuable information, just knowing you're not alone is a help to most.

6.) Encourage your relative to go to TN support group meetings and accompany him or her.

7.) Encourage your relative to stay busy. Idle minds tend to focus on pain more than busy minds.

8.) Be positive. Remind your relative that almost all neuralgians eventually get rid of their pain from one method or another. Don't let him or her lose hope.

9.) Watch for signs of depression. It's common with people in chronic pain, and it's highly treatable – if it's recognized. Chapter 20 lists signs. Depression is a separate condition that needs treatment in a separate way, usually a combination of counseling and antidepressant medication.

10.) Discuss a game plan, preferably when your relative isn't having a pain blowout. That way you'll both be on the same wavelength on what treatments your relative favors and which one he or she doesn't prefer.

11.) Have an emergency plan. If the pain suddenly flares, will you be able to reach your relative's doctor quickly? If that doctor isn't available, who else would be available to help? Do you know where the nearest emergency room is and what, if any, insurance restrictions are involved in ER care in case no other doctor is available?

12.) Be helpful but not over-protective. Getting cold packs or liquefying a meal is one thing. "Babying" your relative to the point where you won't let him or her do anything is another.

13.) Become familiar with your relative's insurance plan. It's best to know what's covered and what's not before you get one of those surprise bills. Also find out if pre-authorization is needed for any treatments being considered in case the pain worsens. If coverage is being denied, you may be able to help gather information, get opinions from doctors and file appeals to have legitimate treatments covered if they're needed.

Continued on next page ...

... Continued from previous page

14.) Be careful about touching your relative. Remember that a simple kiss or a light brush against the face can set off excruciating pain. Know those trigger points. And ask before touching. Prevent others from touching without asking, too.

15.) Help your relative keep track of medication. Make sure he or she doesn't run out of pills. Also make sure he or she is taking the right amounts at the right times. People in pain and on sedating medication may not be thinking clearly.

16.) Keep a list of names and phone numbers of people you may need. This could include doctors, friends, others with TN, insurance contacts and the person at your relative's work who you might need to call if your relative can't make it in.

17.) Understand that sometimes the pain is going to interfere with plans. Be flexible and understanding. Don't get angry and blaming.

18.) Realize that pain and energy levels can change day by day. Just because your relative was able to do something last week doesn't mean he or she will be up to it today.

— *Sources: Trigeminal Neuralgia Association, Audrey Dryden-Parker*

CHAPTER 22

POSSIBILITIES

*"We're seeing a lot of advances in medicine, and I think TN
is going to become one of the gravestones along the way.
This is a problem we're going to lick."*
—Dr. Albert L. Rhoton Jr., Gainesville, Fla., neurosurgeon

Researchers are getting closer than ever to unlocking the intricate mysteries of pain and how it works. The better we can understand the various body chemicals, nerve receptors and brain reactions that go into the many types of pains, the better we'll be able to tailor ways to solve the problem.

Some believe we're on the verge of some major breakthroughs.

"I think we have an opportunity for achievement in the next 10 years that will make achievements of the last 30 years look small," says Dr. David Sirois, chairman of the Department of Oral Medicine at New York University's College of Dentistry.

Much work is going on in pain research around the world, and a lot more is on the drawing board.

Molecular biologists are getting closer and closer to fully understanding how nerve cells work and what's taking place or going wrong when chronic pain results. Several types of cells and hormones already have been isolated as key players.

Pharmaceutical researchers are exploring and trialing new medications that take entirely different approaches to pain control, including ones that stimulate the body's own natural pain-killing chemicals and others that might work as effectively as morphine but without the unwanted sedating and addictive effects.

Surgeons continue to refine current procedures and are looking at new ways to "stimulate" the pain away electrically instead of damaging the nerves.

TN research in particular got a boost in late 2003 when the National Institute of Neurological Disorders and Stroke (NINDS) announced it was committing nearly $4 million in grants for TN research between 2004 and 2006.

The National Institute of Dental and Craniofacial Research also committed another $1.2 million over two years for research in face pain, including TN, migraines, temporomandibular joint disorders and other chronic face pains.

Both fundings were an outgrowth of a 2000 National Institutes of Health scientific meeting on TN – the first time the U.S. government devoted specific attention to TN and its variations.

In one study already in the works, NINDS is seeking a multi-discipline study that will:

• Look into the role the immune system and inflammation plays in face pain.
• Examine the changes that occur in specific genes and proteins during chronic pain.
• Determine the gender, age, ethnic and other demographic factors that might affect face pain.
• And develop techniques to mimic TN and related face pains in animals so future therapies can be tested.

A second study planned for 2005 would seek to identify molecules that might have a specific effect on face pain. The aim is to use these molecules to develop better and more targeted face-pain medications.

Roger Levy, chairman of the Trigeminal Neuralgia Association's board of directors, says the research funding "promises much for tomorrow's patients... Over time, what we hope for is a better understanding of the pain mechanisms that cause face pain, the demographics of those affected, and the means by which pain can be more safely and effectively treated."

A new view of pain

At a more basic level, Western medicine is re-evaluating the whole way it views pain. For a long time, patient studies have found that pain has gone under-treated even though we already have more ways to deal with it than ever before.

As recently as 2004, a survey of U.S. hospital patients found more than 50 percent of patients saying that their pain was not addressed – either in terms of discussion about it or treatment for it.

The nation's new so-called "Pain Care Bill of Rights" hopes to change that, at least in hospital and nursing-home settings. It requires health-care practitioners to regularly ask about and address pain issues, making it as routine of a patient concern as checking blood pressures and temperatures.

Medicine also is beginning to look at chronic pains such as TN in a new light.

"People have thought of pain too much as a symptom," University of Baltimore pain researcher Dr. Ronald Dubner said in interview on NIDCR's web site. "What we're learning now is that pain, in fact, is a disease. This has been suggested for several years, and I think the evidence is quite strong today... Many scientists have assumed that if they identify the root causes of various diseases and cure them, there won't be any more pain. But what I'm saying is pain in itself can be the disease."

Dr. Dubner says that by changing this thinking, researchers can refocus attention on the mechanisms at work in chronic pain and find medications or techniques to interrupt them rather than focusing solely on what might be causing the pain.

What we're learning about pain

"The pain world has come light years in the past 10 years in terms of our understanding," says Dr. Kim Burchiel, a neurosurgeon at Oregon Health Sciences University in Portland and a leading TN researcher.

He says we're now on the brink of turning these new understandings into new treatments for TN and related face pains.

"We're on the forefront of some exciting breakthroughs in the laboratory," Dr. Burchiel says.

PAIN CARE BILL OF RIGHTS

Most hospitals, nursing homes and other health-care facilities are required to assess and treat pain under new U.S. pain-management standards set by the Joint Commission on Accreditation of Healthcare Organizations. The standards went into effect Jan. 1, 2001.

While the law does not require all of the following, the Baltimore-based American Pain Foundation says these are the rights you should expect, and if necessary, demand for your pain care:

• The right to have your report of pain taken seriously and to be treated with dignity and respect by doctors, nurses, pharmacists and other health-care professionals.

• The right to have your pain thoroughly assessed and promptly treated.

• The right to be informed by your doctor about what may be causing your pain, possible treatments and the benefits, risks and costs of each.

• The right to participate actively in decisions about how to manage your pain.

• The right to have your pain reassessed regularly and your treatment adjusted if your pain has not been eased.

• The right to be referred to a pain specialist if your pain persists.

• The right to get clear and prompt answers to your questions, to take time to make decisions and to refuse a particular type of treatment if you choose.

— Source: American Pain Foundation's "Pain Action Guide"

"Things are happening. But basic research takes time and happens in tiny steps."

Let's take a look at some of these "tiny steps" that pain researchers have been taking and how they might translate into future help:

• **Closing pain's gates.** If researchers can identify the exact chemicals and actions that take place when a chronic pain occurs, it stands to reason that medications could be developed to deactivate pain signals or block the chemicals responsible for firing off a pain signal in the first place.

"There are a number of studies looking at how this activity can be cut short to stop pain," says Dr. Parker E. Mahon, professor emeritus at the University of Florida Pain Center. "It's amazing how much research is being done, and one of these days we're going to have an answer."

Much of this work is centering on nerve "receptors" and the "neuro-transmitters" attached to them. Receptors function like little gates along the course of a nerve, opening to let signals through and closing to block them. Each is locked or unlocked by specific body chemicals. Neurotransmitters are the body chemicals that carry nerve impulses from one nerve cell to the next.

One brain chemical called *"glutamate"* has been the focus of a variety of pain studies. Experiments in mice have found that when receptors that respond to glutamate are blocked, pain decreases. The challenge is to determine if that's also the case in humans and whether drugs can be developed to block glutamate receptors.

Other researchers have been trying to isolate chemicals that make another type of receptor that's super-sensitive to pain. Receptors called *"nociceptors"* usually only activate when there's a painful stimulus, such as a pinch or pinprick. But when tissues are injured, body chemicals are released that make nociceptors send off pain signals even in response to gentle stimuli. If these chemicals can be isolated and blocked, that could be a new approach to stopping lightly triggered pains such as TN.

A third receptor being investigated involves the chemical *"acetylcholine."* Researchers have found that a chemical in the skin of an Ecuadorian frog has a marked pain-stopping effect on this receptor. Although that chemical is also highly toxic, researchers are looking into similar compounds that should have a similar effect on the acetylcholine receptors.

• **Disabling pain-related cells.** Another idea is the possibility of disabling nerve cells that transmit unwanted chronic pain signals without undoing the body's ability to perceive acute pain signals (such as the helpful signal that your hand is on a hot stove, for instance).

This might be possible based on the findings in a mice study that used nerve-cell-killing chemicals and Substance P, a neurotransmitter involved in pain. When researchers injected a blend of these agents into mice, the Substance P carried the nerve-toxic chemicals directly to the receptors that communicate pain. Within days, these nerve cells died. As a result, the mice no longer exhibited signs of pain following injury.

The promising part is that the mice otherwise behaved normally and still responded to acute (or "normal") pain. It's unknown if this exact approach will work in treating chronic human pain, but at least it demonstrates that it may be possible to disable unwanted pain without affecting necessary pain.

Researchers at London's Centre for Neuroscience Research also have found a protein that appears to ratchet down the intensity level of neuropathic pain. By injecting this protein into rats with sciatic nerve injuries, researchers found they could desensitize the firing of pain nerve fibers and reduce the rats' pain.

• **Recruiting the body's own painkillers.** One of the most promising areas is in enhancing the production of *"endorphins,"* a type of protein that the body itself produces to reduce pain. Researchers discovered these naturally produced painkillers decades ago while studying how morphine works. (Endorphin means "morphine within.")

Endorphins are released whenever the body is injured. They circulate in the cerebrospinal fluid in the brain and spinal cord and have the ability to quell the firing of the nerve fibers that deliver pain signals to the brain.

By following where the endorphins go, it's been possible to accurately map the exact areas of the brain where pain of various sorts is perceived and what pathways the pain signals followed to get there.

That information has been helpful in several ways:

- It helps locate nerve pathways where pain signals could best be blocked, such as by electrical-stimulation devices.
- It gives clues to which kinds of medications might be most likely to stop a given pain.
- And it identifies the exact area of the brain where surgeons might be able to block the perception of pain, either by disabling targeted brain cells or by interfering with pain signals through the use of surgically implanted electrodes that the patient can activate as needed.

The real hope is that researchers some day will be able to harness endorphins (or something similar) and administer them to people in chronic pain.

According to NINDS, clinical studies have found that chronic-pain patients often have naturally low levels of endorphins in their cerebrospinal fluid.

Whipping up a batch of usable endorphins so far has proved to be more difficult than hoped. Some endorphins break down very quickly after they're released into new cells. Longer-lasting types have been hard to manufacture in enough quantity, and getting them to go to the right place in the brain or spinal cord has been another challenge.

Also a question: What possible unwanted effects might these introduced endorphins cause even if all of the other issues are solved? Besides affecting pain, endorphins help control blood flow. Like narcotic pain-relievers, they also may be addicting.

Besides endorphins, researchers are looking at other body chemicals involved in shutting off the pain switches, including enkephalins, serotonin, norepinephrine and opioid-like chemicals. Drugmakers are looking at all of these as possible agents in future medications.

• **Discouraging the pain-makers.** The opposite of endorphins and the like are body chemicals that kick into action when pain occurs.

Probably the best known are hormones called *"prostaglandins,"* which stimulate nerves at injury sites and cause inflammation, pain and even fever. Some of our most common pain-relievers, including aspirin and ibuprofen, work by blocking the enzyme that's needed to produce prostaglandins.

New research is looking at a similar scenario that may help those with non-classic TN, especially pains that might be related to nerve inflammation or infection. This research focuses on *"proinflammatory cytokines,"* which are immune-system proteins that fight bacterial and viral infections.

The role of cytokines is to cause fever, malaise, pain, fatigue and an increase in white blood cells. That's a good thing in infection-fighting because the increase in body temperature kills germs, and the pain and malaise makes us rest so more energy can be focused on fighting the infection.

But even in chronic, low-grade, non-life-threatening infections, the same cytokines are activated, resulting in varying levels of the same symptoms. Elevated cytokine levels also have been found in the brain and spinal cord following injuries, suggesting that this protein also may play a role in neuropathic and deafferentation pains.

By blocking the release of these cytokines, it's been found that inflammation-related pains can be stopped.

Researchers already have found two agents – thalidomide and interleukin-10 – that seem to block the effects of proinflammatory cytokines. This approach "is ultimately the perfect solution if we learn to harness and utilize it for some of these unusual pains," says Dr. Steven Graff-Radford, a face-pain specialist at Cedars-Sinai Medical Center in Los Angeles.

• **Gene research.** Numerous scientists are at work trying to isolate the exact genes that might be involved in particular nervous-system disorders.

In 1993, scientists isolated the first gene involved in a degenerative neurological disease – Huntingdon's disease. Soon after came the discovery of five genes implicated in Alzheimer's disease, including one that's a predictor of who might be more prone to develop Alzheimer's later in life. A gene also has been identified in spinocerebellar ataxia, a nerve-related movement disorder, and in 2003 scientists were able to reverse Sjogren's disease in mice (a disorder of moisture-producing glands) by attaching the gene for interleukin-10 to a virus and injecting it.

Identifying these genes is important because a cure may hinge on modifying defective genes or introducing new cells that have been genetically altered.

The question is how many disorders involve "bad genes?" Might TN or a related face pain be one of them? If so, which gene or genes? And will it be possible to "reprogram" or treat those genes to stop these pains?

Other researchers are looking at genes' role in producing the body chemicals involved in pain.

One study bred mice that lacked a gene that guides production of a pair of chemicals called "peptides," which are building blocks for proteins. Mice without this gene had a reduced response to severe pain but normal reactions to mild pain. Researchers believe this helped isolate specific chemicals involved in severe pain, which might pave the way for drugs tailored specifically to these kinds of pains.

And another study found that some people lack a gene that makes an enzyme used to break down codeine into morphine. That not only might explain why codeine isn't a very effective pain-reliever for some people but also opens the door to other studies linking genetic defects with the effectiveness of medicines.

Many hurdles remain, not the least of which is getting the genes to go to the right place without causing any unwanted or unexpected other effects. But it's a broad new frontier that could give answers to all sorts of disease, including face pain.

• Recording nerve and brain activity

Dr. Burchiel and Dr. Thomas K. Baumann, a colleague at Oregon Health and Sciences University, recently broke new ground by recording the activity of TN patients' trigeminal nerves while they were undergoing radiofrequency lesioning surgery.

Drs. Burchiel and Baumann made microelectrode recordings of the trigeminal ganglion while the unconscious patients' faces were stroked with a gloved hand and lightly poked with a Q-Tip.

They concluded that not only is it possible to make high-quality recordings of trigeminal nerve activity, but there appears to be abnormal patterns of firing in neuralgians' nerves.

Working with Dr. Priya Chaudhary, Dr. Baumann recently completed another study in rats that may have isolated two of the peptides that are involved in TN when nerve signals "jump tracks" in the trigeminal ganglion and turn a light touch into a stabbing pain.

Other researchers have been focusing more on measuring and deciphering what's going on in the brain when the pain signals are actually delivered.

A functional magnetic resonance imaging (MRI) scan is a fairly new research tool that allows scientists to see what chemical changes are taking place in the brain in response to changes in or around a person.

One researcher used this test to verify that mental and emotional actions have a direct, physical impact on pain. This study specifically looked at changes in an area of the brain called the *"periaqueductal gray,"* which when stimulated causes pain to diminish.

When test subjects had a finger poked with sharp object, this part of the brain lit up under the functional MRI. When another finger was given a mild buzzing stimulus, nothing happened.

When both stimuli were given at the same time, the results varied depending on whether the test subject was focusing on the painful finger or the buzzing one. The more the subjects paid attention to the pain, the more the periaqueductal gray lit up.

Regenerating myelin

Another area of research is figuring out ways to get myelin – the fatty substance that insulates nerves – to regrow. Myelin is at the heart of TN because it's believed that pulsation from compressing blood vessels wears down this protective coating and causes nerve fibers to malfunction, much like an electrical wire short-circuiting after its insulation has been stripped away.

The thinking is that if myelin can be stimulated to grow, the vessel-injured fibers will heal and the pain will stop – perhaps even if vessels continue to beat on them.

Most of the work here is being done in multiple sclerosis, a disorder that results when the body attacks and destroys its own myelin.

Scientists so far have isolated the exact types of cells the body uses to build myelin and are now looking at ways to encourage their growth. Investigators at Cornell University Medical College already have been able to remove myelin-making cells from human brains and transform them in laboratory cultures into mature cells capable of making new myelin.

The next frontier is translating that and similar approaches into ways that stimulate the body to build more myelin (a process called *"remyelination"*). One idea is injecting myelin-making cells into people with myelin-related disorders. Another is searching for drugs that encourage production of these cells.

A type of glial cell called an *"oligodendrocyte"* has been found to be the key player in building myelin in the central nervous system. A second type of glial cell called a *"Schwann cell"* is used to make myelin around all other nerves.

Scientists believe it may be possible to attach myelin-making genes to stem cells and inject these into people with MS, spinal cord injuries and other disorders where myelin has been damaged. Stem cells are found in embryos and are the basic cells from which all other cells develop. Given that basic building block and the right genetic instructions, scientists hope they can cause these injected stem cells to grow into myelin-producing oligodendrocytes.

It may be years until it's determined if that can be done safely and effectively, but preliminary work is under way.

Further along is work that uses a type of antibody to stimulate myelin growth. Dr. Moses Rodriguez, director of the Mayo Clinic's Demyelinating Laboratory in Minnesota, and eight colleagues already have had success with that in mice.

Dr. Rodriguez and his team injected human monoclonal antibodies into mice that had been induced into having symptoms similar to MS. After five weeks of injections, new myelin had repaired about 25 percent of the damaged areas.

"We have secured patents and worked with industry to purify the antibodies and produce them in high concentration," Dr. Rodriguez says. Toxicity studies are under way, and if those check out, clinical testing on humans could be done.

Other researchers are studying the possibility that two immunosuppressant drugs – cyclophosphamide and azathioprine – may stimulate myelin growth. Another study plans to investigate the use of a derivative of progesterone, the female hormone that's produced in the ovaries.

It's still uncertain if any of these will pan out, but Dr. Rodriguez says he's optimistic that one day medicine will be able to offer non-invasive treatments that promote nerve repair.

Medications just for TN

Much of this research lays the groundwork for pharmaceutical scientists to target very specific drugs to very specific problems. After all, pain can originate from muscle, bones, teeth, skin or the nerve itself, so it makes sense that different agents might be needed to address the different pains.

At present, many of our drugs take broad approaches, and the exact way they work is poorly understood. The down side is that while these drugs may help certain disorders, their system-wide approach often brings unwanted side effects. The new approach of using more targeted mechanisms not only holds the promise of giving better results but of cutting down on side effects.

In the case of TN, there's never been a medication that has been developed specifically to target TN pain. Almost all of the medications used today were developed to treat epilepsy. They were then found to work for TN, too, because they simply slowed down the whole central nervous system.

While that might quell TN pain, it also affects other systems and results in unwanted sleepiness, slowed thinking and general lethargy.

Research now is looking not only at more refined anticonvulsants but also at entirely new types of agents that would have a more focused effect on TN and other nerve pains.

"I speculate that within 10 years we won't even be using anticonvulsants (for TN)," says Dr. J. Keith Campbell, emeritus professor of neurology at the Mayo Medical School in Minnesota. "We'll be into other things."

These could include drugs that block certain types of pain-signal channels, drugs that disable particular types of receptors and/or drugs that affect pain-sensing parts of the brain.

Up to now, TN hasn't attracted a lot of pharmaceutical research because it's such an uncommon disorder. After all, it doesn't make sense – if you're a drug company – to sink tons of money into research that would yield a drug that only a relative few people will use.

That's beginning to change. Thanks in large part to NIH's funding, more attention is being given to face-pain drug research.

The National Institute of Dental Research, one of NIH's 23 arms, itself conducted two recent clinical trials to see how effective two existing drugs might be in treating TN and related face pains.

One study involved dextromethorphan, a common, over-the-counter cough-suppressant that some researchers thought might help nerve pain at higher doses. It was implicated because of its apparent ability to block glutamate (a brain chemical involved in pain sensation) and earlier was shown to reduce pain in patients with diabetic neuropathy.

NIDR researchers used doses six to seven times as high as the dose in cough medicine but found it had little effect on face pain.

The other drug being studied is topiramate (Topamax), the anticonvulsant that's already on the market for use in epilepsy. Although doctors may prescribe it for TN, NIDR researchers are optimistic that a controlled trial will prove it's useful in treating TN as well as epilepsy. The study is still in progress as of this writing.

University of Pittsburgh researchers also recently attempted to study a different version of the muscle relaxant baclofen that was thought to be more effective against TN pain and with fewer side effects. However, that study was never completed, partly because the original researcher died and partly because of a difficulty in recruiting patients.

Better delivery of the medicine

Researchers not only are looking for new and better medications, they're exploring more effective ways to put the medicine to use.

In almost all cases, TN patients now take their medications by pill, capsule or liquid – in other words, ingesting it. The medicine then must be digested and absorbed by the digestive system before the active ingredients can go to work.

That not only takes time, but depending on how efficiently your digestive system works, you may not be making optimum use out of the pills. Whatever else happens to be in your stomach – such as milk or antacids – also may affect how much of the medicine you actually are using.

One other way to get medicine to the trigeminal nerve is through *"transconjunctival therapy"* – which is medicalese for using eye drops.

Because the trigeminal nerve supplies the tiny nerve branches that give feeling to the eye, it's possible to transport medicine to the nerve by placing drops in the eye. The conjunctiva in the eye adsorb the medicine and pass it along for the nerve fibers to absorb and use.

The result is medication that goes almost immediately, precisely and directly to where it's needed.

The challenge is to develop forms of medication that are effective for TN pain without irritating or otherwise damaging the eyes.

Neuraxial drug infusion is another approach that is being tried occasionally for severe, chronic cases that haven't responded well to the more common approaches.

This is somewhat akin to an implanted IV drug-infusion line. The device is placed in the sac around the spinal cord, and a battery-operated pump is placed under the skin of the abdomen. The unit then automatically delivers narcotics or other pain-relieving medicine directly to the spinal cord.

It's still an experimental procedure but one that may offer an answer for those with intractable pain. Also on the horizon is infusing the medications directly into selected parts of the brain.

New and improved surgery

Surgeons are always looking for ways to improve results while cutting complication rates.

In the balloon-compression procedure, for example, surgeons have whittled down the chances of dense numbness by settling on 1-minute compression times. In earlier years, some surgeons kept the balloon inflated for as long as 7 minutes before most concluded that 1 minute is just as effective at pain relief with far fewer problems.

Work is now being done on focusing on the exact area of pain by changing the angle of how the compression is done.

Some surgeons also have begun using two through-the-cheek procedures at the same time, such as radiofrequency lesioning and glycerol together in a single surgery. TNA board member Everard Pinneo, who's had this combination done successfully, says his Johns Hopkins surgeon refers to it as a "double whammy."

The theory behind it is that if you "go light" on two procedures, you may end up with better results and longer-lasting pain relief but with less numbness.

New to radiosurgery is a second-generation Gamma Knife called the "Rotating Gamma System." Approved by the U.S. Food and Drug Administration in 1997, this device works in principle much like the original Gamma Knife. The difference is that this unit has 30 rotating cobalt sources instead of one stationary source that's aimed through a helmet with 201 holes.

The goal of the Rotating Gamma System is to better aim and tailor the radiation to the target with even less radiation exposure to the surrounding healthy untargeted tissue.

New types of linac radiosurgery devices also have been introduced that allow radiation to be targeted to the brain with nearly the same accuracy as the Gamma Knife.

MVD advances

Improvements are still being made to the microvascular decompression surgery as well.

Not only are many more neurosurgeons trained in the procedure these days, but their growing experience has led to improved techniques, fewer serious complications, less time to complete the surgery and faster recoveries for patients. All of that is being done with smaller skull openings.

One new tool being used for MVDs at a few centers is the endoscope, a device that employs a fiberoptic tube that's inserted into the skull opening to give a magnified look at the nerves and blood vessels inside. Some are using it instead of the operating microscope, which also lights and magnifies the nerves and vessels but from outside the opening. Others are using it in addition to the conventional microscope.

Backers say the endoscope allows the MVD to be done with a smaller opening, and it doesn't require the cerebellum to be moved.

Dr. Charles Teo, an Australian neurosurgeon who does endoscopic MVDs, says this instrument often gives a better view of the trigeminal nerve because of better lighting, better magnification and the endoscope's ability to rotate and "look around corners."

Dr. Teo says that based on 77 patients he's operated on with an endoscope, he found compressing blood vessels 12 percent of the time that he wouldn't have seen with the standard microscope.

The majority of neurosurgeons aren't yet sold on the tool, though. Some say it gives only an occasional and marginal improvement in view, and it may be slightly more likely to lead to hearing problems. With the smaller opening, there's also less room to work, which could be detrimental in case of a complication, others point out.

Dr. Teo says there is a "learning curve" in adapting to the endoscope. "The more you use it, the more comfortable you become with it."

For now, few neurosurgeons are using it. Most of those who are having good success with the microscope say they are reluctant to start on a new learning curve until they're sure the new technology really will make a significant difference.

Although it's not been used yet in MVDs, an even more advanced computerized operating system is being tried in heart surgery. This system includes the use of robotic arms in addition to endoscopic views.

Through one pencil-sized opening, a camera is inserted into the patient's chest. Through another similar-sized opening, the surgical tools at the end of the robotic arms are inserted. The surgeon sees a high-resolution view inside the chest on a TV monitor that's magnified 12 to 15 times the real size.

Using controls at the computer console, the surgeon guides the robotic arms to make the repairs. The use of robotics greatly improves dexterity and precision because any tremor in the surgeon's hands can be completely filtered out by the computer.

Once it's perfected, it's possible this kind of robotic, endoscopic surgery could be used to move vessels off of trigeminal nerves.

It's also not even that far-fetched anymore to imagine miniature, detached, computer-guided instruments going inside the head to make repairs. After all, NASA scientists have been able to guide robotic equipment millions of miles away on the surface of Mars.

Pittsburgh neurosurgeon Dr. Peter Jannetta says he can envision the day when MVD becomes a "Band-Aid surgery" done with robotic machines so small they can only be seen with the aid of a microscope.

Surgeons also continue to look for better nerve-cushioning materials to use in MVDs and better ways to apply these materials.

Shredded Teflon felt is still most commonly used today, although a few surgeons have been trying other materials, such as Gore-Tex. A few other surgeons use implanted neck muscle, which is soft and natural but has a tendency to break down and be absorbed over time.

Besides inserting these materials between vessels and the nerve, surgeons have tried wrapping the insulating material all the way around the nerve. The idea is to keep vessels from bumping the cushion away and also to protect the nerve at all angles from any vessels that may get near it in the future.

That hasn't proved to be fool-proof either, says Dr. Jannetta. "We've tried that and veins still sneak under there," he says. "Mother Nature is working against us."

Stimulating the pain away?

Surgeons also are looking into new ways of stopping pain without having to damage the trigeminal nerve at all. The main approach is by electrical stimulation of the nerve pathways, a process known as *"neuroaugmentation."*

Rather than burn, radiate, inject or squeeze the trigeminal nerve to stop pain signals from getting through, neuroaugmentation involves overriding these signals with a second, competing signal generated by an implanted or attached electrical stimulation device.

The principle is much like what happens when we rub a body part that hurts. The rubbing sends a different or confusing signal to the brain. The more the pain hurts, the harder we tend to rub.

Surgeons can use this same principle to stimulate the brain with an electrical current. The trigeminal nerve itself can be stimulated (as discussed in the TENS units described in Chapter 15) or the pain-sensing parts of the brain can be stimulated (such as the implanted motor cortex devices described in Chapter 14).

In addition to distracting or confusing the brain, stimulation also seems to release brain chemicals that signal other cells to shut down, which reduces the intensity of signals to the brain.

If the levels and locations of electrical stimulation can be perfected, it's possible that TN surgeries will see a shift from "cutting" to "confusing." Functional MRI tests and positron emission tomography (PET) scans are two newly developed tools that let researchers measure minute chemical changes in the brain that will help perfect stimulation techniques.

Better imaging

Besides the refinements to magnetic resonance imaging (MRI) described in Chapter 8, a new technique called "magnetic resonance tomographic angiography" (MRTA) is showing some of the best pictures yet.

MRTA scans not only show the trigeminal nerve and vessels as small as 1 millimeter, they can even tell the difference between arteries and veins in most cases – especially when gadolinium dye is injected into the patient's bloodstream to enhance the image.

A 1995 British study that compared MRTA scans to actual surgical findings turned out to accurately predict compressing vessels in 50 of 52 cases. While that might not be perfect, it's getting good enough to be a worthwhile tool to help figure out what's going on inside *before* surgery is done.

Obviously, more work needs to be done, but the day may come when we're able to see – affordably – even tiny vessels that could be causing the problem.

More TN education

One of the biggest problems that continues to plague face-pain sufferers is getting an accurate diagnosis in the first place. Although that's been improving, the issue of better, faster diagnoses is high on the Trigeminal Neuralgia Association's list of goals.

"We continue to hear of patients who undergo unnecessary and often harmful procedures before their TN or another related condition is diagnosed," says Roger Levy, chairman of TNA's Board of Directors. "In a recent case, we learned of a child whose health-care costs had amounted to some $500,000 before TN was diagnosed and treated."

TNA's answer: better education of health professionals, especially the "front-line" practitioners such as dentists and family doctors. TNA staff and its Medical Advisory Board already have been getting out the TN message by attending doctor and dentist conventions. Many more are planned.

Neurosurgeon and Medical Advisory Board member Dr. Kenneth Casey has prepared a 90-minute program for professionals on sorting out the various face pains, and dental professor and MAB member Dr. Henry Gremillion is preparing a similar program targeted at dentists. TNA's new Dental Task Force also will focus on ways to incorporate more face-pain instruction at the nation's dental schools.

TNA's biennial national conferences now include teaching sessions for health-care professionals, and additional state and regional sessions are planned.

Also to be targeted for TN educational materials is the growing field of physicians assistants and registered nurse practitioners – professionals who are expected to eventually be responsible for a majority of Americans' primary medical care.

Levy says it's critical that these professionals become familiar with TN and related face pains so patients can get effective treatment much sooner.

TNA also has plans to increase its consumer-awareness programs. In addition to this book, the *TNALERT* newsletter, the biennial conferences and a growing network of local support groups, the Florida-based non-profit is making its www.tna-support.org web site more interactive. This may include setting up forums for patients and doctors to exchange information, adding new links to the latest research, and allowing patients to take part in diagnosis questionnaires and treatment surveys online.

Also on TNA's educational and outreach drawing board:

- Encourage medicine to better classify the various types of face pain and suggest protocols for how to best treat each.
- Discuss drug research with pharmaceutical companies and encourage the industry to develop new and better medicines as well as seek FDA approvals for existing drugs that are now used to treat TN "off-label."
- Produce new patient-education materials and offer regular regional informational meetings.
- Analyze and use information from TNA's "Patient Registry," which is data from the more than 13,000 patient surveys TNA had gathered through 2004. This information not only will be useful in determining which therapies are most effective but also be a potential resource for face-pain researchers.
- Expand the Medical Advisory Board to include representatives of additional pain-management disciplines.
- Encourage additional research grants. TNA was instrumental in seeking the $5.5 million that the National Institutes of Health currently have devoted to TN and face-pain research.
- Coordinate efforts with other organizations that deal with pain conditions, such as the Chronic Pain Association, the Neuropathy Association, the TMJ Association, etc.

Dr. Joanna Zakrzewska, a member of TNA's Medical Advisory Board, says research is sorely needed that gives patients better guidance on which therapies are the best approach at what points.

She says these include: getting a better handle on the expected course of face pains; risk factors involved; the role genetics might play; a better understanding of the causes behind the varying pains; more information *from consumers* on the outcomes of all the therapies, and more clinical trials that look specifically at how well different drugs address TN and related face pains.

"Patient-centered care is what we should be after," Dr. Zakrzewska says.

Lots of hope

If there's one thing on which everyone agrees about TN, it's that medicine today offers more and better treatments than ever before. When one treatment fails, there's always another one to try.

Rarely must surgeons cut the nerve to stop the pain anymore.

With plenty of research still going on, it's likely the TN patient of tomorrow will have even more choices than today. Maybe there even will be a cure.

"There's a lot of hope out there," says TNA founder Claire Patterson. "I never knew anybody was working on this. TN doesn't make head-lines… We may not have major breakthroughs, but every day we can save a patient from suffering needlessly is a victory."

She says the "right" answer may not always be the first thing you try, but "there are options, and you can work with your doctors to find the answer that's right for you. The important thing to keep in mind is that you don't have to learn to live with this pain."

"Doing nothing, being afraid and hoping it'll go away on its own is the worst thing you can do," says Carol James, physician's assistant to Johns Hopkins Hospital neurosurgeon Dr. Benjamin S. Carson Sr. "The best thing you can do is be educated and be informed.

"There's no reason why TN patients should continue in that kind of pain. You have options. You have treatments. Do what's right for you. But do something."

CHAPTER 23

HELPFUL LISTS, QUESTIONNAIRES AND OTHER AIDS

A few other practical bits of information to help you nail down the exact problem and get it treated as quickly and completely as possible:

Questions to diagnose and treat face pain

London face-pain specialist Dr. Joanna Zakrzewska and the American Pain Foundation suggest these 15 questions as clues that doctors can use to help diagnose the different face pains and then decide on a treatment plan that's best tailored to you.

Think about your answers to these before going to your appointment. If your doctor doesn't ask all of the following, it may help to volunteer some of these points that you believe are particularly pertinent.

1.) **Where does it hurt? Does the pain move from one place to another?** Point to exact spots. Show where the pain moves if it travels. Be sure to show all of the places that hurt, not just where it hurts most.
2.) **Do you have more than one spot where it hurts?** If so, point to them. And if the pain is different from one spot to the next, describe the differences. It's possible to have more than one type of disorder at the same time.
3.) **How does the pain behave?** When does it happen? How long does it last? Does it come and go? Or is it constant? When does it begin? When does it end?
4.) **Does the pain keep you from doing all you want to do?** How? What? Describing how pain limits your life will help you and your doctor set treatment goals.
5.) **Does pain interrupt your sleep? Does it change your mood? Affect your appetite?** These are signs the pain is bad enough to affect key parts of your life and threaten your overall health. – physically, mentally, emotionally and/or socially.
6.) **What do you think is causing the pain?** No one knows what it feels like better than you. Your thoughts may help your doctor decide what to look for and where.

7.) **What makes the pain better? What makes it worse?** These clues may help with the diagnosis and assist in developing a treatment plan.

8.) **What have you tried to relieve the pain?** Your doctor may decide to build on things that already have worked and add similar therapies. On the other hand, it'll save time by avoiding types of treatments that already have failed.

9.) **What medicines are you taking for pain right now?** Describe all the medicines you have tried for pain recently. Be prepared to list all other medicines as well, including over-the-counter ones. List the name, amount of medicine, time the medicine was taken, amount of relief, any changes the medicine caused in the pain or its pattern, and any side effects.

10.) **How are you currently taking medications to relieve pain?** Sometimes medications that previously have not worked might be effective if they are taken in a different way or dose. Describe exactly how and when you are taking medicines now.

11.) **Describe how long the medicine takes to work.** How long does pain relief last? Does all of the pain go away after you take the medicine? Does the pain return before the next dose is due? These will help with dosing plans.

12.) **Do you have any side effects from medicines you are taking? Do you have any allergies?** Jot these down. They may provide helpful clues about which exact medications might be the most effective and least troublesome in your particular case.

13.) **Do you have any worries about taking medicines for pain relief?** Many people worry about issues such as addiction and side effects. Your doctor needs to know how you feel about this. Don't hesitate to ask about any concerns you may have.

14.) **How much relief would allow you to get around better? What is your goal for pain relief?** You may be asked to set a goal for pain relief. The goal may be based on a ratings scale or it may focus on activities you would like to carry out. The aim of any treatment plan is to meet the goals you set for pain relief.

15.) Tell the doctor a little about yourself, your work, leisure activities and the people you live with. You don't need to launch into a lengthy history, but a few highlights might help in setting goals, deciding on treatment plans and the like.

SORTING OUT THE EXACT FACE PAIN YOU'VE GOT

Dr. Kim Burchiel, a neurosurgeon at Oregon Health Sciences University, has developed a list of 18 questions to help doctors determine exactly which of the seven proposed new face-pain diagnoses a patient might have.

Those seven diagnoses – TN-1, TN-2, trigeminal neuropathic pain, trigeminal deafferentation pain, post-herpetic neuralgia, symptomatic trigeminal neuralgia and atypical facial pain – are described in detail in Chapter 4.

Following are Dr. Burchiel's diagnostic questions for patients:

- When you have pain, is it predominantly in your face (i.e. forehead, eye, cheek, nose, upper/lower jaw, lips, etc.)?
- Do you have pain just on one side of your face?
- Is your pain either entirely or mostly brief (seconds to minutes) and unpredictable sensations (electrical, shocking, stabbing, shooting)?
- Do you have any constant background facial pain (e.g. aching, burning, throbbing, stinging)?
- Do you have constant background facial pain (aching, burning, throbbing, stinging) for more than half of your waking hours?
- Do you have any constant facial numbness?
- Can your pain start by something touching your face (e.g. by eating, washing your face, shaving, brushing teeth, etc.)?
- Since your pain began, have you ever experienced periods of weeks, months or years when you were pain-free? (This does not include periods after any pain-relieving surgery or while you were on medications for your pain.)
- Have you ever taken Tegretol, Neurontin, baclofen or Trileptal for your pain?

- Did you ever experience any major reduction in facial pain (partial or complete) from taking Tegretol, Neurontin, baclofen or Trileptal?

- Have you ever had trigeminal nerve surgery for your pain? (e.g. neurectomy, radiofrequency lesioning, glycerol injection, balloon compression, rhizotomy, microvascular decompression or radiosurgery)

- Have you ever experienced any major reduction in facial pain (partial or complete) from trigeminal nerve surgery for your pain? (e.g. neurectomy, radiofrequency lesioning, glycerol injection, balloon compression, rhizotomy, microvascular decompression or radiosurgery)

- Did your current pain start only after trigeminal nerve surgery? (e.g. neurectomy, radiofrequency lesioning, glycerol injection, balloon compression, rhizotomy, microvascular decompression or radiosurgery) (If this is a recurrence of your original pain after a successful trigeminal nerve surgery, answer "no.")

- Did your pain start after a facial herpes zoster or "shingles" rash (not merely "fever blisters" around the mouth)?

- Do you have multiple sclerosis?

- Did your pain start after a facial injury?

- Did your pain start only after facial surgery (i.e. oral surgery, ear/nose/throat surgery or plastic surgery)?

- When you place your index finger right in front of your ears on both sides at once and feel your jaw open and close, does the area under your fingers on either side hurt?

THE MCGILL PAIN QUESTIONNAIRE

One of the most respected patient tests to determine the exact nature, location and severity of a person's pain is the McGill Pain Questionnaire.

Written by Dr. Ronald Melzack of Montreal's McGill University in the 1970s, it's widely used by hospitals and health-care professionals all over the world.

The questionnaire has patients mark where their pain is located on figures of different parts of the body. Patients also rate their current pain on a five-level scale ranging from "nil" to "most severe," and in ensuing visits, rate how the frequency and severity of their pain has changed.

To determine the exact nature of a person's pain, the questionnaire includes 20 different groups of pain descriptions, each including anywhere from two to six words that describe how the pain feels. The groups and their descriptors are:

- Group 1: Flickering, quivering, pulsing, throbbing, beating, pounding.
- Group 2: Jumping, flashing, shooting.
- Group 3: Pricking, boring, drilling, stabbing, lancinating.
- Group 4: Sharp, cutting, lacerating.
- Group 5: Pinching, pressing, gnawing, cramping, crushing.
- Group 6: Tugging, pulling, wrenching.
- Group 7: Hot, burning, scalding, searing.
- Group 8: Tingling, itchy, smarting, stinging.
- Group 9: Dull, sore, hurting, aching, heavy.
- Group 10: Tender, taut, rasping, splitting.
- Group 11: Tiring, exhausting.
- Group 12: Sickening, suffocating.
- Group 13: Fearful, frightful, terrifying.
- Group 14: Punishing, grueling, cruel, vicious, killing.
- Group 15: Wretched, blinding.
- Group 16: Annoying, troublesome, miserable, intense, unbearable.
- Group 17: Spreading, radiating, penetrating, piercing.
- Group 18: Tight, numb, drawing, squeezing, tearing.
- Group 19: Cool, cold, freezing.
- Group 20: Nagging, nauseating, agonizing, dreadful, torturing.

Patients can circle the best single descriptor in each group but are instructed to leave out any groups that don't apply.

The "MPQ," as it's often called, not only is helpful in diagnosing disorders, it can be repeated to determine if a particular therapy is helping decrease pain levels.

How is pain affecting your life?

The Pain Research Group at the University of Wisconsin-Madison's Department of Neurology developed a "Brief Pain Inventory" to help determine not only the severity of a person's pain but also how it might be affecting their everyday lives.

This patient survey first asks four questions and has patients answer them by circling numbers on a line that ranges from 0 ("no pain") to 10 ("pain as bad as you can imagine"). These questions are:

1.) Please rate your pain by circling the one number that best describes your pain at its *worst* in the past week.

2.) Please rate your pain by circling the one number that best describes your pain at its *least* in the past week.

3.) Please rate your pain by circling the one number that best describes your pain on the *average.*

4.) Please rate your pain by circling the one number that tells how much pain you have *right now.*

A fifth question is broken down into seven parts dealing with quality-of-life issues. Each of these also is rated on a number line of 0-10 with 0 being "does not interfere" and 10 being "completely interferes."

These seven parts ask patients to tell how much their pain interfered with the following activities in the past week: general activity, mood, walking ability, normal work, relationships with other people, sleep and enjoyment of life.

There's also a follow-up version of the inventory that adds a sixth question asking patients to rate the percentage of relief they've received since treatments were started.

As with the McGill Pain Questionnaire, this Brief Pain Inventory is particularly helpful in gauging a therapy's progress.

Wong-Baker FACES Pain Rating Scale

Dr. Donna Wong, a nurse consultant, and Connie Baker, a child life specialist, were working together in the burn center at Hillcrest Medical Center in Tulsa, Okla., when they developed this test.

What became the Wong-Baker FACES scale began as a way to help child burn victims communicate how bad their pain was. Wong and Baker came up with a simple but effective pain-rating system that uses a series of six faces that range from a smiling "no hurt" face to a deeply frowning face with tears that represents "hurts worst."

Patients select which face best describes the intensity of their pain. Since the test first came out in 1983, it's been used worldwide to gauge all sorts of pain in all age groups, not just children.

Following is what the scale looks like:

WONG-BAKER FACES PAIN RATING SCALE

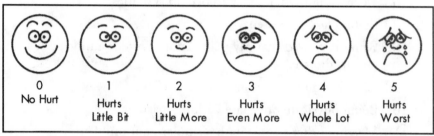

| 0 | 1 | 2 | 3 | 4 | 5 |
| No Hurt | Hurts Little Bit | Hurts Little More | Hurts Even More | Hurts Whole Lot | Hurts Worst |

(From Wong D.L., Hockenberry-Eaton M., Wilson D., Winkelstein M.L., Schwartz P.: *Wong's Essentials of Pediatric Nursing*, ed. 6. St. Louis, 2001, p. 1301. Copyrighted by Mosby Inc. Reprinted by permission.)

ARE YOU AND YOUR DOCTOR ON THE SAME PAGE?

Patients who have chronic pain may not adhere to their doctors' recommendations in as many as 50 percent of the cases, says Dr. Zakrzewska.

That can happen for a variety of reasons: the patient just doesn't agree with the treatment plan; the results aren't as fast or as complete as expected; the patient wants more control over the treatment, and/or the patient had different goals than the doctor.

A lot of this wasted and potentially counter-productive effort could be avoided if doctors and patients talked a bit to make sure they both are shooting for the same treatment goals.

After all, not everyone has the same goals and priorities. Some people want nothing short of complete relief and as soon as possible. Others might be satisfied with enough relief that they can at least carry on their usual activities.

Dr. Zakrzewska has developed a 12-point "Treatment Goals" worksheet that she gives to her face-pain patients. She has patients rate each goal on a four-level scale that includes these ratings: "very important," "moderately important," "slightly important" or "doesn't apply."

Following are the 12 goals:

1.) Returning to work or remaining at work.

2.) Reducing pain medication.

3.) Improving mobility, e.g. walking, sitting, standing.

4.) Feeling less self-conscious in public.

5.) Understanding my pain problem better.

6.) Decreasing my tendency to overdo activities.

7.) Feeling less depressed.

8.) Being reassured that my pain is not a sign of a more serious disease.

9.) Carrying out more household chores.

10.) Being physically intimate with my partner.

11.) Meeting other people with a similar pain problem.

12.) Improving communication with doctors about pain.

At the end of the worksheet, Dr. Zakrzewska asks patients to list the three goals that are most important to them in getting help for their pain. The listings can be from the list or otherwise.

HOW ARE YOU COPING WITH YOUR FACE PAIN?

Dr. Zakrzewska also uses another 12-point questionnaire that helps her assess how patients are coping with their pain.

Besides assessing patients' outlook and progress, this "Coping Strategies Questionnaire" can help determine if counseling or other coping strategies are needed.

The questionnaire asks patients to rate 12 statements on a scale ranging from "never do that" to "sometimes do that" to "always do that." The statements are:

- I tell myself to be brave and carry on despite the pain.

- It is terrible and I feel it is never going to get any better.

- I see it as a challenge and don't let it bother me.

- It is awful and I feel that it overwhelms me.

- I tell myself I can't let the pain stand in the way of what I have to do.

- I feel my life isn't worth living.
- No matter how bad it gets, I know I can handle it.
- I feel like I can't go on.
- I tell myself that I can overcome the pain.
- I feel I can't stand it anymore.
- Although it hurts, I just keep on going.
- I worry all the time about whether it will end.

MEASURES FOR DEPRESSION

TN and related face pains very often go hand-in-hand with depression. When someone begins experiencing symptoms of depression (which can include sleep disruption, loss of appetite, prolonged sadness, loss of interest in usual activities, thoughts of hopelessness or suicide and more), this may signal a need for additional therapies or medicines.

Although any chronic pain can feed depression, these are separate conditions. Most TN medications are not effective for depression.

The most commonly used test to check for depression is the Beck Depression Inventory, a series of questions developed by Dr. Aaron T. Beck at the University of Pennsylvania School of Medicine.

These tests are administered and scored by health-care professionals. Dr. Beck also has developed a battery of other scales that measure anxiety, hopelessness, obsessive-compulsive behavior, suicidal tendencies and more.

Several self-help books also include questionnaires to measure depression along with advice on how to cope with it. One of the best is *"The Feeling Good Handbook"* by Dr. David D. Burns (Plume, 1999), which includes a series of self-administered tests on anxiety and depression.

Depression is usually treated with a combination of antidepressant medications and counseling.

THE ZARIT BURDEN INTERVIEW: HOW ARE OTHERS COPING?

One of the most often used indexes to measure how caregivers are coping with an illness or disability in the family is the Zarit Burden Interview.

This list of 22 questions was developed by Dr. Steven Zarit, head of Penn State University's Department of Human Development and Family Studies.

Caregivers evaluate each question on a five-level scale: 0 for "never," 1 for "rarely," 2 for "sometimes," 3 for "quite frequently," and 4 for "nearly always." The higher the total score, the more stressed and burdened the caregiver is becoming.

Following are the 22 questions, used by permission of Dr. Zarit (copyright 1983 and 1990 by Steven H. Zarit and Judy M. Zarit):

1.) Do you feel that your relative asks for more help than he/she needs?

2.) Do you feel that because of the time you spend with your relative that you don't have enough time for yourself?

3.) Do you feel stressed between caring for your relative and trying to meet other responsibilities for your family or work?

4.) Do you feel embarrassed over your relative's behavior?

5.) Do you feel angry when you are around your relative?

6.) Do you feel that your relative currently affects your relationship with other family members or friends in a negative way?

7.) Are you afraid what the future holds for your relative?

8.) Do you feel your relative is dependent upon you?

9.) Do you feel strained when you are around your relative?

10.) Do you feel your health has suffered because of your involvement with your relative?

11.) Do you feel that you don't have as much privacy as you would like, because of your relative?

12.) Do you feel that your social life has suffered because you are caring for your relative?

13.) Do you feel uncomfortable about having friends over, because of your relative?

14.) Do you feel that your relative seems to expect you to take care of him/her, as if you were the only one he/she could depend on?

15.) Do you feel that you don't have enough money to care for your relative, in addition to the rest of your expenses?

16.) Do you feel that you will be unable to take care of your relative much longer?

17.) Do you feel you have lost control of your life since your relative's illness?

18.) Do you wish you could just leave the care of your relative to someone else?

19.) Do you feel uncertain about what to do about your relative?

20.) Do you feel you should be doing more for your relative?

21.) Do you feel you could do a better job in caring for your relative?

22.) Overall, how burdened do you feel in caring for your relative?

UNDERSTANDING MEDICAL LITERATURE

Not all medical information that you'll come across in libraries, magazines and online is equally reliable. The sources vary widely, and the evidence behind it can range from excellent to non-existent.

Dr. Joanna Zakrzewska and Minnesota neurosurgeon Dr. Stephen Haines, both members of TNA's Medical Advisory Board, offer these tips on researching and evaluating the medical literature.

• **Consider the source.** Be leery of: drug company literature (usually biased in favor of the company's product); free magazines (they are not peer reviewed); testimonials (they are not scientific information), and press releases and reports (these often "jump the gun" and are aimed at promoting particular papers). These sources might be useful for ideas or further research but not as evidence.

• **Screen medical papers.** To assess the value of medical papers, ask yourself the following: Is the purpose of the paper clearly stated? Is the introduction clear? Have the authors chosen a good method to answer the question? Did the authors do what they said they were going to do? What did they actually find?

• **Check the abstract.** The abstract is the beginning summary of a medical paper. It should clearly state the background, the objectives, the methods used, the basic results and a conclusion.

• **Consider the purpose.** The purpose of the paper should ideally be stated as a question, i.e. "Does the first tic accurately diagnose Trigeminal Neuralgia?" or "What is the prognosis of patients with anesthesia dolorosa?"

• **Evaluate diagnosis studies.** If a paper is about helping to decide if you've got a particular condition, it should include both people with and without the condition. There should be discussion of a "gold standard" or commonly used test for comparison. There should be tests of agreement among different observers and among the same observers at different times. Look for diagrams that look like this:

	Disease + (disease present)	Disease - (disease not present)
Test +		
Test -		

• **Evaluate prognosis studies.** If a paper is about what happens to people over a period of time with a condition, the patients should be reliably diagnosed in the first place. The investigation should start at a clearly defined point in their disease, ideally early. Measurements should be taken frequently, objectively and accurately. Every patient must be accounted for. Patients must all be followed long enough to understand their fate.

• **Evaluate treatment studies.** If a paper is about how to treat a condition, does the paper pertain exactly to the condition you're interested in, i.e. trigeminal neuralgia vs. atypical TN vs. anesthesia dolorosa? Are there at least two treatments being compared? (A placebo is unnecessary when other drugs are already effective.) Are the groups being compared truly comparable?

Randomization is the best approach, i.e. there is an equal chance in the two groups that things can be influenced by something you don't know about. For example, the results could be different if one group has HIV and the other doesn't.

Also be sure all the patients are followed in the same way. What did the results show? Keep in mind that the brief conclusion at the end doesn't always accurately represent what the results show. Look for charts like this:

		New Treatment		Standard Treatment
Success		A		B
Failure		C		D

• **Judge with a critical eye.** Ask your doctor what he/she thinks about the study. Look for a critical analysis of the paper by experts. Look at editorials (critiques by peers that are often found at the end of papers). Assess the sources of support (i.e. is the literature funded by a drug company or other entity that might have a biased stake in its outcome?) Look at other research on the same topic and compare with the current paper.

• **Has the work been peer-reviewed?** This means, "Has the paper been subject to review by others in the field?" Keep in mind that some papers are merely "submitted," not reviewed, and that many web sites have information that is little more than opinions. Even many hospitals do not monitor the information their own medical staff posts online. The most reliable, evidence-based information has been reviewed and commented upon by colleagues.

NAVIGATING FOR HEALTH INFORMATION ONLINE

The Internet is loaded with health information. The problem is it's not always accurate, not always complete and not always easy to find either. But millions of people are using it as prime information source, and an estimated 70 percent of them say information obtained online has influenced their treatment decisions.

RAND Health conducted a study of online medical information for the California HealthCare Foundation in 2001 and found that consumers only have a one in five chance of finding relevant health information through search engines.

RAND's searchers found that, on average, it takes 10 to 15 minutes to find the answer to a single question with a high-speed Internet connection.

When consumers are able to find relevant information, much of it is commercial or promotional – in other words, it's coming from sources that are selling a related product or service.

What's more, the RAND researchers found that much of the information is incomplete, hard to understand and that it's not unusual to find conflicting details on different sites – and sometimes within the same site.

On the positive side, RAND found that most web information is fairly current. About half of the dated materials it found on four medical conditions had been updated within the previous year.

And RAND concluded that even if the information is incomplete, it can be helpful as a start and useful in helping consumers develop questions to ask their own doctors.

Some points to ponder when evaluating online medical information:

- Is it clear who has written the information? How qualified is that person or that group?

- Are the aims of the web site spelled out? Who or what is it for?

- Who is behind the web site?

- Does the site offer good, well researched evidence and information or primarily opinions or statements that aren't backed up?

- Is the site up to date?

- Is the information biased or slanted in some way? Or does it attempt to give balanced information from a variety of viewpoints?

- Don't take any one source as gospel. Check information among several resources, especially including your own doctors. Keep in mind, online information can help or hinder your care, depending on the accuracy and reliability of what you're reading.

Several organizations have guidelines for accurate and reliable online health information. Web sites that meet the guidelines will carry seals indicating the guidelines have been met. Among the organizations:

- Health on Net Foundation (HON) (www.hon.ch)
- Health Internet Ethics (www.hiethics.com)
- Medcertain (www.medcertain.org)

A few good online launching points for evidence-based health information are:

- www.guidelines.gov (has summaries of medical topics)
- www.nlm.gov (has a searchable database of medical literature)
- www.intelihealth.com (a searchable database by conditions)
- www.ncbi.nlm.nih.gov/PubMed (a U.S. government link to medical abstracts and papers)
- www.clinicalevidence.com (has a collection of critically reviewed medical articles)

For more details on finding and using health information online, try these web pages:

- www.tna-support.org/Articles/HowTo.html
- www.hopetillman.com/findqual.html

15 POINTS TO LOOK FOR IN A GOOD SURGICAL STUDY

Dr. Zakrzewska and British neurosurgeon Dr. Ben Lopez offer these 15 hallmarks of a well done research paper on TN surgery.

- The abstract should be structured and include key details on background, the objectives, the methods used, the basic results and a conclusion.

- The type of study should be clearly stated, i.e. prospective (begun prior to the procedure), retrospective (evaluates results of past patients), controlled (compared to untreated or differently treated patients), etc.

- The diagnoses should be clearly defined, and if there are those with differing diagnoses, results should be reported separately for each group.

- Basic demographic data should be included, such as age information, gender breakdown, sides and divisions of pain involved, etc.

- Patients should have had detailed sensory testing done both pre- and post-op.

- Details of previous treatments should be spelled out and analyzed, including earlier operations and any sensory problems that already were present from those.

- A brief description of the surgical technique used and the findings at surgery. Any technical failures that prevented the operation from being carried out should be included.

- The follow-up times for evaluation should be spelled out, including both the median time and the range of time.

- Details should be included on how the follow-up was carried out. By whom? By mail? By direct interview? Follow-up should include at least 80 percent of the patients. If a questionnaire was used, it should be provided.

- Outcomes should be reported for complete relief, partial relief and no relief. Details should be spelled out defining each.

- Rates of pain recurrence should be reported and broken down "minor" and "major."

- Complications and rates should be reported and detailed specifically, i.e. permanent vs. temporary or complete numbness vs. mild numbness.

- Kaplan-Meier charts should be used to project success and recurrence rates.

- Complete and partial reliefs should be reported separately. These rates should be broken down by any differences in diagnostic groups, i.e. typical vs. atypical TN or typical vs. multiple-sclerosis-related.

- Drug-related side effects should be reported in cases where surgical relief wasn't complete, and in radiosurgery, the time until maximum pain relief should be analyzed and presented.

"Thoughts to Myself"

Here's a poem neuralgian Jane Fetterly wrote to describe the thoughts that go through a neuralgian's head when the stabbing pain begins:

Zing – "If I concentrate on something else, it will go away."
Zing, Zing – "Did anyone see me grimace?"
Zing, Zing, Zing – "The dreadful roller-coaster ride is beginning again.
I had better leave this place and head for home,
and take the pills and lie in solitude and hope that darkness
will wash over me and carry me to a safer place."

"Do You Know What I Did Today?"

Neuralgian Ron Irons wrote this during one of those sudden remissions from TN:

Do you know what I did this morning? I took a shower.
I not only took a shower, I took the showerhead and put it on pulsating
and let the water beat against my head... let it just vibrate...
let it just massage me from the tip of my head to my whole body.
And it felt so good. Have you ever been able to do that?

Do you know what I did today? I took a nice walk.
It was a blustery day, the wind was blowing, and I didn't wear a hat.
It felt great. I was really brave. I walked directly into the wind.
I conquered the wind today.

Do you know what I did today? I rode in a car, on the passenger side.
I rolled the window down and felt the wind come into the car
and let it caress my head and it felt so good.

Can I tell you what I did today? I gave my wife a hug.
I kissed my wife. She gently caressed my face with her hands.
Let me tell you, it felt so great. Life doesn't get much better than that.

Do you know what I did today? I ate me an apple.
It was a tasty apple, a Red Delicious.
I love Red Delicious apples. Don't you?

Do you know what I did today? I enjoyed a cookout.
Corn on the cob tasted so delicious.
I had a nice porterhouse steak from the grill.
It was a little tough and chewy at one time,
but that's what made it special. I devoured that steak...
even ate the meat close to the bone. What a great cookout.

Do you know what I did today?
I gave a presentation that went really well.
I mean I talked for over an hour. Everybody enjoyed it.
I had practiced, drilled and rehearsed it.
It went as I had planned. It was really great.

Hey! You know what I did today? I brushed my teeth.
I not only brushed them, I took my time.
I brushed up and down, in and out and across the front.
What a joyful experience to just brush one's teeth.

Do you know what I did today? I was working in the yard,
got all sweaty and took out my handkerchief and wiped my brow.
I wiped my upper lip, I wiped my whole face. It felt so good,
I did it again and thought to myself, life is good.

Do you know what I did today?
I approached the day with child-like enthusiasm.
A whole new world is there for me today.
One that I can enjoy and really get into.
Have I told you that I am excited about life?
Excited about living!

Hey! Do you know what makes today so special?
I don't have the pain of yesterday. Isn't that terrific?
With such a great day going for me today,
you would not believe my yesterday.
Or maybe you would!

"TIC DOULOUREUX MY DARLING"

As written and performed by Dr. Peter Jannetta
at the 1996 TNA conference in Cincinnati, Ohio
(To be sung to the tune of "Skip to My Lou, My Darling")

Got my face pain out of the blue,
Got my face pain out of the blue,
Got my face pain out of the blue,
What did I do my darling?

Saw a dentist, as did you,
Saw a dentist, as did you,
Saw a dentist, as did you,
He took my teeth out, darling.

Saw my doctor, as did you,
Saw my doctor, as did you,
Saw my doctor, as did you,
He didn't help, my darling.

Saw a neurologist, as did you,
He diagnosed it, that is true,
He diagnosed it, that is true,
Tic douloureux, my darling.

Tegretol, Dilantin, baclofen,
Dilantin, baclofen, Tegretol,
Baclofen, Tegretol, Dilantin,
Slept all the time, my darling.

Operation is for you,
Operation is for you,
Operation is for you,
Said Dr. So and So, my darling.

All the surgeons do what they do,
Help most of us, hurt a few,
Help most of us, maybe you,
Tic douloureux, my darling.

Tic doulo, tic doulo, tic douloureux,
Tic doulo, tic doulo, tic douloureux,
Tic doulo, tic doulo, tic douloureux,
Tic douloureux, my darling.

RESOURCES

*Some sources for additional information on
trigeminal neuralgia and related face pains:*

TRIGEMINAL NEURALGIA ASSOCIATION

Non-profit association dedicated to helping trigeminal neuralgians and their families through direct patient support. It also provides information on TN and related disorders and promotes research into treatments.

Address: 925 Northwest 56th Terrace, Suite C, Gainesville, FL 32605
Phone: (352) 376-9955
Patient inquiries: (904) 779-0333
Office fax: (352) 376-8688
Patient-inquiry fax: (904) 779-7681
Office e-mail: tnanational@tna-support.org
Patient-inquiry e-mail: tnainfo@aol.com
Web site: www.tna-support.org

ACOUSTIC NEUROMA ASSOCIATION

Non-profit association that offers support and information for those who have acoustic neuromas. These brain tumors sometimes can lead to TN pain.

Address: 600 Peachtree Pkwy, Suite 108, Cumming, GA 30041-6899
Phone: (770) 205-8211
Fax: (770) 205-0239
E-mail: ANAusa@aol.com
Web site: http://anausa.org/

ACADEMY OF UPPER CERVICAL CHIROPRACTIC ORGANIZATION

Coalition of chiropractors and chiropractic organizations that specialize in atlas subluxations. Offers list of doctor referrals.

Address: 1637 Westbridge Drive, Unit H4, Fort Collins, CO 80526
E-mail: auccoweb@yahoo.com
Web site: www.aucco.org

American Academy of Neurology.

Professional organization of neurologists. Offers information on neurological conditions, help finding a neurologist, the latest in neurology news and an on-line newsletter.

Address: 1080 Montreal Ave., St. Paul, MN 55116.
Phone: (800) 879-1960 or (651) 695-2717
E-mail: memberservices@aan.com
Web site: www.aan.com

AMERICAN ACADEMY OF PAIN MEDICINE

Address: 4700 W. Lake Ave., Glenview, IL 60025
Phone: (847)375-4731
Fax: (877)734-8750
E-mail: aapm@amctec.com
Web site: www.painmed.org

AMERICAN ASSOCIATION OF ACUPUNCTURE AND ORIENTAL MEDICINE.
Professional organization that offers educational material on acupuncture and help locating a member acupuncturist.
Address: 5530 Wisconsin Ave., Suite 1210, Chevy Chase, MD 20815
Phone: (888) 500-7999 or (301) 941-1064
Fax: (301) 986-9313
E-mail: info@aaom.org
Web site: www.aaom.org/

AMERICAN ASSOCIATION OF NATUROPATHIC PHYSICIANS
Association of practitioners trained in natural medicine, including herbal and botanical medications.
Address: 3201 New Mexico Ave., NW Suite 350, Washington, DC 20016
Phone: (202) 895-1392 or (866) 538-2267
Fax: (202) 274-1992
E-mail: member.services@naturopathic.org
Web site: www.naturopathic.org

AMERICAN CHIROPRACTIC ASSOCIATION
Professional organization for chiropractors. Provides educational information on chiropractic care, a monthly newsletter and help finding a local member chiropractor.
Address: 1701 Clarendon Blvd., Arlington, VA 22209.
Phone: (800) 986-4636
Fax: (703) 243-2593
E-mail: memberinfo@amerchiro.org
Web site: www.amerchiro.org

AMERICAN CHRONIC PAIN ASSOCIATION
Non-profit organization with 800 chapters worldwide devoted to supporting those with chronic pain. Offers educational and self-help materials as well as an "ACPA Chronicle" newsletter.
Address: P.O. Box 850, Rocklin, CA 95677.
Phone: (800) 533-3231
Fax: (916) 632-3208
E-mail: ACPA@pacbell.net
Web site: www.theacpa.org

AMERICAN HERBALISTS GUILD
Organization of professional and medical herbalists
Address: 1931 Gaddis Road, Canton, GA 30115
Phone:(770) 751-6021
Fax: (770) 751-7472
Email: ahgoffice@earthlink.net
Web site: www.americanherbalistsguild.com

AMERICAN INSTITUTE OF HYPNOTHERAPY
Professional organization that provides training and certification of hypnotherapists. Also offers educational materials.
Address: 16842 Von Karman #475, Irvine, CA 92714.
Phone: (800) 634-9766
E-mail: aih@hypnosis.com
Web site: www.aih.cc

AMERICAN PAIN FOUNDATION
A nonprofit organization that provides information and support for those in pain.
Address: 201 N. Charles Street, Suite 710, Baltimore, Maryland 21201-4111
Phone: 1-888-615-PAIN (7246)
Email: info@painfoundation.org
Website: www.painfoundation.org

AMERICAN PAIN SOCIETY
APS is a multidisciplinary scientific and professional society that seeks to meet the information needs of the general public and especially for people in pain.
Address: 4700 W. Lake Ave., Glenview, IL 60025
Phone: (847) 375-4715
Fax: (877) 734-8758
Website: www.ampainsoc.org
Email: info@ampainsoc.org

AMERICAN SOCIETY OF CLINICAL HYPNOSIS
Professional organization of clinical hypnotists. Offers help finding member hypnotists.
Address: 140 N. Bloomingdale Rd., Bloomingdale, IL 60108-1017
Phone: (630) 980-4740
Fax: (630) 351-8490
Email: info@asch.net

DANA ALLIANCE FOR BRAIN INITIATIVES
A non-profit organization of neuroscientists committed to educating the public about the benefits of brain research. Has educational materials on the brain and contacts to brain-related organizations.
Address: 745 Fifth Ave., Suite 900, New York, NY 10151.
Phone: (212) 223-4040
Fax: (212) 593-7623
E-mail: dabiinfo@dana.org
Web site: www.dana.org

HERB RESEARCH FOUNDATION
Medicinal plant organization that offers news on herbal medicine.
Address: 4140 15th St., Boulder, CO 80304
Phone: (303) 449-2265 or (800) 748-2617
Fax: (303) 449-7849
E-mail: info@herbs.org
Web site: www.herbs.org

INTERNATIONAL ACADEMY OF COMPOUNDING PHARMACISTS
A professional organization whose members are pharmacists who make customized medications.
Address: P.O. Box 1365, Sugar Land, TX 77487
Phone: (281) 933-8400 or 1-800-927-4227
Fax: (281) 495-0602
E-mail: iacpinfo@iacprx.org
Web site: www.iacprx.org

INTERNATIONAL CHIROPRACTERS OF AMERICA
Seeks to advance chiropractic throughout the world as a distinct health care profession predicated upon its unique philosophy, science, and art.
Address: 1110 N. Glebe Road, Suite 1000, Arlington, VA 22201
Phone: (800)423-4690 or (703)528-5000
E-mail: chiro@chiropractic.org
Web site: www.chiropractic.org

INTERNATIONAL RADIOSURGERY SUPPORT ASSOCIATION
Non-profit organization set up to help those considering and those who have undergone radiosurgery treatments, such as the Gamma Knife or Linac. Provides details on these treatments and help finding radiosurgery centers.
Address: 3005 Hoffman St., Harrisburg, PA 17110
Phone: (717) 260-9808
Fax: (717) 260-9809
Web site: www.irsa.org

LYME DISEASE FOUNDATION INC.
Non-profit organization that offers education, treatment information and resources of help for Lyme Disease and other tic-borne diseases. Lyme Disease is sometimes mistaken for TN when a symptom of it is face pain.
Address: 1 Financial Plaza, Hartford, CT 06103.
Phone: (860) 525-2000
Fax: (860) 525-TICK (860-525-8425)
E-mail: lymefnd@aol.com
Web site: www.lyme.org

MULTIPLE SCLEROSIS ASSOCIATION OF AMERICA
Not-for-profit charitable service agency that addresses day-to-day needs of MS patients and their family.
Address: 706 Haddonfield Road, Cherry Hill, NJ 08002.
Phone: (800) 532-7667
Fax: (609) 661-9797
E-mail: msaa@msaa.com
Web site: www.msaa.com

MULTIPLE SCLEROSIS FOUNDATION INC.
Non-profit organization that promotes MS research, publishes a newsletter, offers educational materials, operates a network of 40 local support groups and helps patients find medical help.
Address: 6350 N. Andrews Ave., Fort Lauderdale, FL 33309.
Phone: (888) MSFOCUS (888-673-6287) or (954) 776-6805
E-mail: support@msfocus.org
Web site: www.msfacts.org

NATIONAL AWARENESS CAMPAIGN FOR UPPER CERVICAL CARE
Non-profit organization dedicated to educating the public about upper-cervical chiropractic care. Also offers referrals to upper-cervical chiropractors in inquirers' area.
Address: NACUCC, 5215 Colbert Road, Lakeland, FL 33813.
Phone: (888) 622-8221
E-mail: info@uppercervical.org
Web site: www.uppercervical.org

NATIONAL CENTER FOR COMPLEMENTARY AND ALTERNATIVE MEDICINE
Branch of the National Institutes of Health devoted to research and information on complementary and alternative treatments, including chiropractic, acupuncture, herbal therapy, hypnosis and the like.
Address: NCCAM Clearinghouse, P.O. Box 7923, Gaithersburg, MD 20898
Phone: (888) 644-6226
Fax: (866) 464-3616
E-mail: info@nccam.nih.gov
Web site: nccam.nih.gov

NATIONAL CENTER FOR HOMEOPATHY
Non-profit educational group that publishes a monthly "Homeopathy Today" newsletter and provides other informational material on homeopathic medicine. Also helps individuals find local homeopaths.
Address: 801 N. Fairfax St., Suite 306, Alexandria, VA 22314.
Phone: (703) 548-7790
Fax: (703) 548-7792
E-mail: info@homeopathic.org
Web site: www.homeopathic.org

NATIONAL CHRONIC PAIN OUTREACH ASSOCIATION
Support association that offers a newsletter, articles, book reviews, doctor and support-group referrals and other information on chronic pain of all sorts.
Address: 7979 Old Georgetown Road, Suite 100, Besthesda, MD 20814-2429.
Phone: (301) 652-4948
Fax: (301) 907-0745

NATIONAL INSTITUTE OF NEUROLOGICAL DISORDERS AND STROKES
Government agency that provides funding for research into neurological problems, including TN and other nerve pains.
Address: NIH Neurological Institute, P.O. Box 5801, Bethesda, MD 20824.
  NINDS – Neuroscience Center, Division of Extramural Research,
  6001 Executive Blvd., Suite 3309, Bethesda, MD 20892
Phone: (800) 352-9424 or (301) 496-5751
TTY (for people using adaptive equipment): (301) 468-5981
Web site: www.ninds.nih.gov

NATIONAL MULTIPLE SCLEROSIS SOCIETY
Non-profit organization that offers educational materials, the latest clinical and research information on MS and details on various treatments.
Address: 733 Third Ave., New York, NY 10017
Phone: (800) 344-4867
E-mail: info@nmss.org
Web site: www.nmss.org

SOCIETY OF CHIROPRACTIC ORTHOSPINOLOGY
Non-profit education organization that provides comprehensive information on Orthospinology for doctors, students and patients and as well as insight into the field for everyone.
Phone: (770)517-9921
E-mail: webmaster@orthospinology.org
Web site: www.orthospinology.org

TMJ ASSOCIATION LTD.
Non-profit organization that offers support and help to those with temporomandibular joint disorders and similar joint-related pains. Provides educational materials, help finding treatment and a newsletter.
Address: P.O. Box 26770, Milwaukee, WI 53226-0770.
Phone: (414) 259-3223
Fax: (414) 259-8112
E-mail: info@tmj.org
Web site: http://tmj.org

VZV RESEARCH FOUNDATION INC.
Promotes research and provides information on the virus (Varicella-Zoster) that can cause post-herpetic neuralgia and other diseases.
Address: 40 E. 72nd St., New York, NY 10021.
Phone: (212) 472-3181
Fax: (212) 861-7033
Web site: http://vzvfoundation.org/

OTHER BOOKS ON TN AND FACE PAIN

Foods That Fight Pain: Revolutionary New Strategies for Maximum Pain Relief.
Dr. Neal D. Barnard. Not about TN in particular but discusses the link between diet and pain. Harmony Books. 1999. $14.00. Paperback

The Merck Manual of Medical Information: Second Home Edition.
Robert Berkow, Mark H. Beers and Andrew J. Fletcher. An encyclopedic 1,900 pages on various medicines, their uses, dosages, side effects and precautions. 2003. $37.50. Hardcover.

Medical and Surgical Management of Trigeminal Neuralgia.
Dr. Gerhard H. Fromm, editor. A textbook overview of TN written primarily for doctors. 1987. $22.50. Hardcover.

Neurosurgical and Medical Management of Pain: Trigeminal Neuralgia, Chronic Pain and Cancer Pain. Dr. Ronald Brisman, editor. A medical textbook that details surgical approaches to treating TN, cancer pain and chronic pain in general. Kluwer Academic Publishers. 1989. $222.00. Hardcover.

The Non-Chew Cookbook. J. Randy Wilson. Includes more than 200 recipes for dishes that don't require hard chewing to swallow. Wilson Publishing Inc., P.O. Box 2190, Glenwood Springs, CO 81602. 1986. $29.95. Paperback.

A Pained Life: A Chronic Pain Journey. By Carol Jay Levy. Chronicle of what it's like to have trigeminal neuralgia, written by a Pennsylvania woman who's been there and done that. Xlibris Corp., 2003. $22.99.

The Prevention Pain-Relief System. A 752-page book from the editors of Prevention magazine reviewing a variety of pains, including TN. Also includes information on alternative treatments such as acupuncture, biofeedback, hypnosis, TENS units, etc. Bantam Books. 1994. $6.99. Paperback.

TMJ: Its Many Faces: Second Edition. Dr. Wesley E. Shankland. An overview of temporomandibular joint problems aimed at patients and lay readers. ANADEM Inc. 1998. $19.50. Spiral-bound.

The Truth about Chronic Pain: Patients and Professional on How to Face It, Understand It, Overcome It. Arthur Rosenfeld. 2003. $26.00 Hardcover.

Trigeminal Neuralgia. Dr. Richard L. Rovit. Covers everything from anatomy and diagnosis to surgery. Written by more than a dozen doctors and aimed at other doctors who treat TN. Williams and Wilkins. 1990. $87. Hardcover.

Trigeminal Neuralgia: Current Concepts Regarding Pathogenesis and Treatment.
Dr. Gerhard H. Fromm, author, and Barry J. Sessle, editor. A thorough look at the causes behind TN and the many approaches to treating it. Also aimed primarily at doctors. Heinemann Medical Books. 1990. $75. Hardcover.

<u>Working in a Very Small Place.</u> Mark L. Shelton. A readable biography following the career of Dr. Peter J. Jannetta, the neurosurgeon who popularized the microvascular decompression surgery for TN.
Trigeminal Neuralgia Association. 2004. $19.95. Paperback.

INTERNET SITES WORTH VISITING

Acupuncture.com
http://www.acupuncture.com. Site developed by acupuncturist Al Stone that provides basic information and the latest news on acupuncture plus help finding an acupuncturist and links to Oriental-medicine products.

Allinfo.com
http://www.allinfo.com. Good search engine for trigeminal neuralgia that links to other websites and personal narratives. Very useful in starting a search to get many related sources.

American Association of Neurological Surgeons
http://www.aans.org/pubpages/index.html. Professional organization of neurosurgeons. Offers information on conditions treatable by neurosurgery and help locating a neurosurgeon. Its Web site features monthly live on-line "Chats With a Neurosurgeon."

Apothecary On-Line
http://www.apothecaryon-line.com. An on-line herbal pharmacy sponsored by a Seattle company in the herbal-supplement business. A good index to look up uses of various herbs. Supplements can be ordered on-line.

Atypical Face Pain
http://www.emedicine.com/neuro/topic25.htm. Overview of facial pain diagnoses and treatments, with notes on discriminating between possible sources for chronic face pain. Significant participation by an editorial board of MDs.

BBC Health: Ask the Doctor – Trigeminal Neuralgia
http://www.bbc.co.uk/health/ask_doctor/trigeminal_neuralgia.shtml. A patient with trigeminal neuralgia asks about natural treatments. Dr. Rob Hicks answers in detail about homeopathic treatments.

BioMedNet
http://www.biomednet.com. A research site primarily for medical professionals that offers access to abstracts in hundreds of medical journals plus links to scores of medical journals. Use of the service is free, but there is a fee to order most of the abstracts.

Brain Surgery Information Center
http://www.brain-surgery.com. Mostly geared to tumors but also has a nice glossary of brain-surgery terms, a look at the history and future of brain surgery and specific information on specific types of brain surgery. This site also offers a slide show of a microvascular decompression surgery.

Chronic Pain – Directory for Health, at Google.com
http://directory.google.com/Top/Health/Medicine/Medical_Specialties/Pain_Mana gement/Chronic_Pain/. Organizations, support groups, treatment, connections to resources on fibromyalgia, related disorders sometimes associated with facial pain.

Cluster Headache Help
http://www.chhelp.org. Extensive index to resources and links for information and assistance with cluster headache.

Cluster Headaches Worldwide Support Group
http://www.clusterheadaches.com. An online chat room and support group for those who suffer from clusterheadaches.

CPMC Neurosurgery: Trigeminal Neuralgia
http://cpmcnet.columbia.edu/dept/nsg/NSGCPMC/specialties/trigeminal.html

Consumer Views on Management of Trigeminal Neuralgia
http://www.blackwellsynergy.com/Journals/content/abstracts/hed/2001/41/4/ abstract_hed1067.asp?journal=hed&issueid=5282&artid=101240&cid=hed.2001. 1&ftype=abstracts. J.M. Zakrzewska, MD, in Headache: The Journal of Head and Face Pain, Volume 41 Issue 4 Page 369 - April 2001.

Cranial Nerve V
http://www.sfu.ca/~saunders/l33098/Anatomical%20Glossary/CNV.html. Diagram of the distribution of the three branches of the Trigeminal nerve (5th cranial nerve).

Dennison Memorial Library
http://denison.uchsc.edu/outreach/medbib3.html. Provides an exhaustive overview of Internet medical resources available to librarians and the public.

Drug Information at MedLine-Plus
http://www.nlm.nih.gov/medlineplus/druginformation.html. "Information on thousands of prescription and over-the-counter medications... provided through two drug resources — MedMaster™†, a product of the American Society of Health-System Pharmacists (ASHP), and the USP DI® Advice for the Patient® ‡, a product of the United States Pharmacopeia (USP)."

E-medicine: Instant Access to the Minds of Medicine, Trigeminal Neuralgia
http://www.emedicine.com/emerg/topic617.htm Article on Trigeminal Neuralgia by J. Stephen Huff.

Epilepsy drug information

http://www.neuro.wustl.edu/epilepsy/aed.html. Detailed information on anticonvulsant medications from Washington University Medical Center in St. Louis. Although aimed at epilepsy, these are many of the same drugs used to treat TN.

Facepain.com

http://www.facepain.com. This is the place to start if you've got face pain and an Internet connection. Wonderful wealth of links (4,000 and counting) to articles, face-pain-related Web sites, support groups and anything else that might be useful. Also periodically features live on-line "chats" with doctors, and can help you find a specialist or put you in touch with other people going through the same problem.

Facial Neuralgia Resources

http://facial-neuralgia.org. Don't miss this one! A gold mine of patient-to-patient information including all aspects of face pain — TN, atypical TN, dental pains, glossopharyngeal neuralgia, anesthesia dolorosa... you name it. Also loaded with feedback on various treatments, personal stories, coping tips, support-group information, chat rooms and links to other sources.

Giving Something Back

http://www.erols.com/lawhern#Special. A research specialist and former webmaster of the TN Association website provides links to patient and doctor resources for trigeminal neuralgia, neuropathy, and atypical facial pain. Email inquiries welcomed for personalized research assistance.

Health on the Net Foundation

http://www.hon.ch/. Sets the standards for how healthcare sites on the Internet present their information, their qualifications, and disclosure of who sponsors them. Also provides an excellent healthcare site index and searchable archive.

Healthworld On-Line

http://www.healthy.net/asp/templates/center.asp?centerid=53. Resources for finding practitioners in alternative and complimentary medicine.

Homeopathy Home Page

http://www.homeopathyhome.com. Launching point to all sorts of homeopathy information, including links to research and articles, a directory of organizations, help finding local homeopaths and an online discussion group.

Internet Grateful Med

http://igm.nlm.nih.gov. An on-line search service that offers access to some 9 million abstracts on file at the National Library of Medicine. Also offers links to other on-line medical data.

Lyme Disease and TN

http://www.geocities.com/HotSprings/Spa/6772/tn-index.html. Web page by Art Doherty of California offering information on the connection (and confusion) between Lyme Disease and TN.

Lyme Disease Network Online (LymeNet)
http://www.lymenet.org. A site offering the latest news and articles on Lyme Disease. Also offers a bulletin board for personal messages, links to support groups, a newsletter and pictures of Lyme-caused rashes.

Martindale's Health Science Guide, 2003
http://www.martindalecenter.com/HSGuide.html. See especially, the Brain and Neuro Center at http://www.martindalecenter.com/MedicalBrain.html. Access medical journals, medical dictionaries, a wide variety of research and medical literature.

Massachusetts General Hospital/Harvard Medical School
http://neurosurgery.mgh.harvard.edu/tn-hfshp.htm. Offers details on surgical treatment of TN, glossopharyngeal neuralgia and hemifacial spasm. Also has a "guestbook" that puts TN patients in touch with one another for e-mail messaging.

Massachusetts General Hospital Department of Neurology Web Forum on TN
http://neuro-www.mgh.harvard.edu/forum. A Web page with TN information that offers periodic live on-line "chats" with MassGen neurologists.

Mayo Clinic
http://www.mayoclinic.org/trigeminalneuralgia-rst/
Treatment of Trigeminal Neuralgia at Mayo Clinic in Rochester

Medical College of Ohio
http://www.mco.edu/neuro/tripage.html. Offers information on TN surgery and lets you download a Quicktime movie of a balloon compression procedure.

Medifocus Guide Book: Trigeminal Neuralgia
http://www.medifocus.com. A site that offers guidebooks on over 100 diseases including trigeminal neuralgia.

http://www.medifocus.com/guide_detail.php?gid=NR018. Use this link to get to the trigeminal neuralgia guidebook directly. $29.95

National Center for Complementary and Alternative Medicine
http://nccam.nih.gov/. A center within the National Institutes of Health. Includes extensive information on alternative therapies by name, as well as timely health alerts for doctors and for consumers who use food supplements or herbs as alternatives and complements to mainstream medicine.

National Institutes of Health
http://www.nih.gov. A good gateway to all sorts of government research and information from NIH. Lots of links, including alternative treatments, clinical trials and on-line publications and articles.

Neuropathic Pain: New Insights, New Interventions
http://www.hosppract.com/issues/1998/10/bennett.htm.   Gary J. Bennett, M.D.,
Allegheny University of the Health Sciences.   Overview of research on pain
mechanisms and treatments for neuropathic pain.

Neurosciences on the Internet
http://www.neuroguide.com. A good launching point to look up neurology and
neurosurgery articles on the Internet.

Neurosurgery//On-Call
www.neurosurgery.org/directory/index.html.   The American Association of
Neurological Surgeons and Congress of Neurological Surgeons provides a database
of neurosurgeons which can be searched by location or telephone area code.
Please note: not all neurosurgeons regularly treat trigeminal neuralgia.

See also: "Web Guide", http://www.neurosurgery.org/webguide/index.asp, for
organizations and resources in neurosurgery, world-wide.

Neurosurgery Today
http://www.neurosurgerytoday.org/   A service of the American Association of
Neurological Surgeons.   Provides resources for finding a board certified
neurosurgeon.

See particularly, "What is Neurosurgery?" at
http://www.neurosurgerytoday.org/what/patient_e/adult.asp.

Oreogon Health and Science University
http://www.ohsu.edu/neurosurgery/tgn/index.shtml.   Department of
Neurosurgery posting progress in Trigeminal Neuralgia.

https://neurosurgery.ohsu.edu/tgndiagnosis/TGNPublic.asp.   Diagnostic
questionnaire.

Other Headaches and Facial Pains
http://imigraine.net/other/mout.html. Major overview of information sources and
treatments for facial and headache pain,   by Todd Troost, MD,   Professor and
Chairman of Neurology at Wake Forest University School of Medicine.

Pain Medicine & Palliative Care
http://stoppain.org @ Beth Israel Medical Center. General information on
Trigeminal Neuralgia including who it affects, symptoms, how it occurs, and the
diagnosis and treatment.

Pain Net Inc.
http://www.painnet.com. Primarily a source to educate doctors about pain
treatment but has links to pain books, pain information sources and a state-by-
state listing of pain specialists.

Patient's Guide to Healthcare Information on the Internet

http://www3.bc.sympatico.ca/me/patientsguide/. Provides gateways to on-line searchable databases, medical dictionaries, support groups and more. Not currently maintained, but still a gold mine for those who can spend some time.

Pharmaceutical Information Network

http://www.pharminfo.com/pubs/msb. Aimed at keeping pharmacists up to date on the latest in medication news. Offers Medical Sciences Bulletins on various medications as published by Pharmaceutical Information Associates.

PharmInfoNet

http://pharminfo.com/drugdb. Provides latest news about medications, including pharmaceutical press releases, journal articles and basic information on medications and their uses. Handy way to look up any medication.

Pub Med

http://www.ncbi.nlm.nih.gov/entrez/query.fcgi. The National Institutes of Health and the National Library of Medicine provide a direct-access gateway to *PubMed,* the abstract search engine on which the well-known Internet Grateful Med was originally layered. This resource allows keyword search on millions of medical abstracts dating from 1960 to the present. NLM is gradually adding links to full-text articles, though the numbers are still relatively small. There is an article delivery service for printouts, generally costing in excess of $10 dollars per full-text article. However, most libraries can obtain articles for you via inter-library loan, free or at duplication cost.

Quackwatch

http://www.quackwatch.org. A consumer-alert site that blows the whistle on fraudulent health claims and offers research-based counterpoints to alternative and complementary medicine issues.

RxList.Com

http://www.rxlist.com RX-List," is a searchable database of FDA-approved information on over 4000 commonly used drugs. Includes info on drug interactions and side effects based on controlled clinical trials.

TMJ and Facial Pain Center

http://www.drshankland.com. A site primarily about TMJ, its causes and its treatment by Ohio oral surgeon and face-pain specialist Dr. Wesley Shankland. Also offers information on other face pains and provides links to other helpful Web sites.

Trigeminal Neuralgia

http://www.neurosurgery.ucsd.edu/cnd/trigeminal_neuralgia.htm. Some useful information on Trigeminal Neuralgia.

Trigeminal Neuralgia: Evaluation and Treatment

http://www.albany.net/~tjc/trigeminal-neuralgia.html. This tutorial provides a logical approach to the diagnosis of Trigeminal Neuralgia (TN), and helps avoid common pitfalls in the treatment of this painful condition.

Trigeminal Neuralgia / Hemifacial Spasms Wake Forest University School of Medicine

http://www.bgsm.edu/bgsm/surg-sci/ns/tn-hfs.html Links to information about trigeminal neuralgia, glossopharyngeal neuralgia, vagal neuralgia, superior laryngeal neuralgia, nervus intermedius or geniculate neuralgia, and hemifacial spasm, with special emphasis on surgical treatments such as microvascular decompression, Gamma Knife stereotactic radiosurgery, and radiofrequency lesioning.

Trigeminal Neuralgia: Homeopathic Treatment

http://www.trigeminalneuralgia.us. Asia's leading center offers effective homeopathic options online.

Trigeminal Neuralgia Resources

http://neurosurgery.mgh.harvard.edu/tnr. The forerunner to Facial Neuralgia Resources. Loaded with great information and links elsewhere. Focuses mainly on classic TN instead of related face pains. Includes articles, treatment information, alternatives to traditional treatment, personal experiences, coping tips, links to support groups and more.

Trigeminal Neuralgia Association UK

http://www.tna.org.uk/ . The Trigeminal Neuralgia Association patient support home site for the United Kingdom.

Trigeminal Neuralgia, CCND Winnipeg

http://www.umanitoba.ca/cranial_nerves/trigeminal_neuralgia/tutorial.html. Offers an interactive tutorial on trigeminal neuralgia. It includes general information, medication, and overviews.

University of Pittsburgh Neuronet

http://www.neurosurgery.pitt.edu. Neurosurgery site from the University of Pittsburgh, one of the world's leaders in TN research and treatment. Includes articles and research findings by Dr. Peter Jannetta and staff plus links to other TN resources, links to support groups and detailed information on Pitt's experience with the Gamma Knife.

Vimy Park Pharmacy

http://www.vimy-park.mb.ca/herb.html. A good herbal reference site designed to inform pharmacists about herbs. Good for separating the known and proven from the anecdotes, myths and unproven claims. Done by a Canadian pharmacy.

Worldwide Congress on Pain

http://www.pain.com. Offers a searchable archive of more than 2,500 pain articles plus a newsletter, interviews with pain experts and help finding local pain clinics.

Your Complete Guide to Trigeminal Neuralgia; A.M. Kaufmann & M. Patel CCND Winnipeg

http://www.umanitoba.ca/cranial_nerves/trigeminal_neuralgia/manuscript/index.html

"You're Not Alone"

http://www.creps.org/tn. Site set up by Deborah Creps of San Jose, Calif., as kind of an on-line support group for TN patients. Offers basic information on treatments and links to regional support groups and other Web sites of interest to neuralgians.

GLOSSARY

ACOUSTIC NEUROMA. A tumor growing on the acoustic or hearing nerve. This can sometimes cause TN when the nearby tumor pushes a blood vessel onto the trigeminal nerve.

ADHESIONS. Fibrous growths similar to scar tissue that forms at the site of tissue damage.

ANALGESICS. Medications that relieve pain.

ANESTHESIA DOLOROSA. A hard-to-treat condition that feels like a combination of pain and numbness. Sometimes occurs as unwanted side effect of some surgical TN treatments.

ANEURYSM. Weakness in a blood vessel that allows vessel to bulge and possibly rupture.

ANTICONVULSANT. Medication that prevents convulsions or seizures.

APLASTIC ANEMIA. Potentially fatal blood disorder caused by damage to bone marrow. Rare but potential side effect of some anticonvulsant medications.

ARACHNOID. A membrane of the brain. When abnormally thickened, it is a potential cause of compression on the trigeminal nerve.

ARTERIOVENOUS MALFORMATION (AVM). An abnormal growth of blood vessels that sometimes rupture without warning. These vessels can cause TN if they grow near and compress the trigeminal nerve.

ATLAS. The top-most bone of the spine.

ATYPICAL FACE PAIN. Facial pain with mixed symptoms and of unknown origin. May have some of the symptoms of TN but also others, maybe even outside the areas served by the trigeminal nerve. A newer proposed definition is "face pain of psychogenic origin," or pain that is originating in the brain.

ATYPICAL TRIGEMINAL NEURALGIA. A type of facial pain that may have some of the characteristics of classic TN (i.e. sharp stabs and trigger points) but also symptoms that aren't common to classic TN (i.e. constant, aching or burning pain in addition to the stabs). Sometimes referred to as "TN-2."

AVULSION. Tearing away of a structure, as in removing or cutting away a section of nerve.

BILATERAL. Referring to both sides. Bilateral TN means pain on both sides of the face.

BIOFEEDBACK. A technique in which people learn to control body functions such as breathing rate, blood pressure and body temperature by responding to feedback from electrodes that monitor changing body conditions.

BOTOX. A purified form of the botulinum toxin that, when injected, can partially paralyze muscles. Usually used in tightening wrinkled skin but it's also being tried as a temporary TN pain-relief measure.

CT SCAN. An internal picture of the body constructed by a computer by piecing together a series of X-rays. Sometimes used in detecting tumors. CT stands for *"computed tomography."*

CAPSAICIN. The chemical that makes hot peppers hot. Used in a topical cream, it sometimes is used to treat TN.

CAUTERIZE. To seal off, as in sealing off sections of blood vessels to stop or prevent bleeding.

CATHETER. A tube used to drain fluids from the body, to introduce liquids to the body, or in the case of TN, to allow passage of a balloon to the site of the trigeminal nerve.

CEREBELLUM. Part of the brain that controls movements.

CEREBRAL CORTEX. Part of the brain that analyzes nerve signals and sends out responses.

CEREBROSPINAL FLUID (CSF). A fluid composed mostly of water, glucose, salt and proteins that surrounds, cushions and provides nutrients to the brain and spinal cord.

CERVIX. The top vertebrae of the spine where the trigeminal nerve originates and through which the spinal cord passes to connect to the brainstem.

CLUSTER HEADACHE. Searing, boring, come-and-go pain in the face or forehead thought to be caused by dilation of the blood vessels in the skull. Sometimes confused with trigeminal neuralgia.

CLUSTER TIC SYNDROME. Combination of cluster headaches and trigeminal neuralgia.

COMPOUNDING. A pharmacy technique in which medications are custom-prepared to meet specific needs of individual customers. Those who offer this service are called "compounding pharmacists."

CRANIAL NERVES. Twelve pairs of nerves that serve various areas and functions of the head. The trigeminal nerve is one of these nerves.

CRANIECTOMY. Surgical opening of the skull necessary for brain surgery. The bone is not replaced after surgery.

CRANIOSACRAL THERAPY. Gentle manipulation technique somewhat similar to light massage that's aimed at freeing the flow of cerebrospinal fluid. Some believe impeded flow of this fluid can cause face pain.

CRANIOTOMY. Surgical opening of the skull necessary for brain surgery. The bone is replaced after surgery.

CRYOTHERAPY. Using cold agents to deaden or kill nerve fibers. Sometimes used to treat TN.

DEAFFERENTATION PAIN. Pain that occurs when parts of a nerve are injured to the point where they're disabled. It's usually a constant, burning type of pain.

DEEP BRAIN STIMULATION. An experimental procedure in which surgeons insert a thin electrode through a small opening in the skull into the thalamus, a part of the brain where pain sensation occurs. A stimulation device attached to the electrode delivers low-grade electrical signals in an attempt to override pain signals.

DEMYELINATION. The process of losing or destroying myelin, the protective sheath around nerve fibers.

DURA. The waterproof covering that surrounds the brain.

DREZ. Acronym for *"dorsal root entry zone,"* a surgical procedure done in the neck region to disable the origin of the trigeminal nerve in the upper spine.

DYSESTHESIA. A numbness or abnormal sensation severe enough that a patient considers it disturbing.

ELECTRODE. Small pointed tool used to deliver controlled charges of electricity or radiowaves.

ENDOSCOPE. A new surgical instrument that uses a tiny camera to project brightened and magnified images from inside the body.

EPILEPSY. Disorder of the nervous system marked by seizures and temporary losses of consciousness or concentration.

ENDORPHINS. Pain-killing proteins produced naturally by the body.

FACIAL NERVE. A cranial nerve that controls most of the muscles in the face. This is a separate nerve from the trigeminal nerve, which controls sensation in the face and some of the muscles that control chewing.

FLUOROSCOPE. A fluorescent X-ray device that surgeons use to guide a needle or catheter to the right location in the body.

FORAMEN OVALE. The opening in the skull through which the trigeminal nerve passes on its way into the face.

FOTHERGILL'S DISEASE. Another name for TN. Comes from 18th-century English physician John Fothergill. Seldom used anymore.

GAMMA KNIFE. A non-incision surgical device that uses Gamma radiation to cause precisely aimed damage to targeted tissue. Used to create lesions on the root of the trigeminal nerve.

GANGLION. A cluster of nerve cells.

GANGLIOLYSIS. A surgery to create targeted damage to a ganglion, usually to stop pain signals from getting to the brain.

GASSERIAN GANGLION. The cluster of nerve cells where the trigeminal nerve branches out into its three divisions and exits the skull.

GLIAL CELLS. Type of cells that the body uses to build myelin, the insulating sheath around nerves. Also see oligodendrocytes and Schwann cells.

GLOSSOPHARYNGEAL NEURALGIA. Similar condition to TN, only this pain is in the throat and neck. Causes are thought to be similar to TN but involving the glossopharyngeal nerve.

GLYCEROL. An oily alcohol substance that damages nerve fibers when in direct contact with the fibers.

HERPES ZOSTER. Also known as shingles, this is a viral infection caused by the same virus that causes chickenpox. When it strikes the face, it can cause burning pain.

HYPESTHESIA. Medical term for numbness.

HYPONATREMIA. Abnormally low levels of blood sodium. Can be a side effect of some TN medications.

LESION. An area of tissue damage.

LEUKOPENIA. A deficiency in white blood cells, which protect the body against disease-causing microorganisms. Can be a side effect of some TN medications.

LILT. Acronym for *"low-intensity laser therapy."* It's a therapy using beams of highly focused laser light that's being tried as a pain-relief measure.

LINAC. Acronym for linear accelerator, a non-incision surgical device that uses high-energy X-rays to cause precisely aimed damage to targeted. Often used for tumors but sometimes for TN.

MAGNETIC RESONANCE IMAGING (MRI). A device that creates computerized images of the body's interior. Instead of using radiation as in an X-ray, MRIs involves a rapid series of pictures taken while the subject is inside a magnetized chamber. An MRI brain scan is painless and is useful in detecting multiple sclerosis and brain tumors.

MAGNETIC RESONANCE TOMOGRAPHIC ANGIOGRAPHY (MRTA). A type of imaging similar to MRI that can pick up even very small blood vessels. Gadolinium dye is injected into the patient's bloodstream to enhance the image.

MANDIBULAR. Area referring to the lower jaw region of the face.

MAXILLARY. Area referring to the upper jaw and cheek region of the face.

MENINGITIS. An inflammation of the membrane that covers the brain and spinal cord. It's a potential complication of brain surgery.

MENINGIOMA. A tumor of the meninges, the membrane that covers the brain and spinal cord. This can cause TN if the tumor pushes a blood vessel against the trigeminal nerve.

MICROVASCULAR DECOMPRESSION (MVD). A type of brain surgery in which the aim is to lift a compressing blood vessel off the trigeminal nerve and insulate the two with a small cushion.

MOTOR CORTEX STIMULATION. A surgical procedure in which one or two small contact plates – attached to an electrical stimulation device – are placed on the surface of the brain over the cortex region. Stimulating this region with low-grade electrical current reduces activity in the thalamus, where pain is felt.

MULTIPLE SCLEROSIS (MS). A degenerative disease affecting the central nervous system. MS causes scarring of nerve fibers and leads to such symptoms as arm and leg weakness, numbness, double vision and impaired coordination and movement. Trigeminal neuralgia also sometimes develops when MS scars the trigeminal nerve.

MYELIN. The protective coating that surrounds nerve fibers. It's made out of a layer of proteins packed between two layers of lipids (fats).

MYOFASCIAL PAIN. Dull, aching muscle pain of uncertain cause. When it occurs in the facial muscles, it's sometimes confused with TN because the pain can be triggered by touching the area.

NERVE BLOCK. Use of a drug, chemical or surgery to stop a nerve signal from getting through to the brain. In the case of TN, these can be used for temporary pain relief or as a way to diagnose the exact nature and location of a pain.

NERVE FIBER. A strand of tissue made up of nerve cells that carries nerve impulses (biochemical signals to and from the brain).

NERVUS INTERMEDIUS. A branch of the geniculate nerve. When compressed by a blood vessel, it can cause pain deep in the ear.

NEURAXIAL DRUG INFUSION. A way to deliver pain-relieving medicine directly to the spinal cord, using a battery-operated pump implanted under the skin.

NEURECTOMY. Surgical removal of a nerve or nerve branch.

NEUROAUGMENTATION. Attempting to block pain signals by overriding them with a competing signal generated by an implanted or attached electrical stimulation device.

NEUROMA. A tangle of poorly developed nerve endings that resprout following a nerve injury.

NEUROPATHIC PAIN. Pain that originates in the nerve, usually due to injury or disease.

NEURONS. Cells that send and receive electrical signals to and from parts of the body. These are the nerve cells that are stimulated to send impulses (messages) to and from the brain.

NEUROTRANSMITTER. A body chemical that's used to transmit nerve impulses from one nerve cell to another. Sodium and calcium are two of the most common.

NEUTROPENIA. A diminished number of neutrophils, a type of white blood cell needed to fight infections. Can be a side effect of some TN medications.

NICO. Acronym for *"neuralgia-inducing cavitational osteonecrosis,"* a controversial type of facial pain that may be confused with TN. Presumed cause is a chronic infection of bone in the jaw that can damage the nerve branches in the affected bone.

NOCICEPTOR. A type of nerve receptor that activate when there's a painful stimulus.

OLIGODENDROCYTE. A specific type of glial cell that the body uses to build myelin in the central nervous system.

OPHTHALMIC. Area referring to the region of the face around the eyes.

OPIOIDS. Pain-killing agents that originate from the poppy flower and its product opium. Morphine and codeine were two of the earliest. These are sometimes used to treat persistent face pains that haven't responded to other therapies.

OROFACIAL. Area of the face around the mouth.

PAIN THRESHOLD. The point at which an applied, escalating sensory stimulus (heat, cold, pressure, pin-prick, etc.) is reported by a person as pain.

PAIN TOLERANCE. The reaction of a person to reported pain after it has crossed the pain threshold.

PANCYTOPENIA. Abnormal decrease in all types of blood cells. Can be a side effect of some TN medications.

PARATRIGEMINAL NEURALGIA. Throbbing headache-like pain in the upper branch of the trigeminal nerve, thought to be caused either by an inflammation or infection of the nerve. Also called *"Raeder's syndrome."*

PARESTHESIA. An unusual sensation that may be described as "tingling," "crawling" or "pins and needles." Often accompanies mild numbness.

PEMF. Acronym for *"pulsed electromagnetic field."* This is a device that generates wave-like charges called electromagnetic fields. The changing polarity of this magnetic device has been shown to help fractured bones heal and is being tried in treating pain.

PERCUTANEOUS. Through the skin. When referring to "percutaneous procedures" in treating TN, it means a type of surgery in which the surgeon inserts a needle or electrode through the cheek as opposed to entering the skull.

PERIPHERAL NERVES. Nerves outside the brain and spinal cord. In the case of TN, these include the many branches of the trigeminal nerve that serve the teeth, gums and other parts of the face.

PONS. Part of the brain to which the trigeminal nerve is connected.

POST-HERPETIC NEURALGIA. A type of facial pain caused by damage from the herpes zoster (chicken-pox) virus. Can occur after a bout of shingles.

POST-TRAUMATIC NEURALGIA. A type of facial pain caused by physical damage to the trigeminal nerve and/or its branches.

PRETRIGEMINAL NEURALGIA. A precursor to TN marked by more of a constant ache than sharp, stabbing attacks that are triggered by light touches to the face.

PROSTAGLANDINS. Hormones that kick into action to help fight infections, specifically by creating pain, inflammation and fever that causes us to reduce activity and allow our body's energy to focus on stopping the infection.

PSYCHOGENIC. Pain that originates in the brain.

RADIOFREQUENCY. Use of generated heat through an electrode to cause selected damage to tissue. One type of surgical treatment for TN.

RADIOSURGERY. The use of radiation devices to treat diseases and disorders without having to cut into tissue. Two examples of devices used in treating TN are Gamma Knife and Linac.

RECEPTORS. Cells that are attached to nerve fibers that monitor the environment in, on and around the body for changes.

REMYELINATION. The process of rebuilding lost or damaged myelin, the protective sheath around nerve fibers.

ROOT CANAL. An oral surgery in which the nerve is removed from an inflamed tooth.

RHIZOTOMY. A surgery to cut or damage a nerve root so as to interfere with the transmission of pain signals to the brain.

SCHWANN CELL. A type of glial cell that the body uses to build myelin in nerves outside the central nervous system.

SUBLUXATION. Chiropractic term that means one or more vertebrae are out of their proper alignment.

STEREOTACTIC. Guided by X-ray view or similar scanning device. A way for TN surgeons to be guided to precise, three-dimensional locations in the skull and face.

SUNCT. Acronym for *"short-lasting, unilateral, neuralgiform headaches with conjunctival injection and tearing."* Sometimes confused with TN, it's a sharp, come-and-go pain centering around the eye along with a red eye, tearing and a runny nose. Believed to be caused by an inflammation of blood vessels around the eye.

SYMPTOMATIC TRIGEMINAL NEURALGIA. Trigeminal nerve pain that occurs as a result of another condition, such as multiple sclerosis or a tumor.

SYNAPSE. Gaps between nerve fibers that nerve impulses must jump to continue on.

TEMPORAL ARTERITIS. Aching, throbbing and sometimes burning pain in the temple area caused by an inflamed artery in that area. Sometimes confused with TN.

TENS UNIT. A device that delivers regular, low-grade electrical signals that distract or override pain signals. TENS stands for "transcutaneous electrical stimulation."

THERMOCOAGULATION. Using heat to create tissue injury. It's the technique used in the radiofrequency lesioning surgery used to treat TN.

THALAMUS. The part of the brain that relays messages between various parts of the body and the appropriate other part of the brain. It's kind of the brain's "central switching station."

THROMBOCYTOPENIA. Abnormally low blood platelets, which are needed for clotting. Can be a side effect of some TN medications.

TIC DOULOUREUX. Another name for trigeminal neuralgia. Means "painful spasm" in French.

TMJ/TMD. Pain in the jaw joint sometimes confused with TN. The jaw joint is the temporomandibular joint.

TRANSCONJUNCTIVAL THERAPY. Medicine that's delivered by drops or creams in the eye. The conjunctiva is the tissue around the eye.

TRIGEMINAL NEURITIS. An inflammation of the trigeminal nerve and/or its branches.

TRIGEMINAL NUCLEUS. The origin of the trigeminal nerve in the top three bones of the spinal column (the upper-cervical spine).

REFERENCES

Adler, Roberta J. "Trigeminal Glycerol Chemoneurolysis: Nursing Implications." *Journal of Neuroscience Nursing*. December 1989.

Alberca, Dr. Roman and Ochoa, Dr. Juan Jose. "Cluster Tic Syndrome." *Journal of Neurology*. June 1994.

American Chemical Society. "Hot Stuff: Peppers May Stop Pain." *What's Happening in Chemistry?* 1994.

American Dietetic Association. "Vitamin and Mineral Supplementation." *Journal of the American Dietetic Association*. 2001.

American Pain Foundation. "Pain Action Guide." Brochure published by American Pain Foundation, Baltimore, Md. 2001.

Angell, Dr. Marcia and Kassirer, Dr. Jerome P. "Alternative Medicine: The Risk of Untested and Unregulated Remedies." *New England Journal of Medicine*. Sept. 17, 1998.

Apfelbaum, Dr. Ronald I. "Glycerol Trigeminal Neurolysis." *Techniques in Neurosurgery*. Lippincott Williams and Wilkins Inc. 1999.

Appleton, Dr. Stanton S. and Kawai, Dr. Tsuneo K. "Trigeminal Neuralgia." *General Dentistry*. May-June 1991.

Astin, Dr. John A. "Why Patients Use Alternative Medicine: Results of a National Study." *Journal of the American Medical Association*. May 20, 1998.

Aviles, Dr. Jennifer et al. "Intercessory Prayer and Cardiovascular Disease Progression in a Coronary Care Unit Population: A Randomized Controlled Trial." *Mayo Clinic Proceedings*. December 2001.

Barker, Dr. Fred G., Jannetta, Dr. Peter J., Bissonette, David J., Larkins, Dr. Mark V. and Jho, Dr. Hae Dong. "The Long-Term Outcome of Microvascular Decompression for Trigeminal Neuralgia." *New England Journal of Medicine*. April 25, 1996.

Barnard, Dr. Neal. "Foods That Fight Pain." Harmony Books. 1998.

Barrett, Dr. Stephen. "Acupuncture, Qigong and Chinese Medicine." www.quackwatch.org. 2004.

Barrett, Dr. Stephen. "Be Wary of 'Alternative' Health Methods." www.quackwatch.org. 2004.

Barrett, Dr. Stephen. "Magnet Therapy." www.quackwatch.org. 2004.

Barrett, Dr. Stephen. "Orthomolecular Therapy." www.quackwatch.org. 2004.

Barrett, Dr. Stephen. "Therapeutic Touch." www.quackwatch.org. 2004.

Barrett, Dr. Stephen. "Twenty-Five Ways to Spot Quacks and Vitamin Pushers." www.quackwatch.org. 2004.

Baumann, Dr. Thomas K. and Burchiel, Dr. Kim J. "A Method for Intraoperative Microneurographic Recording of Unitary Activity in the Trigeminal Ganglion of Patients with Trigeminal Neuralgia." *Journal of Neuroscience Methods*. 2003.

Bernat, Dr. James L. and Sullivan, Dr. John Kelly. "Trigeminal Neuralgia from Digitalis Intoxication." *Journal of the American Medical Association*. Jan. 12, 1979.

Bittar, Dr. Geber T. and Graff-Radford, Dr. Steven B. "The Effects of Streptomycin/Lidocaine Block on Trigeminal Neuralgia: A Double Blind Crossover Placebo Controlled Study." Headache Journal. March 1993.

Blakeslee, Sandra. "Dentists May Rush to Treat a Toothache That Isn't One." *New York Times*. May 6, 1992.

Borodic, Dr. Gary E. and Acquadro, Dr. Martin A. "The Use of Botulinum Toxin for the Treatment of Chronic Face Pain." *The Journal of Pain*. February 2002.

Bouquot, Dr. Jerry E. and Christian, Dr. James. "Long-Term Effects of Jawbone Curettage on the Pain of Facial Neuralgia." *Journal of Oral Maxillofacial Surgery*. 1995.

Bouquot, Dr. Jerry E., Roberts, Dr. A.M., Person, Dr. P., Christian, Dr. James. "Neuralgia Inducing Cavitational Osteonecrosis." *Oral Surgery Oral Medicine Oral Pathology*. March 1992.

Bouquot, Dr. Jerry E. and McMahon, Dr. Robert E. "Maxillofacial Osteonecrosis: Part 1, A Review of NICO." The Maxillofacial Center, Morgantown, W.Va. 1998.

Brazeau, Dr. Gayle, et al. "The Role of Pharmacy in the Management of Patients With Temporomandibular Disorders and Orofacial Pain." *Journal of the American Pharmaceutical Association*. 1998.

Brisman, Dr. Ronald. "Bilateral Trigeminal Neuralgia." *Journal of Neurosurgery*. July 1987.

Brown, Dr. Jeffrey A., McDaniel, Matthew D. and Weaver, Michael T. "Percutaneous Trigeminal Nerve Compression for Treatment of Trigeminal Neuralgia: Results in 50 Patients." *Neurosurgery*, Volume 32, No. 4, April 1993.

Brown, Dr. Jeffrey A. and Gouda, Dr. Jan J. "Percutaneous Balloon Compression Treatment for Trigeminal Neuralgia." *Techniques in Neurosurgery*. Lippincott Williams and Wilkins Inc. 1999.

Burrascano, Dr. Joseph J. Jr. "Managing Lyme Disease: Diagnostic Hints and Treatment Guidelines for Lyme Borreliosis." *Lyme Disease Network Online*, 1998.

Campbell, Dr. Robert L., Trentacosti, Dr. Cynthia D., Eschenroeder, Dr. Thomas A. and Harkins, Dr. Stephen W. "An Evaluation of Sensory Changes and Pain Relief in Trigeminal Neuralgia Following Intracranial Microvascular Decompression and/or Trigeminal Glycerol Rhizotomy." *Journal of Oral Maxillofacial Surgery*. 1990.

Canavero, Dr. Sergio and Bonicalzi, Dr. Vincenzo. "Lamotrigine Control of Trigeminal Neuralgia: An Expanded Study." *Journal of Neurology*. 1997.

Castleman, Michael. "The Healing Herbs." Bantam Books. 1995.

Chapman, Diana L. "Surgery Ends RPV Councilman's Strange, Painful, Enduring Ordeal." *The Daily Breeze*, Torrance, Calif. Sept. 30, 1990.

Chaudhary, Dr. Priya and Baumann, Dr. Thomas K. "Expression of VPAC2 Receptor and PAC1 Receptor Splice Variants in the Trigeminal Ganglion of the Adult Rat." *Molecular Brain Research*. 2002.

Cheng, Dr. Theresa M.W., Cascino, Dr. Terrence L. and Onofrio, Dr. Burton M. "Comprehensive Study of Diagnosis and Treatment of Trigeminal Neuralgia Secondary to Tumors." *Journal of Neurology*. November 1993.

Cheshire, Dr. William P. Jr. "The Shocking Tooth About Trigeminal Neuralgia." Letter to *The New England Journal of Medicine*. June 29, 2000.

Chevallier, Andrew. "The Encyclopedia of Medicinal Plants." DK Publishing Inc. 1996.

Chronic Pain Letter. "Self-Help Groups: Talking and Sharing With Like-Minded Others Can Ease Pain." 1990.

Chronic Pain Letter. "TENS Technique for Face, Head, Neck Pain." 1990.

Chronic Pain Letter. "More on Eye Anesthetic's Relieving Trigeminal Neuralgia." 1991.

Chronic Pain Letter. "Pain and Suffering Are Not Synonymous: It Is Important That Both Be Addressed." 1991.

Chronic Pain Letter. "Preventing and Alleviating Pain Patients' Helplessness: Reduction of Pain, Success of Therapies May Be at Stake." 1994.

Connell, Sherri L. "But You LOOK Good!" *Invisible Disabilities Advocate.* 2003.

Consumer Reports. "Acupuncture." January 1994.

Consumer Reports. "The Mainstreaming of Alternative Medicine." May 2000.

Consumer Reports Books. "Complete Drug Reference." Consumers Union. 1996.

Cronin, Steven. "Barnegat Woman Helps Sufferers of TN Face Pain." *The Press* of Atlantic City, N.J. 1993.

Dalessio, Dr. Donald J. "Diagnosis and Treatment of Cranial Neuralgias." *Headache.* May 1991.

Dam, Dr. Mogens. "Practical Aspects of Oxcarbazepine Treatment." *Epilepsia.* 1994.

Dana Alliance for Brain Initiatives. "An Agenda: The Progress of Brain Research in the Next Five Years." Briefing paper, Oct. 20, 1997.

Dana Alliance for Brain Initiatives. "Visions of the Brain." The Dana Press. 2002.

Darlow, Dr. Lloyd A., Brooks, Dr. Michael L. and Quinn, Dr. Peter D. "Magnetic Resonance Imaging in the Diagnosis of Trigeminal Neuralgia." *Journal of Oral Maxillofacial Surgery.* 1992.

Daum, Mary. "Gene Therapy Shows Promise in Treating Sjogren's Syndrome in an Animal Model." *National Institute of Dental and Craniofacial Research* press release, Oct. 21, 2003.

Davis, Jeanie Lerche. "The Power of Prayer in Medicine." *WebMD Medical News* Archive. Nov. 6, 2001. www.mywebmd.com.

Dodes, Dr. John E. and Schissel, Dr. Marvin. "The Whole Tooth: How to Find a Good Dentist, Keep Healthy Teeth and Avoid the Incompetents, Quacks and Frauds." St. Martin's Press. 1997.

Douglas, Elizabeth. "Early Intervention of Amitriptyline Prevents Neuropathic Pain." *Pain Medicine News.* January/February 2003.

Duffy, James A. "MDs Confirm Rising Use of Alternative Medicine." *Knight-Ridder News Service.* Nov. 11, 1998.

Duke, Dr. James A. "The Green Pharmacy." St. Martins Paperbacks. 1997.

Eckerdal, Arne and Bastian, Lehmann. "Can Low Reactive-Level Laser Therapy Be Used in the Treatment of Neurogenic Facial Pain?" *Laser Therapy.* 1996.

Editors of Prevention Magazine Health Books. "The Prevention Pain-Relief System." Bantam Books. 1992.

Editors of Time-Life Books. "The Medical Advisor: The Complete Guide to Alternate and Conventional Treatments." *Time-Life Books.* 1996.

Eisenberg, Dr. David M. et al. "Trends in Alternative Medicine Use in the United States, 1990-1997: Results of a Follow-Up National Survey." *Journal of the American Medical Association.* Nov. 11, 1998.

Escott-Stump, Sylvia. "Nutrition and Diagnosis-Related Care." Williams and Wilkins. 1998.

Fackelmann, Kathleen. "The Power of Prayer: Six-Year Study Suggests People Can Be Blessed with Longer Lives." *USA Today.* July 18, 2000.

Fromm, Dr. Gerhard H. "Trigeminal Neuralgia and Related Disorders." *Neurologic Clinics*. May 1989.

Fromm, Dr. Gerhard, Graff-Radford, Dr. Steven B., Terrence, Dr. Christopher and Sweet, Dr. William H. "Pretrigeminal Neuralgia." *Journal of Neurology*. 1990.

Fromm, Dr. Gerhard H. "Clinical Pharmacology of Drugs Used to Treat Head and Face Pain." *Neurologic Clinics*. February 1990.

Fromm, Dr. Gerhard. "Neuralgias of the Face and Oral Cavity." Pain Digest. 1991.

Fujimaki, Dr. Takamitsu, Fukushima, Dr. Takanori and Miyazaki, Dr. Shinichiro. "Percutaneous Retrogasserian Glycerol Injection in the Management of Trigeminal Neuralgia: Long-Term Follow-Up Results." *Journal of Neurosurgery*. August 1990.

Fusco, Dr. Bruno M. and Alessandri, Dr. Massimo. "Analgesic Effect of Capsaicin in Idiopathic Trigeminal Neuralgia." *International Anesthesia Research Society*. 1992.

Glore, Dr. Stephen and Ricker, Arlene. "Trigeminal Neuralgia: Case Study of Pain Cessation With a Low-Caffeine Diet." *Journal of the American Dietetic Association*. September 1991.

Goss, Dr. B.W. et al. "Linear Accelerator Radiosurgery Using 90 Gray for Essential Trigeminal Neuralgia: Results and Dose Volume Histogram Analysis." *Neurosurgery*. October 2003.

Graff-Radford, Dr. Steven B. "Headache Problems That Can Present As Toothache." *Dental Clinics of North America*. January 1991.

Graff-Radford, Dr. Steven B. "The Differential Diagnosis of Orofacial Pain." *Clark's Clinical Dentistry*. 1993.

Graff-Radford, Dr. Steven B. et al. "Thermographic Assessment of Neuropathic Facial Pain." *Journal of Orofacial Pain*. Volume 9, No. 2, 1995.

Grant, Susan M. and Faulds, Diana. "Oxcarbazepine. A Review of Its Pharmacology and Therapeutic Potential in Epilepsy, Trigeminal Neuralgia and Affective Disorders." *Drugs*. 1992.

Green, Dr. Mark W. and Selman, Dr. Jay E. "Review Article: The Medical Management of Trigeminal Neuralgia." *Headache*. October 1991.

Grostic, Dr. John D. "Dentate Ligament—Cord Distortion Hypothesis." *Chiropractic Research Journal*. Spring 1988.

Hamlyn, Dr. Peter J. and King, Dr. Thomas T. "Neurovascular Compression in Trigeminal Neuralgia: A Clinical and Anatomical Study." *Journal of Neurosurgery*. June 1992.

Hannemann, Holger. "Magnet Therapy: Balancing Your Body's Energy Flow for Self-Healing." Sterling Publishing Co. Inc. 1990.

Hausman, Patricia. "The Right Dose: How to Take Vitamins and Minerals Safely." Ballantine Books. 1987.

Health Watch. "Methylcobalamin: A Potential Breakthrough in Neurological Disease." www.ImmuneSupport.com. Feb. 1, 1999.

Hoffer, Dr. Abram and Walker, Dr. Morton. "Putting It All Together: The New Orthomolecular Nutrition." McGraw-Hill. 1998.

Hutchins, Dr. Lawrence G., Harnsberger, Dr. H. Ric, Jacobs, Dr. John M. and Apfelbaum, Dr. Ronald I. "Trigeminal Neuralgia (Tic Douloureux): MR Imaging Assessment." *Radiology*. 1990.

Jannetta, Dr. Peter J. "Vascular Compression Is the Cause of Trigeminal Neuralgia." *APS Journal.* 1993.

Jannetta, Dr. Peter J. and Bissonette, David J. "Management of the Failed Patient With Trigeminal Neuralgia." *Clinical Neurosurgery.* Date unknown.

Jannetta, Dr. Peter J. "Microsurgical Management of Trigeminal Neuralgia." *Archives of Neurology.* August 1985.

Johnson, Dr. Lenworth N. "Digoxin Toxicity Presenting With Visual Disturbance and Trigeminal Neuralgia." *Journal of Neurology.* September 1990.

Kalauokalani, D. et al. "Acupuncture for Chronic Low Back Pain: Diagnosis and Treatment Patterns Among Acupuncturists Evaluating the Same Patient." *Southern Medical Journal.* 2001.

Kasuya, Dr. Richard T., Polgar-Bailey, Patricia, and Takeuchi, Robbyn. "Caregiver Burden and Burnout." *Postgraduate Medicine.* December 2000.

Katusic, Dr. Slavica, Beard, Mary, Bergstralh, Erik and Kurland, Dr. Leonard T. "Incidence and Clinical Features of Trigeminal Neuralgia, Rochester, Minn., 1945-1984." *Annals of Neurology.* January 1990.

Kondziolka, Dr. Douglas et al. "The Effect of Single-Application Topical Ophthalmic Anesthesia in Patients With Trigeminal Neuralgia." *Journal of Neurosurgery.* June 1994.

Kondziolka, Dr. Douglas et al. "Stereotactic Radiosurgery for Trigeminal Neuralgia: A Multi-Institutional Study Using the Gamma Unit." *Journal of Neurosurgery.* June 1996.

Kondziolka, Dr. Douglas et al. "Gamma Knife Radiosurgery for Trigeminal Neuralgia: Results and Expectations." University of Pittsburgh Medical Center Web site report. February 1999.

Kondziolka, Dr. Douglas et al. "Histological Effects of Trigeminal Nerve Radiosurgery in a Primate Model: Implications for Trigeminal Neuralgia Radiosurgery." *Neurosurgery.* April 2000.

Lee, Dr. Sun H. et al. "Recurrent Trigeminal Neuralgia Attributable to Veins After Microvascular Decompression." *Neurosurgery.* February 2000.

Lee, K.P., Carlini, W.G., McCormick, G.F. and Albers, G.W. "Neurologic Complications Following Chiropractic Manipulation: A Survey of California Neurologists." *Neurology.* June 1995.

Lobato, Dr. Ramiro D., Rivas, Dr. Juan J., Sarabia, Dr. Rosario and Lama, Dr. Eduardo. "Percutaneous Microcompression of the Gasserian Ganglion for Trigeminal Neuralgia." *Journal of Neurosurgery.* April 1990.

Loeser, Dr. John D. "Chronic Neuralgias." *The Management of Pain.* Volume 1, Second Edition. Lea and Febiger. 1990.

Love, Dr. Seth and Coakham, Dr. Hugh B. "Trigeminal Neuralgia: Pathology and Pathogenesis." *Brain: A Journal of Neurology.* December 2001.

Lunsford, Dr. Dade L. and Apfelbaum, Dr. Ronald I. "Choice of Surgical Therapeutic Modalities for Treatment of Trigeminal Neuralgia." *Journal of Clinical Neurosurgery.* 1985.

Luxton, Dr. G. et al. "Stereotactic Radiosurgery: Principles and Comparison of Treatment Methods." *Neurosurgery.* February 1993.

MacPherson, H. et al. "York Acupuncture Safety Study: Prospective Survey of 24,000 Treatments by Traditional Acupuncturists." *British Medical Journal.* 2001.

Marbach, Dr. Joseph J. "Temporomandibular Pain and Dysfunction Syndrome." *Musculoskeletal Medicine.* August 1996.

McConaghy, Dorothy J. "Trigeminal Neuralgia: A Personal Review and Nursing Implications." *Journal of Neuroscience Nursing.* April 1994.

McGhee, Dr. Paul. "Humor and Health." An Internet course offered by Corexcel at www.corexcel.com/html/body.humor.htm. January 2004.

McLaughlin, Dr. Mark R., Jannetta, Dr. Peter J. and Lovely, Dr. Thomas J. "Microvascular Decompression and Rhizotomy for Trigeminal Neuralgia." *Techniques in Neurosurgery.* Lippincott Williams and Wilkins Inc. 1999.

Meaney, Dr. James F.M. et al. "Demonstration of Neurovascular Compression in Trigeminal Neuralgia With Magnetic Resonance Imaging." *Journal of Neurosurgery.* November 1995.

Megerian, Dr. C.A., Busaba, Dr. N.Y., McKenna, Dr. M.J. and Ojemann, Dr. R.G. "Teflon Granuloma Presenting as an Enlarging, Gadolinium Enhancing, Posterior Fossa Mass With Progressive Hearing Loss Following Microvascular Decompression." *American Journal of Otolaryngology.* November 1995.

Merrill, Dr. Robert L. and Graff-Radford, Dr. Steven B. "Trigeminal Neuralgia: How to Rule Out the Wrong Treatment." *Journal of the American Dental Association.* February 1992.

Moraci, Dr. A. et al. "Trigeminal Neuralgia Treated by Percutaneous Thermocoagulation: Comparative Analysis of Percutaneous Thermocoagulation and Other Surgical Procedures." *Neurochirurgia.* 1992.

Morley, Dr. Thomas P. "Case Against Microvascular Decompression in the Treatment of Trigeminal Neuralgia." *Archives of Neurology.* August 1985.

Murphy, Dr. Gerald D. "Utilization of Transcutaneous Electrical Nerve Stimulation in Managing Craniofacial Pain." *Clinical Journal of Pain.* 1990.

National Center for Complementary and Alternative Medicine. "What Is Complementary and Alternative Medicine?" www.nccam.nih.org. January 2004.

National Center for Complementary and Alternative Medicine. "Selecting a Complementary and Alternative Medicine Practitioner." www.nccam.nih.org. January, 2004.

National Institute of Dental and Craniofacial Research. "Pain Research: Past, Present and Future." Interview with Dr. Ronald Dubner. www.nidcr.nih.gov. October 2003.

National Institute of Neurological Disorders and Stroke. "SUNCT Headache Information Page." www.ninds.nih.gov. Reviewed Sept. 23, 2003.

National Institute of Neurological Disorders and Stroke. "Pain: Hope Through Research." NINDS Office of Communications and Public Liaison booklet. September 2001.

Neims, Dr. Allen H. "Why I Would Recommend Complementary or Alternative Therapies: A Physician's Perspective." *Complementary and Alternative Therapies for Rheumatic Diseases.* November 1999.

Newton-John, Dr. Toby. "Strategies for Coping with Pain." Trigeminal Neuralgia Association United Kingdom newsletter. June 2002.

Norheim, J.A., and Fennebe, V. "Adverse Effects of Acupuncture." Lancet. 1995.

North, Dr. Richard B., Kidd, David H., Piantadosi, Dr. Steven and Carson, Dr. Benjamin S. "Percutaneous Retrogasserian Glycerol Rhizotomy." *Journal of Neurosurgery.* June 1990.

Nurmikko, Dr. Turo J. "Altered Cutaneous Sensation in Trigeminal Neuralgia." *Archives of Neurology.* May 1991.

"Nursing 2003 Drug Handbook." 23rd edition. Lippincott, Williams and Wilkins. 2003.

Olin, Dr. Richard J. "The Etiologies of Tic Douloureux: Trigeminal Neuralgia." *Journal of Craniomandibular Practice.* October 1990.

Osborn, Wren. "A Case for Alternative Treatments." Facial Neuralgia Resources web site (http://facial-neuralgia.org). 2002.

Padilla, Dr. Mariela, Clark, Dr. Glenn T. and Merrill, Dr. Robert L. "Topical Medications for Orofacial Neuropathic Pain: A Review." *Journal of the American Dental Association.* February 2000.

Pain Medicine News. "Non-Medical Therapies Alleviate Chronic Migraine Pain." (McMahon Publishing Group). January/February 2003.

Pareja, Dr. Juan A. and Sjaastad, Dr. Ottar. "SUNCT Syndrome: A Clinical Review." *Headache: The Journal of Head and Face Pain.* April 1997.

Pawluk, Dr. William. "Medical Magnetic Fields." www.naturalhealthweb.com. 2004.

Pollack, Dr. Ian F., Jannetta, Dr. Peter J. and Bissonette, David J. "Bilateral Trigeminal Neuralgia: A 14-Year Experience With Microvascular Decompression." *Journal of Neurosurgery.* April 1988.

Pradel, Dr. W. et al. "Cryosurgical treatment of genuine trigeminal neuralgia." *Journal of Oral and Maxillofacial Surgery.* June 20002.

Premsagar, Dr. I.C., Moss. Dr. T., and Coakham, Dr. Hugh B. "Teflon-Induced Granuloma Following Treatment of Trigeminal Neuralgia by Microvascular Decompression: Report of Two Cases." *Journal of Neurosurgery.* 1997.

Rand, Dr. R.W. et al. "Leksell Gamma Knife Treatment of Tic Douloureux." *Stereotactic Functional Neurosurgery.* 1993.

Rappaport, Dr. Z. Harry and Devor, Dr. Marshall. "Trigeminal Neuralgia: The Role of Self-Sustaining Discharge in the Trigeminal Ganglion." *Pain.* 1994.

Rhoton, Dr. Albert L. Jr. "The Surgical Treatment of Trigeminal Neuralgia and Hemifacial Spasm." Patient booklet from the University of Florida's Shands Neurological Center. 1995.

Rosa, Linda, Rosa, Emily, Sarner, L. and Barrett, Dr. Stephen. "A Close Look at Therapeutic Touch." *Journal of the American Medical Association*, 1998.

Riley, Harris D. Jr. "Jefferson Davis and His Health." *Journal of Mississippi History.* August 1987 and November 1987.

Remillard, Dr. Guy. "Oxcarbazepine and Intractable Trigeminal Neuralgia." Paper delivered at symposium on Trileptal in Norway. July 1993.

Rosenkopf, Dr. Kenneth L. "Current Concepts Concerning the Etiology and Treatment of Trigeminal Neuralgia." *Journal of Craniomandibular Practice.* October 1989.

Rovit, Dr. Richard L. "Trigeminal Neuralgia." *Comprehensive Therapy.* 1992.

Sahni, Dr. K. Singh, Pieper, Dr. Daniel R., Anderson, Randy and Baldwin, Dr. Nevan G. "Relation of Hypesthesia to the Outcome of Glycerol Rhizolysis for Trigeminal Neuralgia." *Journal of Neurosurgery.* January 1990.

Shankland, Dr. Wesley E. II. "Trigeminal Neuralgia: Typical or Atypical?" *Journal of Craniomandibular Practice.* April 1993.

Shuhan, G., Benren, X. and Yuhuan, Z. "Treatment of Primary Trigeminal Neuralgia With Acupuncture in 1,500 Cases." *Journal of Traditional Chinese Medicine.* 1991.

Sime, Andrea. "Case Study of Trigeminal Neuralgia Using Neurofeedback and Peripheral Biofeedback." First Step Wellness Center, Lincoln, Neb. www.eegspectrum.com. 2004.

Smith, Dr. Z.A. et al. "Dedicated Linear Accelerator Radiosurgery for the Treatment of Trigeminal Neuralgia." *Journal of Neurosurgery.* September 2003.

Smyth, Angela. "The Complete Home Healer." HarperCollins. 1994.

Solomon, Dr. S., Apfelbaum, Dr. Ronald I. and Guglielmo, Dr. K.M. "The Cluster Tic Syndrome and Its Surgical Therapy." *Cephalalgia.* June, 1985.

Spence, Alexander P. and Mason, Elliott B. "Human Anatomy and Physiology." Second edition. The Benjamin/Cummings Publishing Co. Inc. 1983.

Sweet, Dr. William H. "The Treatment of Trigeminal Neuralgia." *New England Journal of Medicine.* July 17, 1986.

Sweet, Dr. William H. "Faciocephalic Pain." In "Brain Surgery: Complication Avoidance and Management." 1993.

Taha, Dr. Jamal M. and Tew, Dr. John M. Jr. "Therapeutic Decisions in Facial Pain." *Clinical Neurosurgery,* Volume 46. 1998.

Taha, Dr. Jamal M. and Tew, Dr. John M. Jr. "Radiofrequency Trigeminal Rhizolysis." *Techniques in Neurosurgery.* Lippincott Williams and Wilkins Inc. 1999.

Tang, J.-L., Zhan, S.-Y. and Ernst, E. "Review of Randomized Controlled Trials of Traditional Chinese Medicine." *British Medical Journal.* 1999.

Taylor, Dr. Danette and Mankowki, Dr. Ken. "Tolosa-Hunt Syndrome." www.eMedicine.com. March 21, 2003.

Tekkok, Dr. Ismail H. and Brown, Dr. Jeffrey A. "The Neurosurgical Management of Trigeminal Neuralgia." *Neurosurgery Quarterly.* Volume 6, No. 2. 1996.

Tew, Dr. John M. and Van Loveren, Dr. Harry. "Surgical Treatment of Trigeminal Neuralgia." *American Family Physician.* May 1985.

The Medical Letter Inc. "Spinal Manipulation." The Medical Letter on Drugs and Therapeutics newsletter. May 27, 2002.

Tyler-Kabara, Dr. E.C. et al. "Predictors of Outcome in Surgically Managed Patients with Typical and Atypical Trigeminal Neuralgia: Comparison of Results Following Microvascular Decompression." *Journal of Neurosurgery.* March 2002.

Velasco-Siles, Dr. Jose Manuel et al. "Bilateral Trigeminal Neuralgia." *Surgical Neurology.* August 1981.

Vogel Enterprises Inc. "Atlas Orthogonal Chiropractic." Third edition. 1990.

Voorhies, Dr. Rand and Patterson, Dr. Russel H. "Management of Trigeminal Neuralgia (Tic Douloureux)." *Journal of the American Medical Association.* June 26, 1981.

Walchenbach, Dr. R., Voormolen, Dr. J.H.C. and Hermans, Dr. J. "Microvascular Decompression for Trigeminal Neuralgia: A Critical Reappraisal." *Clinical Neurology Neurosurgery.* 1994.

Walker, Dr. J.B. et al. "Laser Therapy for Pain of Trigeminal Neuralgia." *Clinical Journal of Pain.* 1987.

Weiss, Rick. "Medicine's Latest Miracle." *Health magazine.* January/February 1995.

White, A. et al. "Adverse Events Following Acupuncture: Prospective Surgery of 32,000 Consultations With Doctors and Physiotherapists." *British Medical Journal.* 2001.

Wilkins, Dr. Robert H. "Historical Overview of Surgical Techniques for Trigeminal Neuralgia." *Techniques in Neurosurgery.* Lippincott Williams and Wilkins Inc. 1999.

Woodham, Anne and Peters, Dr. David. "Encyclopedia of Healing Therapies." Dorling Kindersley. 1997.

Yamaki, Dr. T. et al. "Results of Reoperation for Failed Microvascular Decompression." *Acta Neurochirurgica.* 1992.

Yamashita, H. et al. "Adverse Events Related to Acupuncture." *Journal of the American Medical Association.* 1998.

Yiu, Heung-Hung and Tam, Dr. Kwong-Chuen. "Acupuncture for Several Functional Disorders." *American Journal of Chinese Medicine.* 1976.

Youmans, Dr. Julian R. "Neurological Surgery." Fourth edition. W.B. Saunders Co. 1996.

Young, Dr. Ronald F. "Radiosurgery vs. Microsurgery for Trigeminal Neuralgia." *Current Techniques in Neurosurgery.* Current Medicine Inc. 1998.

Yoshishige, Dr. Nagaseki et al. "Oblique Sagittal Magnetic Resonance Imaging Visualizing Vascular Compression of the Trigeminal or Facial Nerve." *Journal of Neurosurgery.* September 1992.

Zakrzewska, Dr. J.M. "Medical Management of Trigeminal Neuralgia." *British Dental Journal.* 1990.

Zakrzewska, Dr. J.M. "Surgical Management of Trigeminal Neuralgia." *British Dental Journal.* 1991.

Zakrzewska, Dr. J.M. "Trigeminal Neuralgia." W.B. Saunders Co. Ltd. 1995.

Zakrzewska, Dr. J.M. and Harrison, Dr. S.D. "Pain Research and Clinical Management: Assessment and Management of Orofacial Pain." *Elsevier Science.* 2002.

Zakrzewska, Dr. J.M. and Patsalos, Dr. P.N. "Oxcarbazepine: A New Drug in the Management of Intractable Trigeminal Neuralgia." *Journal of Neurology, Neurosurgery and Psychiatry.* 1989.

Zakrzewska, Dr. J.M. and Patsalos, Dr. P.N. "Drugs Used in the Management of Trigeminal Neuralgia." *Oral Surgery Oral Medicine Oral Pathology.* October 1992.

Zakrzewska, Dr. J.M. and Thomas, Dr. D.G.T. "Patient's Assessment of Outcome After Three Surgical Procedures for the Management of Trigeminal Neuralgia." *Acta-Neurochirurgica.* 1993.

Zamora, Dulce. "Self-Help: Popular, but Effective?" WebMD, www.mywebmd.com, June 16, 2003.

Zhang, Dr. Kai Wen, Zhao, Dr. Yong Hong, Shun, Dr. Zi Ting and Li, Dr. Ping. "Microvascular Decompression by Retrosigmoid Approach for Trigeminal Neuralgia: Experience in 200 Patients." *Annals of Otolaryngology, Rhinology and Laryngology.* 1990.

Authors' note: Many of the comments by doctors quoted in this book were made during presentations at the Trigeminal Neuralgia Association conferences in Cincinnati, Ohio, in October 1996; in Orlando, Fla., in November 1998; in Pittsburgh, Pa., in October 2000, and in San Diego, Calif., in November 2002. Other comments were made by various doctors' presentations at TNA support group meetings around the country. The remaining quoted comments were obtained from published papers and by personal contacts.

INDEX

Abducens nerve, 42
Accessory nerve, 42
Acetaminophen (Tylenol), 108, 114, 152
Acetylcholine, 301, 430
Acidophilus, 85, 348
Acoustic neuroma, 44, 463, 479
Acquadro, Dr. Martin A., 301-302, 488
Actiq, 152
Acupressure, 321
Acupuncture, VI, IX, XVII, 10, 16, 92, 93,
    100, 114, 167, 170, 178, 180, 269, 281,
    284, 288, 291, 292, 304, 314, 316, 319,
    320, 321, 322, 323, 324, 325, 326, 327,
    328, 340, 358, 361, 368, 464, 467, 469,
    470, 487, 489, 491, 492, 494, 495
Acute alveolar osteitis, 69
Acyclovir (Zovirax), 195
Adhesions, 244, 250, 263, 479
Agranulocytosis, 136, 141, 144
Alcohol, 7, 22, 56, 71, 79-80, 82, 85, 90,
    95, 118, 153, 185, 213-214, 270-275,
    351, 365, 481
Alfalfa, 310, 348
Alksne, Dr. John, XVII, 14, 51, 174, 176,
    185-186, 191, 193, 263, 265
Almotriptan (Axert), 82, 105
Alveolar osteitis, 69
Amantadine, 85
Amerge (naratriptan), 82
Amethopterin (methotrexate), 96
Amiodarone, 136
Amitriptyline (Elavil), IV, 54, 88, 91-92, 97,
    110, 112, 142-145, 147, 149, 156, 158,
    168, 194-196, 268, 489
Amoxicillin, 85
Anafranil (clomipramine), 91
Analgesics, 108, 479
Anbesol, 75, 366
Andre, Nicolaus, 6
Anesthesia dolorosa, 57, 151, 177, 202,
    210-211, 215, 218, 221, 223-224, 233,
    238, 248, 256-257, 263, 266-269, 273,
    277-278, 342, 424, 455-456, 472, 479
Aneurysm, 24, 479
Antacids, 114, 130, 135, 158, 437
Antibiotics, 46, 69, 83-85, 94, 100, 102,
    104, 113, 149, 158, 160, 212, 257, 274
Anticonvulsant, 10, 48, 54, 63, 81-82, 86-
    87, 90, 97-98, 107-110, 115, 119, 121,
    127, 132, 138, 140, 142, 146-147, 150,
    156, 166, 199, 211, 281, 311, 361, 367,
    416, 437, 472, 479
Antidepressants, 48, 54, 61, 85, 88, 91-92,

97-98, 100, 102, 104, 110, 114, 126,
    130, 134, 138, 139, 140, 142, 143, 144,
    145, 147, 148, 149, 150, 151, 153, 158,
    160, 162, 194, 195, 196, 211, 267, 268,
    269, 383
Antihistamines, 94, 100, 102, 104, 130,
    134, 138, 139, 140, 144, 147, 153
Anxiety, 115, 130, 134, 138, 144, 147-148,
    158, 160, 171, 182, 282, 288, 291, 314,
    352, 377, 379-380, 382-383, 386, 388-
    389, 391-393, 395, 397, 412, 415, 453
Apfelbaum, Dr. Ronald I., XVII, 86, 174,
    193, 213, 216-217, 253, 261, 487, 490-
    491, 494
Aplastic anemia, 126, 128, 141, 479
Arachnoid, 44-45, 209, 479
Arginine, 347
Aromatherapy, VI, 179, 283, 309, 311
Arsenic, 7
Arteriovenous malformation, 60, 479
Artery, 6, 8, 40, 89, 93, 100, 102, 104, 185,
    193, 218, 224, 241, 245, 246, 257, 262,
    341, 342, 351, 417, 485
Aspartame (NutraSweet, Equal), 179, 347,
    362
Aspirin, 94, 108, 126, 152, 387, 397, 432
Asplundh, Gwen, XVIII, 3, 358, 360
Astin, Dr. John A., 286-288, 487
Atlas, 330-331, 333-334, 337, 339, 463,
    479, 494
Atlas Orthogonality, 333
Atypical, III, IV, VIX, 4, 18, 48, 49, 50, 51,
    52, 53, 54, 61, 70, 71, 85, 97, 99, 100,
    102, 104, 112, 142, 180, 181, 182, 186,
    187, 193, 194, 195, 202, 216, 222, 231,
    237, 247, 263, 277, 278, 279, 288, 299,
    301, 303, 321, 328, 339, 340, 342, 382,
    383, 403, 424, 447, 456, 460, 470, 472,
    479, 494
Atypical odontalgia, IV, 97, 142
Auditory nerve, 60, 187, 241-242, 251
Axert (almotriptan), 82
Ayurveda, 177, 283, 309, 316
Azathioprine (Imuran), 96, 436
Azithromycin, 85

Backonja, Dr. Miroslav, 129
Baclofen (Lioresal), IV, 9, 110-111, 115,
    121, 139, 145-148, 156, 158, 160, 163,
    168, 269, 376, 437, 447, 448, 462
Ballew, Doris, 340

ABOUT THE AUTHORS

George Weigel is a veteran newspaper journalist and trigeminal neuralgia sufferer. He was a TN support group leader in central Pennsylvania for many years and was the founding editor of "TNAlert," the newsletter of the Trigeminal Neuralgia Association.

Dr. Kenneth Casey is a neurosurgeon who specializes in treating face pain. He is a lieutenant colonel in the U.S. Army Reserves and has served on the staffs of several major teaching hospitals, including those at the universities of Colorado, Connecticut, Pennsylvania and Detroit. He also is the author of numerous medical abstracts and journal articles.